Coping with Chronic Disease

RESEARCH AND APPLICATIONS

Coping with Chronic Disease

RESEARCH AND APPLICATIONS

EDITED BY

THOMAS G. BURISH

Department of Psychology
Vanderbilt University
Nashville, Tennessee

LAURENCE A. BRADLEY

Section on Medical Psychology
Bowman Gray School of Medicine of Wake Forest University
Winston-Salem, North Carolina

WITH A FOREWORD BY W. DOYLE GENTRY

1983

CALIFORNIA SCHOOL OF PROFESSIONAL PSYCHOLOGY LOS ANGELES

ACADEMIC PRESS

A Subsidiary of Harcourt Brace Jovanovich, Publishers
New York   London
Paris   San Diego   San Francisco   São Paulo   Sydney   Tokyo   Toronto

ACADEMIC PRESS, INC.
111 Fifth Avenue, New York, New York 10003

United Kingdom Edition published by
ACADEMIC PRESS, INC. (LONDON) LTD.
24/28 Oval Road, London NW1 7DX

Library of Congress Cataloging in Publication Data

Main entry under title:

Coping with chronic disease.

 Includes bibliographies and indexes.
 1. Chronic diseases--Psychological aspects.
2. Adjustment (Psychology) 3. Behavior therapy.
4. Chronic diseases--Social aspects. I. Burish,
Thomas G. II. Bradley, Laurence A. [DNLM:
1. Behavior therapy. 2. Chronic disease--
Rehabilitation. 3. Chronic disease--Therapy.
4. Long term care. WT 30 C783]
RC108.C66 1983 616 82-24457
ISBN 0-12-144450-3

PRINTED IN THE UNITED STATES OF AMERICA

83 84 85 86   9 8 7 6 5 4 3 2 1

Contents

8. Diabetes Mellitus: A Cognitive-Functional Analysis of Stress

DENNIS C. TURK AND MARJORIE A. SPEERS

9. Coping with Obesity

MARGRET K. STRAW

10. Coping with Epilepsy

BONNIE J. KAPLAN AND ALLEN R. WYLER

11. Spinal Cord Injuries

BERNARD S. BRUCKER

Contributors

Numbers in parentheses indicate the pages on which the authors' contributions begin.

Laurence A. Bradley (3, 339, 475), Section on Medical Psychology, Bowman Gray School of Medicine of Wake Forest University, Winston-Salem, North Carolina 27103

Bernard S. Brucker (285), Department of Orthopedics and Rehabilitation, University of Miami School of Medicine, Miami, Florida 33101

Thomas G. Burish (3, 159, 475), Department of Psychology, Vanderbilt University, Nashville, Tennessee 37240

Mary C. Cerreto (381), Department of Pediatrics, University of Texas Medical Branch, Galveston, Texas 77550

Thomas L. Creer (313), Department of Psychology, Ohio University, Athens, Ohio 45701

A. Wallace Deckel[1] (85), Uniformed Services University of the Health Sciences, Department of Medical Psychology, School of Medicine, Bethesda, Maryland 20814

Leonard Diller (113), Department of Rehabilitation Medicine, New York University Medical Center, New York, New York 10016

Wayne A. Gordon (113), Department of Rehabilitation Medicine, New York University Medical Center, New York, New York 10016

Richard L. Heinrich (137), Department of Psychiatry and Biobehavioral Sciences, University of California at Los Angeles, Los Angeles, California 90024; and Behavioral Rehabilitation Research Laboratory, Sepulveda Veterans Medical Center, Sepulveda, California 91343

Ruth B. Hoppe (447), Department of Medicine, Michigan State University, East Lansing, Michigan 48824

Bonnie J. Kaplan (259), Department of Psychology, University of Calgary, Calgary, Alberta T2N 1N4, Canada; and Behavioural Research Unit, Alberta Children's Hospital Research Centre, Calgary, Alberta T2T 5C7, Canada

Philip C. Kendall (39), Department of Psychology, University of Minnesota, Minneapolis, Minnesota 55455

David S. Krantz (85), Uniformed Services University of the Health Sci-

[1]Present address: Division of Medical Psychology, Johns Hopkins Hospital, Baltimore, Maryland 21218.

ences, Department of Medical Psychology, School of Medicine, Bethesda, Maryland 20814

Howard Leventhal (13), Department of Psychology, University of Wisconsin, Madison, Wisconsin 53706

Sandra M. Levy (425), Behavioral Medicine Branch, National Cancer Institute, National Institutes of Health, Silver Spring, Maryland 20205

Jeanne Naramore Lyles (159), Department of Psychology, Vanderbilt University, Nashville, Tennessee 37240

John C. Masters (381), Department of Psychology, Vanderbilt University, Nashville, Tennessee 37240

Debra R. Mendlowitz (381), Peabody College, Vanderbilt University, Nashville, Tennessee 37203

Beth E. Meyerowitz (137), Department of Psychology, Vanderbilt University, Nashville, Tennessee 37240

David R. Nerenz[2] (13), Department of Psychology, University of Wisconsin, Madison, Wisconsin 53706

Ada G. Rogers (409), Analgesic Studies Section, Sloan-Kettering Institute for Cancer Research, New York, New York 10021

Cyndie Coscarelli Schag (137), Department of Psychiatry and Biobehavioral Sciences, University of California at Los Angeles, Los Angeles, California 90024; and Behavioral Rehabilitation Research Laboratory, Sepulveda Veterans Medical Center, Sepulveda, California 91343

Marjorie A. Speers (191), Department of Psychology, Yale University, New Haven, Connecticut 06520

Thomas Stachnik (447), Department of Psychiatry, Michigan State University, East Lansing, Michigan 48824

Bertram Stoffelmayr (447), Department of Psychiatry, Michigan State University, East Lansing, Michigan 48824

Margret K. Straw (219), Department of Psychiatry and Behavioral Medicine, Section on Medical Psychology, Bowman Gray School of Medicine of Wake Forest University, Winston-Salem, North Carolina 27103

Dennis C. Turk (191), Department of Psychology, Yale University, New Haven, Connecticut 06520

David Watson (39), Department of Psychiatry, Washington University School of Medicine, St. Louis, Missouri 63110

Allen R. Wyler (259), Department of Neurological Surgery, University of Washington School of Medicine, Seattle, Washington 98195

[2]Present address: William S. Middleton Memorial Veterans Hospital, Madison, Wisconsin 53705.

Foreword

This volume serves as a welcome addition to the literature characterizing the emerging fields of health psychology and behavioral medicine. It deals with a topic that has received surprisingly little attention to date—chronic disease—and yet seemingly represents a major challenge to millions of the U.S. population. Recent trends in morbidity and mortality in this country show that we are living longer these days, to the point where medical and social scientists are beginning to distinguish between young-oldsters (between 60 and 75 years of age) and old-oldsters (those over 75 years). In large part, this is due to the sharp decline in premature death from acute infectious diseases and illnesses such as influenza, pneumonia, tuberculosis, gastroenteritis, and chronic nephritis, all of which represented leading causes of death in the early 1900s. Instead, Americans are now living with and dying of chronic diseases such as ischemic heart disease, cancers, cerebrovascular disease, diabetes mellitus, and respiratory diseases including asthma and emphysema. To illustrate this further, one need only consider the fact that the 15 most common diagnoses at physicians' office visits include essential benign hypertension (fourth), chronic heart disease (eighth), obesity (twelfth), chronic dermatitis (fourteenth), and diabetes (fifteenth). Moreover, from the patients' standpoint, the majority of complaints presented involve some type of self-reported pain associated with chronic disease(s), (e.g., originating in the upper and lower extremities, back, abdomen, chest, and head). In short, at least 10% of all physician diagnoses and 20% of all patient complaints stem from chronic disease of one sort or another. This is the scope of the problem facing health psychology and behavioral medicine practitioners and researchers.

Those of us who provide services to and collect research data from persons suffering from chronic disease(s) are well acquainted with their common problems. To begin with, many individuals simply cannot seem to accept the new, and often shattering, realities of diagnosed diabetes, cancer, and/or ischemic heart disease. Because of this basic denial that they have a chronic, and perhaps progressive, disease, such individuals generally fail to comply fully with the prescribed medical regimen, often evidence exaggerated and unwarranted disability (e.g., a chronic pain patient who avoids all work, sex, and recreational activities in hopes that the "acute" pain problem will go away), and repeatedly become anxious or depressed when faced with recurring symptoms. Such individuals vacillate emotionally, at times appearing extremely anxious and uncertain, angry, depressed, and confused. Their attitudes about their illness and life itself can range from false optimism to an abiding sense of hopelessness. More importantly, although certain aspects of coping with chronic disease are consistent across the various types of illness (e.g., depression resulting from loss of function), others are not. For instance, patients suffering from multiple sclerosis are faced with two problems not encountered by persons with other types of chronic disease: they are diagnosed "by default" when their persistent symptoms cannot be explained by other diseases, and there is no uniform pattern of symptoms that affect all MS victims. Because of this, persons with MS have particular difficulty in accepting the fact that they have the disease (and thus should mentally prepare for certain types of changes in their personality and level of functional ability) and have a profound sense of uncertainty and apprehension about what will happen next.

This volume presents a wealth of information for both the novice and experienced practitioner, as well as the researcher looking for new frontiers to conquer. As noted, its various chapters deal specifically with the major categories of chronic disease facing Americans today: heart disease, stroke, cancer, diabetes, obesity, pain, epilepsy, and respiratory diseases. By and large, the contributors offer a consistent approach toward the chronically ill patient; that is, an emphasis on self and individual responsibility for learning to live with illness (coping), a pragmatic behavioral strategy for defining and dealing with what R. H. Moos and others have referred to as "major adaptive tasks," and a focus on the patient attitudes and cognitions that often precede and guide patient behavior.

This volume clearly extends and expands the boundaries of health psychology and behavioral medicine beyond the scope of prevention or what J. D. Matarazzo has called "behavioral health" (i.e., concerns about smoking cessation, weight reduction, and Type A behavior that presumably serve to reduce an otherwise healthy person's risk for acute or chronic illness). It provides both a rationale and basis for assisting millions of Americans in their efforts to escape the burden of illness resulting from chronic disease. It goes that necessary step beyond understanding behavioral contributions to the etiology and pathogenesis of chronic disease, which has heretofore consumed most of the attention of behavioral scientists operating in these fields. Finally, by highlighting the important roles played by family and care-givers in coping with disease, it reinforces the trend away from "psychological individualism" that has too long characterized our approach to seriously ill persons; that is, they *alone* shoulder the responsibility for coping effectively with illness. Clearly, this responsibility must be shared by all of us, if we are to be successful in this regard. The social support available to certain patients with chronic disease may, in fact, make the difference in how well these individuals cope.

Along with the editors, I fully expect that this volume will provide a point of integration for psychosocial issues in coping with chronic disease, will act as a catalyst for behavioral medicine research in areas other than prevention and etiology-pathogenesis, and will further enhance the already important place of the behavioral scientist in the mainstream of American medicine.

W. Doyle Gentry
University of Virginia School of Medicine, Charlottesville

Preface

A number of very important changes in the health status of the U.S. population have occurred since the mid-1960s. For example, since 1968 there has been a steady reduction of deaths due to a wide variety of infectious diseases. This decrease, in turn, has caused the annual death rate to decrease from approximately 7.5 per 1000 in 1960 to 6 per 1000 in 1980. Concomitantly, the rate of long-term disability among inhabitants of the United States has increased from about 250 per 10,000 in 1968 to over 400 per 10,000 in 1980. This increase has been associated with a sharp increase in per capita health care expenditures, from nearly $250 in 1968 to more than $1000 in 1980. These data make it clear that the U.S. medical community has had tremendous success in controlling the infectious diseases that have been the major causes of death in the nation. However, the extension of life produced by medical advances has been accompanied by an increase in the number of persons with chronic illnesses that require long-term, expensive care. This change requires that physicians, allied health personnel, and medical or health psychologists devote a major portion of their time to developing the strategies and technology necessary to help persons with chronic disease cope successfully with their impairments—that is, to function at maximum attainable levels both psychologically and in their activities of daily living.

Despite recognition by many scholars, textbook authors, and federal and private funding agencies of the importance of coping with chronic disease, the current volume represents the first attempt to prepare a state of the art review of the theories, methods, and practical concerns of researchers and clinicians working in the area.

Part I begins with an introduction to several important issues in the study of coping with chronic disease. The introductory chapter is followed by the presentation of a theoretical model of how people may attempt to cope with chronic disease and a discussion of methodological issues relevant to research on the topic. Part II consists of critical reviews of research in the area of coping with various chronic diseases or their treatments. Part III, the final part, includes discussions of several issues and problems that are common to nearly all chronic diseases. These include discussions of pain control, the promotion of health maintenance, the role of the nurse and family in coping with chronic disease, and issues surrounding death and dying. This part also includes a summary chapter that attempts to integrate several theoretical, empirical, and practical concerns. The diseases included in this volume do not represent all of the chronic conditions that afflict individuals and present management difficulties for health care professionals; they do, however, comprise the chronic diseases about which there is a substantial research literature.

This volume is designed to serve as an advanced undergraduate- or graduate-level text for behavioral medicine and medical or health psychology courses that either are exclusively devoted to the topic of coping with chronic disease or reserve a major portion of time to the discussion of this topic. In addition, the volume may be used as an adjunct text in courses for medical students, physician assistants, nurses, and other allied health personnel. Finally, the book will serve as a reference text for psychologists and other health professionals interested in research and applied issues in coping with chronic disease.

We gratefully acknowledge the cooperation and support of the Department of Psychology at Vanderbilt University and the Section on Medical Psychology of the Bowman Gray School of Medicine of Wake Forest University. Invaluable assistance in the preparation of this volume was provided by Nancy Garwood, Sherry Baird, Mary N. White, and Ruth Houck. We also would like to thank our families for their support and patience during the production of the book. Finally, we would like to sincerely thank Academic Press and all of our contributors for their encouragement, as well as their expertise and effort.

Coping with Chronic Disease

RESEARCH AND APPLICATIONS

PART I

Overview and Perspective

1

Coping with Chronic Disease: Definitions and Issues

THOMAS G. BURISH

LAURENCE A. BRADLEY

Introduction

Most people reading this book will probably die of a chronic disease. Indeed, 8 of the 10 most common causes of death in the United States are chronic diseases, including the 3 leading causes of death—heart disease, cancer, and cerebrovascular diseases (Matarazzo, 1982; Sexton, 1979; Stachnik, Stoffelmayr, & Hoppe, Chapter 17).

The pernicious increase of chronic disease in our country is a relatively recent phenomenon. In 1900, 6 of the 10 leading causes of death were infectious diseases or diseases related to infectious processes, e.g., tuberculosis, influenza–pneumonia, and diphtheria (Matarazzo, 1982; Stachnik *et al.*, Chapter 17). The discovery of sulpha drugs and major advances in medical research based upon the one-germ–one-disease–one-treatment model eventually brought most infectious diseases under control. As a result, the rate of death from infectious disease decreased from about 36 per 100 deaths in the year 1900 to the 1980 level of approximately 6 per 100. In contrast, the rate of death from chronic disease increased during the first 8 decades of this century from about 20 per 100 deaths to nearly 70 per 100 (Matarazzo, 1982).

Chronic and infectious diseases may be differentiated from one another along a number of dimensions. Although many dimensions might be discussed, we will examine only the four dimensions that make up patients' subjective definitions of their illnesses. One dimension consists of the *causes* of chronic and infectious diseases. There are a number of causes that are shared by both chronic and infectious diseases; for instance, genetic, nutritional, and psychosocial factors can play an etiological role in both types of disease (see Plaut & Friedman, 1981). However, the onset of infectious disease requires exposure to infectious agents such as viruses, whereas the major causes of chronic diseases often are related to persons' lifestyles (e.g., exercise levels, salt intake, use of tobacco and alcohol; Stachnik *et al.*, Chapter 17).

A second dimension that differentiates chronic from infectious diseases is the *time-line* associated with each of them. That is, infectious diseases are acute in onset and usually last for a brief and relatively predictable length of time, whereas chronic diseases often have a slow, insidious onset and endure over a long and indefinite period.

A third dimension that distinguishes chronic from infectious diseases is the *identity* of the two forms of disease. The identity of a disease refers to patients' ideas regarding what is actually wrong with their bodies or functioning. Infectious diseases may be attributed to various infectious agents or, at the very least, may be associated with some clearly identifiable symptoms that are viewed by patients as concrete causes. Chronic diseases, however, usually are not attributed to single causal agents. With several chronic diseases there may not even be observable symptoms present (e.g., symptoms of cancer and rheumatoid arthritis may disappear during periods of remission; there may be no observable symptoms associated with hypertension or coronary heart disease until the disease has reached an advanced stage).

Finally, a fourth dimension consists of the *outcomes* associated with chronic and infectious diseases. Given proper treatment, most persons today with infectious diseases will recover within a reasonably limited length of time. In contrast, most persons with chronic diseases usually remain ill for long periods—often the rest of their lives.

Leventhal and Nerenz (Leventhal, Meyer, & Nerenz, 1980; Leventhal & Nerenz, 1981; Nerenz & Leventhal, Chapter 2) have suggested that individuals develop an organized, commonsense theory for the regulation of their behavioral responses to illness based on their beliefs about the four dimensions just described, their beliefs about treatment, and their symptoms. Unfortunately, it appears that many individuals attempt to regulate their responses to chronic diseases in a manner appropriate only for more acute illnesses (e.g., those persons with diabetes mellitus who do not comply with their medication regimens; those persons with asthma who ignore their symptoms until they must seek help at the local emergency room). As the average age of the American population rises and the incidence and prevalence of chronic disease increase, there will be greater numbers of people who require help in effectively adapting to and living with their chronic illnesses. These people will need to learn new coping skills if they are to lead maximally fulfilling lives.[1]

Helping individuals to cope with chronic disease requires attention to a series of issues that often are not considered in dealing with relatively acute diseases or the traditional behavior disorders. All of these issues are discussed to varying degrees in the chapters of this book. Initially, however, it may be helpful to outline several salient considerations in order to provide a general context in which to consider the problem of coping with chronic disease.

Issues in Coping with Chronic Disease

DEFINITION OF COPING

It seems obvious that the first task confronting any investigator who wishes to examine persons' attempts to cope with chronic disease is to provide a definition of *coping*. Providing a definition of coping, however, is not easy, and some researchers simply have avoided offering one. For example, Moos (1977), who edited one of the first volumes devoted solely to the ways in which people cope with physical illness, decided not to provide a definition of coping, but rather attempted to delineate various illness-related and general adaptive tasks confronted by patients and the major coping skills that patients may use in response to their illnesses (Moos & Tsu, 1977). Other investigators (e.g., Haan, 1977) have attempted to distinguish between coping responses and defense mechanisms. These individuals have viewed defense mechanisms as rigid patterns of behavior that ultimately may be maladaptive. Coping behaviors, on the other hand, were seen as flexible and adaptive responses to illness or other stressors. Nevertheless, the behavior shown by persons with chronic disease in treatment or rehabilitation settings may not be regarded as equivalent to the same behavior displayed in other contexts by physically healthy individuals (e.g., Barofsky, 1981; Barth & Boll, 1981). Displays of denial among psychiatric patients, for example, usually are regarded as maladaptive by their psychotherapists, whereas the use of denial by persons following a myocardial infarction might actually be associated with good adjustment (see Krantz & Deckel, Chapter 4). Also, in

---

[1]It also will be necessary to help physicians and other biomedical professionals, including medical students, to increase their involvement in fostering preventive and health maintenance skills among their patients (Bradley, Prokop, & Clayman, 1981; Stachnik *et al.*, Chapter 17).

some cases of central nervous system dysfunction, denial is a response that may be common among patients with visual information processing disorders resulting from right hemisphere brain damage (see Gordon & Diller, Chapter 5).

We have adopted the definition of coping originally offered by Lazarus and Launier (1978), namely, "efforts, both action-oriented and intrapsychic, to manage (i.e., master, tolerate, reduce, minimize) environmental and internal demands, and conflicts among them, which tax or exceed a person's resources [p. 311]." Although the definition proposed by Lazarus and Launier is not directly addressed by the contributors to this volume, the views advocated by the contributors are consistent with this definition.

ASSESSMENT OF COPING

Barofsky (1981) has noted that "the measurement of coping is critically dependent on its definition [p. 60]." Based on the definition of coping used in this volume, in which coping is assumed to be manifested by *purposeful* and *intentional acts*, the authors of the various chapters have attempted to assess coping in terms of overt and covert behaviors. Nonetheless, there are many unresolved difficulties within the chronic disease literature regarding the assessment of coping (Barofsky, 1981; Cohen & Lazarus, 1979). These difficulties include the following:

1. Coping may be evaluated either as a relatively stable disposition or as a process.
2. The measurement of coping is confounded by the fact that acts of coping change in response to environmental demands over time.
3. Little is known regarding relationships among various measures of coping (e.g., self-report, observer-report, and physiological measures).
4. Judgments of coping effectiveness may vary within different domains (e.g., social versus vocational domains) or across different time periods (e.g., immediately following a myocardial infarction or during the subsequent rehabilitation period).
5. Most investigations have assessed coping in only one specific situation, and it may not be appropriate to generalize their findings to other situations.

These difficulties are discussed in many of the chapters in the present volume. Watson and Kendall's review (Chapter 3) provides an especially detailed discussion of most of the difficulties involved in the assessment of coping as well as of several other methodological issues relevant to research on chronic disease.

PERSONAL RESPONSIBILITY FOR HEALTH

Chronic disease patients face problems associated with the issue of personal responsibility for their state of health. As noted earlier, the causes of the chronic diseases are often closely related to individuals' life-styles—for example, their typical patterns of eating, exercise, stress management, and alcohol intake. Every individual, therefore, has a great deal of responsibility for maintaining—or losing—his or her health. Knowles (1977) poignantly summarized the situation:

> Over 99 percent of us are born healthy and suffer premature death and disability only as a result of personal misbehavior and environmental conditions. . . . The individual has the power—indeed, the moral responsibility—to maintain his own health by the observance of simple, prudent rules of behavior relating to sleep, exercise, diet and weight, alcohol, and smoking. . . . He should be aware of the dangers of stress and the need for precautionary measures during periods of sudden change [pp. 79–80].

In other words, chronic illness is largely a *behavioral* problem for which each individual bears considerable *responsibility*. At least one useful and one damaging consequence can result from the realization that people influence their own states of health. On the positive side, people can take concrete steps to preserve their health and avoid disease, especially chronic disease. This fact is at the heart of the preventive approach to medicine (or behavioral health as defined by Matarazzo, 1980, 1982) that has gained popularity across the country. On the negative side, the constant reminder of responsibility for one's own health frequently causes considerable guilt in victims of chronic disease. For example, lung cancer patients may feel that they, rather than an uncontrollable illness with no known cause, are ultimately responsible for the financial and emotional hardships borne by their family and friends. Many chronically ill patients therefore bear not only the suffering caused to themselves by their disease and treatment, but also the suffering imposed upon their loved ones. The burden can be tremendous. Low self-esteem, anxiety, depression, increased sensitivity to rejection, and reduced attempts to engage in the usual activities of daily living often result, posing major but common coping problems.

THE ROLE OF THE PATIENT'S FAMILY AND FRIENDS

The family and friends of chronically ill patients often exert a major influence on the patient's ability to cope. Chronic disease, much more than infectious disease, is a social phenomenon. The outcome of the patient's coping behaviors depend not only upon his or her efforts and psychological state, but also upon the manner in which family members and friends (as well as health professionals) react to those coping behaviors (Masters, Cerreto, & Mendlowitz, Chapter 14). Family members and friends often do not realize their importance in helping the patient adapt to chronic illness, and often they are not properly informed about how they can aid in the rehabilitation process. For example, families and friends can cause considerable damage by being overly protective or indulgent, by abruptly reducing intimate contact, or by socially excluding the patient (see Lavigne & Burns, 1981). Family members and friends also may have personal difficulties in coping with the patient's chronic disease, and these problems may have to be dealt with before these individuals can concentrate on helping the patient. Mechanic (1977) has provided a cogent summary of the situation:

> Families often have their own problems in coping with the sick or disabled family member and may require information and assistance from the clinical team. Moreover, family members can become a very effective extension of the clinical team by providing support for active coping, encouraging conformity with medical instructions, and facilitating through joint participation those patterns of behavior most consistent with minimizing the patient's disability. . . . The fact is that many family members feel excluded from the care process, have difficulty obtaining needed information, and rarely receive adequate instruction as to what they might do and how to do it [p. 83].

One of the major problems that usually requires considerable preparation and change by the family is the increased dependency caused by chronic diseases. Difficult as it is for some adult patients, they must now depend on others for financial assistance and for such things as helping with personal hygiene, meeting new dietary requirements, and assuming some of their chores and responsibilities. In some cases, the roles of the husband or wife, father or mother, must be largely taken over by others, which reduces many of the pleasures and increases the guilt of the patient. The increased dependency produced by chronic illness among pediatric patients also may disrupt relationships within the family (Lavigne & Burns, 1981). Unless both the patient and family are prepared for such changes, they may present major obstacles to effective coping.

PAIN CONTROL

Pain control is an area of concern for almost all chronically ill patients. The experience of chronic pain may result from diverse causes such as diabetes mellitus, rheumatoid arthritis, coronary heart disease, spinal cord injuries, and various cancers. In addition, the experience of chronic benign pain (i.e., long-term pain that is not the result of a malignant process) may itself become a disease characterized by drug misuse, decreases in physical activity, depression, and disability (Brena, 1978; Fordyce, 1976). It is also important to note that pain is affected by psychological factors such as attention, suggestion, anxiety, modeling, and conditioning (Weisenberg, 1980). Hence, the ability of many chronically ill patients to withstand pain and reduce its influence on their life-styles depends upon their psychological coping abilities. Bradley (Chapter 13) provides a discussion of the research concerning self-regulation of pain among chronically ill patients.

COMPLIANCE

Abundant data exist that suggest many chronically ill patients will not comply with their physicians' orders despite the overall satisfaction that most patients express with their medical care (Rachman & Phillips, 1980). The extent of noncompliance is so great that it has been suggested that funds spent specifically on improving compliance with hypertension, for example, would reduce more deaths than would an equal amount of money spent on the detection of new cases of the disease and the subsequent initiation of treatment (Weinstein & Stason, 1976). Patients' failure to comply with their treatment regimens not only reduces the likelihood of a timely and complete recovery, but also may interfere with the patient–doctor relationship—a relationship that can be crucial to successful coping. Noncompliance also may compromise the potential benefits of any treatment protocol and may lead to misinterpretations of treatment outcome studies (i.e., when compliance rates vary across treatments; Bradley & Prokop, 1982). Unfortunately, little well-controlled research has been conducted to test hypotheses regarding the factors that affect patient compliance with specific treatments at particular stages of various chronic diseases as well as techniques for enhancing compliance.

THE MEDICAL MODEL

Inherent in all of the issues noted previously is the fact that the medical model alone is largely inadequate to promote positive adaptation to chronic disease. In fact, it has been suggested that there is a crisis in medical practice; the technology of medicine and health care appears to be best suited for the treatment of acute infectious diseases, and offers little to people with chronic disease. Glazier (1973) has described this crisis:

> The medical system of the U.S. is able to meet with high efficiency the kind of medical problem that was dominant until about 40 years ago, namely infectious disease. It also deals effectively with episodes of acute illness and with accidents that call for advanced, hospital-based biomedical knowledge and technology. The system is much less effective in delivering the kind of care that is more often needed today: primary (first-contact) care and the kind of care needed at a time when chronic illnesses predominate. . . . For these diseases medicine has few measures and not even much comfort [p. 13].

Glazier (1973) has noted that the prevalent medical system is deficient in dealing with chronic disease for three reasons. First, the medical system is passive; it is based on the assumption that patients will quickly seek treatment after observing symptoms. Yet patients do not observe symptoms until very late in the progress of many chronic diseases, and many patients may not even seek treatment immediately after observing their symptoms. Second, the medical system generally uses a one-to-one, episodic relationship in which a patient visits a physician, receives an examination or treatment, and pays a fee. The system, therefore, has tended to produce physicians who are primarily interested in administering treatment to patients and observing positive and relatively rapid results. Unfortunately, this type of physician behavior is often inappropriate for chronic care. In addition, the medical system does not encourage physicians to attempt to foster health maintenance behaviors among their patients, as third-party reimbursements for the provision of health-behavior change efforts generally are difficult to obtain (Stachnik *et al.*, Chapter 17). Finally, and perhaps most important, medicine as a discipline is ill equipped to deal with problems of psychological coping (including those involving patient behaviors and attitudes) and of family support and involvement in treatment.

Clearly, given the deficiencies of the current medical model, traditional physician care can be only one part of the overall effort necessary to help patients cope adequately with chronic disease. The remainder of the effort requires the skills of a variety of additional health professionals, including nurses, physical therapists, physician assistants, social workers, dietitians, and psychologists.

Coping with Chronic Disease: Research and Applications

The purpose of the present volume is to present, clearly and comprehensively, a description of the practical, theoretical, and empirical issues involved in helping persons to cope with various chronic diseases. A theoretical model for the study of coping with chronic disease is first presented in Chapter 2; the third chapter then provides a comprehensive review of the major methodological issues (including the assessment of coping) involved in chronic disease research. The next nine chapters examine the empirical work that has been carried out on the process of coping with various specific chronic diseases or their treatments. In addition, most of these chapters provide practitioners with suggestions for facilitating the coping process among their chronically ill patients. The volume concludes with six chapters devoted to general issues relevant to all chronic diseases such as the promotion of health maintenance, the control of chronic pain, death and dying, and the important roles played by nurses and by patients' families in the coping process. Overall, the volume attempts to integrate theory and research in the area of chronic disease and to provide descriptions of practical approaches for helping patients cope better with their chronic illnesses.

The existing research on the topic of coping with chronic diseases raises many more questions than it provides answers. It is hoped that this volume will both help to integrate what is now known about the field and provide a stimulus for further theory construction and empirical research. Both of these goals seem of urgent importance, for coping with chronic disease is not an insignificant problem affecting a minority of people. Rather, it represents one of the greatest challenges for health care professionals.

References

Barofsky, I. Issues and approaches to the psychosocial assessment of the cancer patient. In C. K. Prokop & L. A. Bradley (Eds.), *Medical psychology: Contributions to behavioral medicine.* New York: Academic Press, 1981.

Barth, J. T., & Boll, T. J. Rehabilitation and treatment of central nervous system dysfunction: A behavioral medicine perspective. In C. K. Prokop & L. A. Bradley (Eds.), *Medical psychology: Contributions to behavioral medicine.* New York: Academic Press, 1981.

Brena, S. F. (Ed.). *Chronic pain: America's hidden epidemic: Behavior modification as an alternative to drugs and surgery.* New York: Atheneum, 1978.

Bradley, L. A., & Prokop, C. K. Research methods in contemporary medical psychology. In P. C. Kendall & J. N. Butcher (Eds.), *Handbook of research methods in clinical psychology.* New York: Wiley, 1982.

Bradley, L. A., Prokop, C. K., & Clayman, D. A. Medical psychology in behavioral medicine: Summary and future concerns. In C. K. Prokop & L. A. Bradley (Eds.), *Medical psychology: Contributions to behavioral medicine.* New York: Academic Press, 1981.

Cohen, F., & Lazarus, R. S. Coping with the stresses of illness. In G. C. Stone, F. Cohen, & N. E. Adler (Eds.), *Health psychology: A handbook.* San Francisco: Jossey-Bass, 1979.

Fordyce, W. E. *Behavioral methods for chronic pain and illness.* St. Louis, Mo.: C. V. Mosby, 1976.

Glazier, W. H. The task of medicine. *Scientific American,* 1973, *228,* 13–17.

Haan, N. *Coping and defending: Processes of self-environment organization.* New York: Academic Press, 1977.

Knowles, J. H. The responsibility of the individual. In J. H. Knowles (Ed.), *Doing better and feeling worse: Health in the United States.* New York: W. W. Norton, 1977.

Lavigne, J. V., & Burns, W. J. *Pediatric psychology: An introduction for pediatricians and psychologists.* New York: Grune & Stratton, 1981.

Lazarus, R. S., & Launier, R. Stress-related transactions between person and environment. In L. A. Pervin & M. Lewis (Eds.), *Perspectives in interactional psychology.* New York: Plenum Press, 1978.

Leventhal, H., Meyer, D., & Nerenz, D. The common sense representation of illness danger. In S. Rachman (Ed.), *Contributions of medical psychology* (Vol. 2). Elmsford, N.Y.: Pergamon Press, 1980.

Leventhal, H., & Nerenz, D. R. *Illness cognitions as a source of distress and treatment.* Paper presented at the meeting of the American Psychological Association, Los Angeles, August 1981.

Matarazzo, J. D. Behavioral health and behavioral medicine: Frontiers for a new health psychology. *American Psychologist*, 1980, 35, 807–817.

Matarazzo, J. D. Behavioral health's challenge to academic, scientific, and professional psychology. *American Psychologist*, 1982, 37, 1–14.

Mechanic, D. Illness behavior, social adaptation, and medical models. *Journal of Nervous and Mental Disease*, 1977, 165, 79–89.

Moos, R. H. (Ed.). *Coping with physical illness.* New York: Plenum Press, 1977.

Moos, R. H., & Tsu, V. D. The crisis of physical illness: An overview. In R. H. Moos (Ed.), *Coping with physical illness.* New York: Plenum Press, 1977.

Plaut, S. M., and Friedman, S. B. Psychosocial factors in infectious disease. In R. Ader (Ed.), *Psychoneuroimmunology.* New York: Academic Press, 1981.

Rachman, S. J., & Phillips, C. *Psychology and behavioral medicine.* New York: Cambridge University Press, 1980.

Sexton, M. M. Behavioral epidemiology. In O. F. Pomerleau & J. P. Brady (Eds.), *Behavioral medicine: Theory and practice.* Baltimore: Williams & Wilkins, 1979.

Weinstein, M. C., & Stason, W. *Hypertension: A policy perspective.* Cambridge, Mass.: Harvard University Press, 1976.

Weisenberg, M. Understanding pain phenomena. In S. Rachman (Ed.), *Contributions to medical psychology* (Vol. 2). Elmsford, N.Y.: Pergamon Press, 1980.

2

Self-Regulation Theory in Chronic Illness*

DAVID R. NERENZ
HOWARD LEVENTHAL

Introduction

Over the past several years we have been developing a model to describe
and predict how people cope with stressful health threats. The efforts began
with a series of studies of fear messages warning people to take health-
promotive actions such as quitting smoking, taking tetanus shots, making use
of seat belts, and driving safely (Leventhal, 1970). Our aim was to study the
way fearful warnings led to changes in people's knowledge, attitudes, intentions, and actions. We wanted to understand better the effects of fear on
mental and behavioral processes and to do so using messages about topics
that were of practical significance—hence our focus on health and safety.
Encouraged by the finding that different types of information were needed
to influence attitudes and actions, we decided to apply the model to situations where people were actively coping with a noxious event, for example,
ischemic pain and distress induced by cold water or pressure in a laboratory
situation (Johnson, 1975; Leventhal & Everhart, 1979), or pain and distress
induced by an endoscopic examination (Johnson & Leventhal, 1974), by
childbirth (Leventhal, Shacham, Boothe, & Leventhal, 1981), or by surgery
in a hospital setting (Johnson, Rice, Fuller & Endress, 1978). We used
messages both to prepare people for the sensory aspects of these procedures

*Preparation of this chapter was facilitated by Grant CA 26235 from the National Cancer
Institute and by Grant HL24530 from the National Heart, Lung, and Blood Institute.

(for example, what it would feel like when one's hand was in cold water or when one was swallowing the flexible endoscopic fiber-optic tube) and to prepare them to perform specific coping reactions. The results supported our initial assumption that different types of information are critical for defining the nature of a threat setting and for developing the skills needed to cope with it.

All of our prior efforts focused on adaptation over relatively short periods of time; for example, 6 minutes in a cold pressor, 1 or 2 hours for endoscopy, 5 or sometimes 12 or even 24 hours for labor, 3–12 days for surgery, and 1–4 weeks for tetanus shots. Many illnesses, however, require repeated adaptive efforts over relatively long periods of time, perhaps many months and years. Can our conceptual framework generalize to these situations? And what changes, if any, will be needed in our model for it to describe coping with long-term chronic illness? The goal of this chapter is first to present our conceptual formulation as it emerged from the study of adaptation to acute episodes and then to expand it to deal with the longer-term adaptation required by chronic illness.

Overview of the Self-Regulation Model

Our model can be characterized in several ways; we have at various times called it a self-regulation model, an information-processing model, a commonsense model of illness representations, and a parallel-processing model. Nearly all of these terms (except for the last, which refers to a particular structural feature of the model) convey a common theme: we view the patient as actively constructing a definition or representation of his or her illness (or stress) episode (hence the information-processing, illness-cognition, and commonsense model of illness labels) and basing or regulating his or her behavior in terms of this representation (the self-regulation, or coping, aspect of the model). It is clear, therefore, that we share earlier views of people as active information processors who construct representations of problems and construct plans and actions for coping (Kelly, 1955; Neisser, 1967).

The multiplicity of labels used to describe the same model tells us that the model is complex. We are not offering a hypothesis about adaptation—for example, that feelings of control reduce distress—but rather a model of an adaptive system. *This is a crucial issue.* In our framework, adaptation to stressful situations is the product of a system of mediating factors. When we use the terms *coping resource* or *coping response*, we are referring to one of several factors that make up this mediating system. Coping is the skill component, the planning and response execution part of a set of mediating factors that together determine the success or failure of the individual's adaptive efforts.

Another aspect of the model (which is also alluded to by its names) is that it describes, in part, our conscious experience of health threats and our conscious experience of our efforts to cope with these threats. But although the model does indeed reflect the contents of consciousness and the form or content of behavior, its primary function is to identify the variables or factors that underlie experience and action. This chapter focuses primarily on the underlying system and its links to the external and internal environment. If at times it seems that we are describing the contents of consciousness or the contents of observable behavior, that may be due to the similarity of their form and content to the form and content of the underlying processing system. We shall try to be clear, however, about when we are merely describing the form and content of behavior and when we are describing the form and content of the underlying self-regulating (adaptive) system.

BASIC COMPONENTS OF THE MODEL

A primary feature of our model is the idea that the underlying system is composed of a series of stages for guiding adaptive action. The first of these stages, the *representation*, involves the reception and interpretation of information for the definition of the potential or actual health threat. The second stage, *action planning* or *coping*, involves the assembly, selection, sequencing, and performance of response alternatives. The third stage, the *appraisal* or *monitoring* stage, involves the setting of criteria for evaluating responses and appraising one's coping efforts against them. The basic structure of the model is not substantially different, therefore, from many earlier feedback models for behavioral self-regulation such as those suggested by Carver and Scheier (1978, 1981); Lazarus (1966); Miller, Galanter, and Pribram (1960); Powers (1973); and von Bertalanffy (1968).

A second important feature of our model is the postulate of parallel processing, or the assumption that at least two types of feedback loops are active in self-regulation in most illness or stress situations—one for the regulation of danger (*danger control*), the other for the regulation of emotion (*emotion control*). Each regulatory system has somewhat separate components. The danger-control system consists of representations of the health threat as objectively perceived and of plans and reactions for modifying the impact of the threat on the individual. The emotion control system consists of the representation of the subjective feeling state and the cognitions specific to it and of plans and reactions for modifying the emotional state of the individual.

The need for this distinction became clear in early work on the persuasive impact of fear communications. These studies showed that high-fear messages, in comparison to less fearful messages, produced a variety of short-term reactions including (a) the fear response itself (e.g., autonomic change; averting gaze from fearful slides; subjective feelings of fear, anger, and distress), (b) unfavorable attitudes toward the threat (e.g., smoking is harmful, tetanus dangerous), (c) favorable attitudes toward the recommended actions (e.g., take a tetanus shot, quit smoking, use seat belts), and (d) intentions to engage in the recommended practices (see Leventhal, 1970; Rogers, 1982). These responses usually lasted no longer than 24–48 hours. The longer-term reactions, such as taking a tetanus shot during the following 2 weeks or quitting smoking for a period of 3 months, were based on the combination of two components: the subjects' understanding of the danger and their plans for action or coping skills. Both were required for successful protective action. The knowledge component was clearly some type of cognitive representation of the threat along with the skills (action plans) appropriate for its regulation. The action plans needed for emotional regulation were usually different from those needed for regulation of the danger, often overlapping with behaviors that might be labeled as defenses. The two types of reactions could compete with one another or could complement one another depending on the specifics of the situation. The important issue at this point is to note the existence of both types of regulatory systems and their potential for interaction.

The third important feature of the underlying processing system is that it is hierarchically organized. Each stage, the representation, action plans, and appraisal, can be thought of as a series of hierarchically arranged layers going from highly abstract material at the top end to more concrete, situationally bound material at the bottom. The concrete level of representing danger and the concrete level of coping involve perceptual and attentional processes that combine incoming information with perceptual memories or perceptual schemata (see Broadbent, 1977, for a discussion of perceptual categorization). Combining stimuli with perceptual categories or perceptual schemata produces perceptions of illness and perceptions of feelings (e.g., "I see and feel that I have a swollen and infected arm and I feel pained, distressed, and angry because of it"). The memories or schematic structures that combine with new information can be memories of specific prior episodes of illness or generalized prototypes of classes of illness. Either way these perceptual memories combine with information to give rise to concrete experiences of ongoing events.

Abstract or conceptual processing, on the other hand, is more like what we typically regard as cognitive processing or cognitive interpretations of situations that are close to consciousness. For example, if I have severe pain in the arm, I may suspect it is very seriously injured. This conclusion reflects two abstract rules. The first is a *pain–injury* rule, or the assumption that pain follows injury or mechanical damage. The second is a *magnitude* rule, or the assumption that the more severe the pain the more severe the injury (see Leventhal & Everhart, 1979). Although both concrete-perceptual and abstract-conceptual processing may be automatic, it is clear that perceptual processing is nearly always so whereas conceptual processing may be either automatic or deliberate, volitional, and controlled (Shiffrin & Schneider, 1977).

The different levels of processing may generate similar and mutually supportive outputs or dissimilar and conflicting outputs. Discrepancies between seeing and thinking—for example between feeling well and being told you do not look well, or between feeling pain in an arm and knowing the arm is amputated (as is the case in phantom pain)—are likely to stimulate emotional arousal and intensive efforts at resolution. These reactions may include powerful emotions such as fear, depression, a sense of bewilderment, doubt about one's sanity (Melzack, 1973), and a sense of alienation or detachment of the mind from the body, a process labeled *depersonalization* (see Leventhal, 1975). These affective reactions are likely to have important consequences for coping.

ADAPTATION TO ACUTE ILLNESS EPISODES

In order to understand the model, to identify the variables that operate at each of the stages, and to see how it can help us discover and account for unexpected findings, we shall describe its operation for an acute illness episode. Our example is drawn from interview protocols of several patients we have studied who were coping either with treatment for acute conditions or for chronic illnesses such as hypertension and cancer.

The Illness Episode

Imagine for a moment a case of a 38-year-old white male who notices a higher level of tension or nervousness in himself during a particularly stressful workday. Having an external explanation for this experience, he attributes little significance to it until the following day, when he again notices tension and some heart palpitations even though the stress episode is now "over." He may also notice fatigue and a headachy feeling. Because of his dysphoric state, he is now tuned to his body and a bit concerned that something may be wrong. Our hypothetical patient may engage in a variety of appraisal behaviors. He may read the health column in the paper, take a wait-and-see attitude, assume the dysphoric, headachy feelings will go away after a good night's sleep, and he may mention his feelings to his wife or friends to find out if they feel the same.

We have labelled this part of the illness episode an *appraisal delay*—the first of several periods with potential for delay in the seeking of medical care. During this period, our hypothetical person is elaborating upon or developing his *representation* of the illness problem. Planning and action—that is, *coping*—are not the most visible aspects of thought and/or behavior. This delay period, therefore, is characterized by the observation of a discrepancy or departure from normal, everyday feelings, and by efforts to attribute the departure to various environmental events. These appraisal reactions—reading, observing outer pressures, talking to others—may be more or less automatic. They provide some sense of the contingency between the discrepant feelings and potential causes (Safer, Tharps, Jackson, & Leventhal, 1979; Suchman, 1965).

The appraisal reactions allow the individual to assess the potential meaning or significance of departures from normal. It is clear, however, that appraisal reactions usually do not occur if the symptoms are severe (Suchman, 1965); intense pain and bleeding are likely to bring the individual into the medical care system without delay. Many of our breast cancer patients report experiencing an immediate emotional response, "chills up and down my spine," "my stomach turning to lead," or "nearly passing out" when noticing a lump in the breast. Cognitive activity that extends over hours, days, or weeks before seeking care (including wondering what is wrong and checking with books and other people) seems more likely with vague, amorphous symptoms.

It is also clear that the cognitive activity involved in appraisal reactions includes a process of comparing the observed symptomatic state to a variety of implicit templates. These templates include one's own past concrete experiences with illness, ideas gleaned from others, and the experiences of other people who share one's environment. For example, Gutmann, Pollock, Schmidt, and Dudek (1981) found that bypass patients who had interpreted their cardiac distress as gastric pain had delayed an average of 2 years before seeking help! The sensations of gastric illness and cardiac disease were so similar that it was difficult for these individuals to tell one from the other, something that can be readily understood because they had never before experienced a coronary attack. But even a person who has had a coronary may have difficulty telling a second episode from gastrointestinal upset if he expects the second attack to be exactly like the first. Fears of recurrence may lead to overemphasis of minor deviations between the two, to the individual's ultimate detriment. The similarity in the sensory experience between gastric upset and coronary disease provides a substantial basis for confusion. Thus, one should not be too quick to explain the misreading of such illness episodes as a type of denial of threat.

Comparing a current state of bodily experience with that of others is also very common. An individual may notice abdominal pain or discomfort and inquire whether his or her spouse is experiencing similar upset. Assuming a more or less similar set of exposures, the individual can interpret or attribute the upset to some specific event they were both exposed to or to an event that only one of them was exposed to: "It was the cheesecake I had that caused this upset."

To get back to our example: having experienced symptoms for several days, our 38-year-old male may begin to suspect that something is really wrong. He now believes he is in trouble, that he is ill. And he has probably narrowed his hypotheses to two or three alternatives: he might suspect he has a stress-induced ulcer or perhaps he has the makings of coronary artery disease. Our subject has begun to fill out the conceptual part of his representation by applying labels to the symptomatology. The symptoms plus the label are the *identity* of the representation. Other hypotheses being formulated with respect to the *cause, consequences,* and potential *duration* or time-line of the problem complete the attributes of the representation. Perhaps he can recall the experience of a somewhat older office-mate who thought he had an ulcer and wound up with the diagnosis of cardiovascular disease, a lengthy hospitalization, painful surgery, and a recovery that was at best only partial. Indeed, he may see a vivid image of his friend wheezing in pain as he tries to walk or perform other everyday tasks. The fear stimulated by this image may create a good deal of hesitation about visiting his physician and may lead him to think he would rather "die in his sleep than undergo painful surgery for so little benefit." In time, however, he may decide to make an appointment with his doctor and find out what really is the matter. He may be driven to the decision because he can no longer live with his anxiety, because he realizes it is the rational thing to do, or because his wife or someone else pressures him into arranging an appointment.

We have labeled the delay from the point of recognition that he is ill to the decision to make use of the medical care system as the period of *illness delay.* Its length is a function of factors such as fear of treatment, socially generated definitions of the problem, and social pressures to seek care. We have labelled the period of time from the decision to seek care to entering the medical care system *utilization delay.* The period of utilization delay is brief in the case we are discussing because our patient has medical insurance and has no difficulty obtaining time off from work for the visit.

Our hypothetical patient has moved from an appraisal step through two additional steps in seeking care: illness delay and utilization delay. Illness delay was increased by anxiety resulting from fear of the consequences of the illness and from a view of its possible chronicity; a long-term, debilitating illness is frightening and depressing to contemplate. Utilization delay was brief as he has the resources needed to use the medical care system. Now that he is in the system, our patient will be exposed to a wide range of tests during which he will experience a variety of events in his body and receive a good deal of information from his health care provider. In the case we envision, the patient is examined and told he has no current sign of coronary artery disease and that his "chest" pains are probably of gastrointestinal origin, due perhaps to the unusual levels of stress he reports at his work.

For the most part his acute episode has ended. However, he does not have a clean bill of health because his blood pressure is somewhat elevated, which is not too surprising because he smokes and is under pressure. Our patient is now reasonably convinced that his heart palpitations and headache were caused by his elevated blood pressure, or hypertension, and that both his hypertension and his gastric symptomatology, which may foretell ulcers, are due to work stress. His physician may recommend antihypertensive medication and that he quit smoking. As our patient is a self-made man who prides himself on his autonomy and ability to regulate his life, he is willing to undertake treatment and to quit smoking in the firm expectation this will lead to a complete cure. He throws off the smoking habit, takes medications for a couple of months, notices that most of his symptoms clear up (though the headaches recur whenever there is stress at the office), and finally decides he should find a line of work that is less harassing. He makes a major life change, finds himself headache-free, assumes he is cured, and stops his medications.

Though coping and appraisal are the most salient features at these later points in time, it is clear that the representation of hypertension is still playing a central role in guiding his behavior. Our patient has redefined his illness problem as stress-induced gastric upset and stress-induced hypertension. He has identified his high blood pressure with headaches and used headaches to guide his treatment. Finally, he has not only made use of medical advice and treatment, he has also generated his own treatment regimen and used it in combination with his medically based treatment until he assumed he was cured; at that point he dropped out of the medical care system.

Conceptual Formulation of the Episode

Episodes of this sort illustrate essentially all the features we have studied with respect to adaptation to illness. First, the episode extended over time and unfolded as a series of steps. These steps—from appraisal, to illness, to use of the medical care system, to sick role (taking-medication behavior), and finally to cure—are not of primary concern to us at this moment. Of concern now is the mechanism underlying the individual's self-regulation. The individual moved from the recognition of vague body disturbances to a decision that he was ill, and finally to labeling himself as having high blood pressure. His representation of high blood pressure had a clear *identity*—it had a name (hypertension) and an associated set of symptoms (initially, heart palpitations, later, headache)—and a presumed *cause*, externally induced stress. The representation also had imagined *consequences*, in this instance his friend's coronary surgery and poor postsurgical rehabilitation. The seriousness of these consequences and their associated *time-line* or duration (i.e., his friend would always be sick) led to a rather dramatic commitment to cope with the threat both by following the doctor's prescribed regimen and by making a major life change—moving to a new position.

The example illustrates the basic components of illness representations: causes, time-lines, consequences, and identities. Affect (fear and depression) also appears in the representation in response to imagery of a colleague's pain and distress, illustrating that emotion as well as objective perceptual factors enter into the meaning of the illness. It is extremely important to note that the representation was both abstract and concrete: the identity of high blood pressure was both the label and the headaches, the consequences were both abstract information given by his practitioner and the vivid images of his colleague's illness.

It is also clear that the representation, the symptoms, and feared consequences guided this man's coping, as did the more abstract information provided by his practitioner.

EMPIRICAL FINDINGS OF SPECIAL RELEVANCE TO THE MODEL

We assembled the case history to illustrate our basic model. Now we present some empirical examples of its validity. The data has been selected to illustrate the three aspects of the model that we believe to be of greatest importance for understanding long-term adaptation to chronic illness. These are (*a*) the hierarchical feature of processing; (*b*) the dependence of coping on one's representation of illness; and (*c*) the appearance of specific models of illness, particularly the organization of illness behavior around an *acute* behavioral schema. We will briefly review evidence pertaining to each of these notions before discussing broader issues peculiar to chronic illness.

Hierarchical Processing

We have argued that representations of illness problems are both abstract and concrete. Thus, each feature of the representation (cause, identity, consequences, and even time-line) is processed and retained in both abstract and concrete memory codes. This is seen in several striking outcomes in the study of patients with hypertension. For example, Meyer (1981) found that 80% of those in treatment for 6 months or longer believed that people in general could not tell when their blood pressure was elevated. On the other hand, when asked if *they* could tell when their blood pressure was elevated, 88% indicated they could. It appears that hypertensives try to forge a link between their diagnostic label (abstract) and specific symptoms (concrete). When patients observe symptoms, they seek to label or to diagnose and explain them. On the other hand, when patients are given a label or diagnosis, they search for concrete symptoms to serve as indicators of the disease process.

Equally striking examples of hierarchical processing appeared in our studies of the adaptation of cancer patients to chemotherapy treatment. In one study, Nerenz (1979) assessed the levels of distress during chemotherapy for patients with malignant lymphoma. He was able to divide his patient population into a group that could feel and monitor cancerous lymph nodes, approximately two-thirds of his 59 cases, and those who could not. He divided the patients who could monitor nodes into one group whose nodes disappeared rapidly with treatment and another whose nodes shrank slowly, in graded steps, with continuing treatment. Nerenz found the first group of patients far more distressed with chemotherapy than the second! From the perspective of common sense, one might expect those patients whose cancerous nodes disappear in a month or two to be more favorable toward chemotherapy. On the other hand, from the point of view of the integration of labels (lymphoma) with concrete symptoms (cancerous nodes), it is clear that treatment created a discrepancy between labels and symptoms when it eliminated the concrete sign that disease was present. From the point of view of the patient's perceptual or concrete experience, he or she is well and no longer in need of treatment. Yet treatment continues and produces a wide range of distressing experiences ranging from specific and well-defined symptoms such as nausea, vomiting, and hair loss on one extreme to vague and ill-defined symptoms such as fatigue, pain, and tiredness on the other. Treatment is making the person feel ill! Reassurance from the practitioner apparently fails to reduce the distress induced by these circumstances.

A second example is seen in Ringler's (1981) study of breast cancer patients. Ringler found that patients who were in treatment for preventive reasons were more upset by the side effects of nausea and vomiting than patients with disseminated disease. (Preventive chemotherapy is given women who have had successful surgery for breast cancer and is used to destroy cancerous cells that may have wandered to other parts of the body and are undetected.) On the other hand, women with disseminated disease were more distressed by the vague symptoms of treatment: tiredness, fatigue, and weakness of the limbs. These symptoms are readily confused with the outcomes of recurrent metastatic disease and are very threatening to severely ill women.

In all of the instances reviewed, patients attempt to integrate concrete and abstract material. They invent or find symptoms to match labels and are distressed by the absence of symptoms when they are labeled as ill and undergoing treatment; when they are labeled as seriously ill, they are disturbed by those symptoms that are most readily experienced as illness (fatigue, tiredness, and weakness) and pay less attention to concrete symptoms that are clearly attributable to treatment. We believe the same processes are crucial for the understanding of chronic illness. When a patient adopts a label of him- or herself as "chronically" ill, there is a strong possibility that the person will find and experience ongoing symptoms consistent with the label. And it is likely that those symptoms most closely resembling those of illness in general, such as fatigue, weakness, or tiredness, will generate the conviction that one is indeed chronically, uncurably, and hopelessly ill. The illness label leads the individual to search his or her present and past concrete experiences for validating signs or symptoms, and those signs that are common to all illness episodes, such as fatigue and tiredness, are most available and most likely to be incorporated into the illness representation. The label, therefore, serves as an organizing device in integrating more specific, concrete information into the illness picture.

Coping Is Directed by the Illness Representation

Our studies of the behavior of hypertensive patients make clear that action is directed by the illness representation. In Meyer's data (Meyer, Leventhal, & Gutmann, in press) on compliance with medical regimens, hypertensives who had entered and remained in treatment were more compliant and had better blood pressure control if they believed that treatment had favorable effects on their "symptoms." Seventy-one percent of those patients were taking medications as prescribed. In contrast, only 30% of those whose treatment had no effects on symptoms were compliant. Using symptoms to monitor blood pressure may not be a good strategy, as there was no relationship between symptom reporting and blood pressure in this sample of subjects. A similar effort to find correlations between blood pressure levels and symptoms by Baumann (1982) was also unsuccessful. She used a within-subject design that included 20 occasions on which subjects predicted pressures and had pressures measured. She found that people most confident about their ability to predict pressure changes were least likely to be accurate.

The data support the conclusion that representations are important factors in directing or guiding coping. Representations are a map for coping efforts.

And it is the most readily available, concrete aspect of the representation, the presumed illness symptoms, that guide moment-by-moment coping.

Meyer's data and data from our studies of cancer patients (Nerenz, 1979; Ringler, 1981), point to another way representations direct coping. In all of these studies we have found individual cases in which people have initiated self-treatment to supplement ongoing medical care. Self-treatments may be additive (introduce new foods, exercise routines) or subtractive (remove stresses and strains), and are intended to enhance or improve upon medical treatment and prevent recurrences of disease by removing the factors presumed to have initiated disease in the first place.

Models of Illness Representations

Our observations suggest that illness representations fall into classes which define three specific commonsense models of illness based on the expected duration or time-line of the episode: *acute* (symptomatic and curable), *cyclic* (symptomatic, removable, but recurrent), and *chronic* (a stable part of the self regardless of their symptomatic nature). Temporal expectations associated with these models have important effects upon behavior. This was clear in Meyer's (1981) data. He observed a smaller percentage of patients believing hypertension an acute disorder when he compared his "Newly Treated" patients to his "Reentry" (those who had been in treatment, left, and re-entered) and "Continuing Treatment" cases (40% versus 18% and 13%). The percentage of patients holding a chronic or long-term outlook increased, going from "Newly Treated" to "Continuing Treatment" (28% through 43% to 65%). These changes could be due to learning (as people participate in treatment they learn that hypertension is a chronic and not an acute disorder) or to selective sampling, as individuals with acute models of hypertension should be much more likely to drop out of treatment either if their symptoms clear (at which point they can assume they are cured) or if their symptoms do not clear (at which point they can assume their treatment is ineffective). Meyer found evidence for both effects: 58% of his "Newly Treated" sample dropped out of treatment by the 6-month follow-up interview if they initially represented hypertension as an acute disorder. By contrast, of those "Newly Treated" patients whose initial representation of hypertension was that of a chronic or long-lasting disorder, only 17% dropped out. Learning also took place, as those patients who shifted from an acute to a chronic representation of the disorder remained in treatment.

We suspect that nearly all illness episodes are initially represented as acute, even when people fall ill with diseases which are known to be chronic and fatal. For example, many of the cancer patients studied by Nerenz (1979) spoke of their cancers as acute diseases. Zimmerman and his associates

(Zimmerman, Linz, Leventhal, & Penrod, 1982) provided a different type of demonstration of the strength of this tendency. They conducted a laboratory study in which subjects were randomly assigned to one of two conditions following an elaborate and carefully recorded measure of their blood pressure. Following the measurement, half the subjects were told their readings were normal (in the 120/80 range) and the other half were told their readings were elevated (in the 145/95 range). (Subjects were assigned to one of the two conditions only if their actual reading was normal; those few with elevated readings were excluded from the study.) After sitting a few minutes alone in the laboratory, each subject completed several questionnaires with items asking about the number of symptoms experienced during the past 3 months, expectations about the duration of the elevated readings, and so on. In comparison to subjects given normal readings, those given high readings reported significantly more symptoms and were more certain that elevated blood pressures were temporary. Providing a label such as "your blood pressure is elevated" led subjects to scan and recall concrete symptoms and to generate an acute temporal representation.

SUMMARY

The evidence from our studies of people with hypertension, cancer, diabetes, and other such disorders suggests that our model provides a reasonably accurate picture of the mechanisms underlying behavior during illness episodes. People construct representations that are both abstract (conceptually processed) and concrete (schematically processed) and these representations serve as maps to guide coping. The hierarchical aspect of representations is obviously critical, as both the concrete and the abstract levels of the representation guide coping, sometimes in different and conflicting ways. Moreover, discrepancies between abstract and concrete levels of the representation can be distress-inducing. Finally, we discerned a degree of organization or structuring in representations suggesting it may be possible to classify or group them in categories such a acute, cyclic, and chronic. These labels are based primarily on the temporal aspect of representations, but appear to incorporate symptomatology as well.

There are two important qualifications to be made about patients' temporal expectations and illness cognition models. First, the models held by most patients are not well organized. They cannot label their thoughts as acute, cyclic, and/or chronic. Moreover, their representations are not necessarily complete and well integrated. Only some of the attributes of representations may be present, and they may fail to point to a clearly specified coping strategy with precise criteria for the appraisal of coping outcomes.

Even when an individual has included all or nearly all of the attributes in his or her disease picture, the attributes need not be consistent. The time-line may disagree with the label and both may be at odds with the perceived cause. One should not expect illness cognitions to be logically organized or biomedically valid.

A second qualification to the picture we have presented is the dearth of information on how illness models form and change. We are not well informed as to what factors change the time-line, and we have yet to identify the process and the factors involved in moving from acute to cyclic to chronic views of illness. Patients appear to resist such change, but we have said little about the factors that operate to retard the acceptance of new ways of formulating the illness problem. This and related issues are the main focus of the following section in which we discuss the application of illness cognition theory to chronic disease.

Illness Cognition and Chronic Illness

To apply our model to the broader range of problems associated with chronic disease, such as psychological disability and life disruption caused by prolonged illness, we must address two important questions, "How do people make the psychological transition from acute to cyclic and/or to chronic representations of illness?" and "What are the implications of this change for emotional response and for coping?"

THE TRANSITION TO CHRONICITY

The self-regulation model that we have proposed was designed to deal with moment by moment behavior. The patient's representation of an illness at a given moment, his or her coping skills, and the criteria he or she sets for appraising coping outcomes regulate moment by moment behavior. To generalize the model to long-term illness and illness-related disability and dependence, we will need to add concepts in addition to those involved in our basic stages of representation, coping, and appraisal, and suggest how the total system processes information and how it is changed and can be changed by external information.

The Self and the Episodic Structure of Behavior

Representations, coping, and appraisal change from situation to situation because they are products of the interaction of current stimulus information with the underlying processing system. Situational stimuli interact with the underlying conceptual and schematic memory systems to generate the representation. Once the representation is formed, a set of underlying memory structures constructs plans for coping and coping responses. The latter operations are dependent, as we have seen, upon the former (the representation). As situations change, they call into action different underlying structures, generate different representations and coping plans, and lead to different types of behavior.

This point is not introduced as a theoretical disgression. It is essential for an understanding of illness behavior as it suggests that all behavior is episodic. In the classroom we are teachers or students; in the home, we are spouses, parents, or children; in cars we are drivers or passengers; when in hospitals we are practitioners or patients, and when we are patients we are tired, frightened, and impotent. Representations, coping, and appraisals (our phenomenology and overt acts) change as we move from place to place and from role to role. Continuity is established and maintained across varied occasions by the perception in all representations of a stable set of contextual factors consisting of the environment at large and the continued presence of the self-system (Epstein, 1973). Different aspects of self are involved in different settings, but the "same" self, physically and psychologically, is experienced in all settings.

Perhaps the central issue in chronic illness is how the representation of the illness is related to the underlying self-system. This relationship is likely to explain whether the illness remains episodic (something to be dealt with when symptomatic or when in the practitioner's office) or chronic (something that must be dealt with regardless of the situation in which the self appears and acts). How does the illness become part of the self? How does it retain its independence as a situationally specific event? Can the illness be represented as an independent entity and be seen as cyclic or chronic?

It is clear that the acute representation of illness reflects the episodic organization of everyday life. We also believe that one overriding feature of adjustment to illness, acute or chronic, is the striving to deal with the disease as a series of recurrent episodes. Hypertension is salient when the patient is in for a check on blood pressure or to have medications refilled. It may also be somewhat salient when the patient is taking pills or choosing food in a restaurant. Cancer is salient when the patient is coming to the hospital for chemotherapy, or when the disease imposes limitations on specific, everyday activities. When the illness moves beyond these boundaries into other areas of life, the time-line may become cyclic or chronic and the illness seen as increasingly permanent.

Types of Self–Illness Relationships

Gutmann et al. (1981) conducted an intensive series of interviews with a series of coronary bypass patients and observed changes in the time-lines or models they used to represent their disorders. Gutmann *et al.* found a gradual shift from acute through cyclic to chronic representations. There was an added complexity to their findings. Patients who developed a permanent time-line actually fell into two different categories: *chronic* and *at-risk*. Patients holding a chronic representation saw themselves as ill, appeared depressed, and showed little inclination to engage in rehabilitative activities. Patients holding an at-risk representation, on the other hand, felt it important to participate in rehabilitative and preventive activities to avoid recurrence of the acute, symptomatic phase of their coronary disease. Those in the first of these two groups of "surgically cured" patients still saw themselves as permanently ill. The latter patients saw themselves as permanently exposed to the risk of acute illness episodes. Their adaptations were vastly different.

After some reflection on Gutmann *et al.*'s findings and an examination of the variety of reactions of our cancer patients, we would suggest at least three different ways in which the illness representation can relate to the self-system. The first is *total:* the self is the disease, the disease is the self. The second is *encapsulated:* a component of the self is diseased but large areas of the self are disease-free. The third is *risk:* the self (total or part) faces a constant threat of outbursts of acute, symptomatic illness. All three involve chronic or stable relationships, i.e., the total self or a portion of the self is constantly afflicted by the disease or is constantly threatened by the potential for an acute outbreak of the disease.

Total involvement with the disease is a condition where every aspect of human activity incorporates illness. No matter what the situation, no matter what problem is represented in awareness, and no matter what coping skills are called for, the representation and coping system include the concept and the concrete experience and emotion that one is a diseased person. Hence, every person–situation interaction becomes a disease–situation interaction. The uniqueness of life's varied episodes disintegrates and all life is a life of cancer, a life of heart disease, and so on.

Encapsulation of the disease to a segment of the self is seen in many of our most successfully adapted cancer patients. They are people who have cancer, but they are not living, walking cancer. Cancer is in their bodies, some part of the body, and it sets limits on activities and longevity. But limits are defined: one works, socializes, and conducts life as usual; indeed, one places special value on the important, interpersonal affectional and work opportunities of life and keeps them cancer-free.

The third type, at-risk, involves the recognition of a permanent state of threat or potential for acute outbreaks of disease. The at-risk person acts to block the recurrence of illness. It is an active orientation where a reasonably high level of vigilance is sustained in minimizing threat.

DETERMINANTS OF THE RELATIONSHIP OF SELF
AND ILLNESS

It is relatively easy to find a case example of a living heart attack, a person whose every physical and mental act is tempered by fear of sudden coronary death, or a living cancer, a person whose family and work relationships and everyday activities are infused with depression and fear of pain and death. And it is possible to find such examples among former heart disease patients who could live near-normal lives and among cancer patients for whom disease-produced death is years away and for whom disease-produced disability is objectively minimal. In sharp contrast, one can find people who are plagued with frequent bouts of one or another illness while energetically pursuing the tasks of daily life. A case in point is a youngster who was a respondent in one of our studies of health behavior in schoolchildren (Glynne, Hirschman, & Leventhal, 1982). When asked how many colds he had the past school year, he replied "Twelve." When asked if he was as healthy as most of his peers, he replied "Sure, I'm more healthy than most." The interviewer's observation of the respondent's running nose and buoyant reactions provided validation of his seemingly contradictory responses. As for most people at most ages, except perhaps the elderly, colds and injuries are temporary inflictions from without; they are not permanent attributes of self (Herzlich, 1973). What variables can account for the sharp contrasts outlined in these examples and for the three types of adaptation outlined in our theroretical analysis?

Our search for the determinants of self–illness relationships and for the process by which these relationships are wrought can be helped by application of our model of self-regulation to illness episodes (e.g., the stages of representation, coping, and appraisal) and by our hypotheses about the underlying processing mechanism as hierarchical and parallel. The model helps identify specific ways in which the environment can interact with the processing system to join self and illness. We can also consider three types of environmental influence, *cultural, interpersonal communication,* and *private experience,* that interact with the processing system to link illness representations to the self-system.

Cultural Influences

At least two kinds of cultural factors can be identified that play an important role in the structuring of illness representations and coping and that link the illness regulatory system to the self: linguistic labels and institutional structures. Both factors direct attention and structure coping in ways that encourage the development of acute or chronic conceptions of illness and then link these conceptions in one or another way to the self-system. For example, the term *hypertension* influences the way individuals search for confirming, concrete symptomatic evidence to bolster a representation of the disorder as stress-induced (see Leventhal, Nerenz, & Steele, 1983). Mental illness labels provide yet another example. Cultural lore suggests mental illness is chronic and characteristic of the self. In the social perception of everyday life neurotic and psychotic acts are viewed as expressions of permanent, underlying traits, much the way acts of kindness, honesty, intelligence, and cultured behavior are viewed (Nisbett & Ross, 1980). As a consequence, Mosbach (1982) found, a very high proportion of patients appearing for the first time at a mental health clinic reported concrete evidence for their current problems as far back as 5 or more years, a retrospective search that contrasts sharply with the retrospective search of a few days or weeks that is characteristic of patients coming to a medical outpatient clinic. The labels define different time frames. They also define different causes. In a study using multidimensional scaling on ratings of similarity between pairs of disease labels, Linz, Penrod, and Leventhal (1981) found mental illness labels ranked high on a dimension of self-causation (as did ulcers, alcoholism, and heart attack), whereas cancers ranked very low on this dimension.

The structure of the medical care system also directs attention and coping to encourage specific types of illness representations and self-illness linkages. The system is designed to deal with emergencies and acute care. It orients one to symptoms and external causes (contacts with sick others, ingested foods, etc.) and teaches short-term self-maintenance coping strategies, rewarding them with "cures." The structure reinforces the view of illness as due to "alien" invading forces to be destroyed by miracle drugs and surgery.

The power of the system in shaping illness cognition resides in its providing an integrated view: it relates labels to symptom experience (the abstract to the concrete), provides coping regimens for representations, and ameliorates the emotional distress and fear that parallel the illness representation and coping system (emotional reactions have the same acute time-line and symptomatic property as illness itself, hence treatment cures emotion as well as illness). Our examples should also help show that our three types of environmental factors—cultural, social communication, and private experience—are closely intertwined: the activity of the processing system integrates all sources of information into a common representational and coping structure. Our separation of these sources is strictly for convenience of exposition.

Social Communication

The social environment does much to structure representations, coping, and appraisals both by direct instruction and by example. Elsewhere we have discussed how the practitioner can foster the connection of symptoms to labels and the development of acute time-lines. For example, patients coming for blood pressure checks and medication refills are typically queried about symptoms. The questions may be motivated by the desire to identify side effects of drugs or locate potential damage from prolonged hypertension. The reason for questioning is seldom communicated to the patient, and it is not surprising that the patient assumes the doctor is asking about symptoms of high blood pressure that can be used as potential clues to changes in his condition and the need for treatment.

While we have not investigated this issue in detail, it is our impression that many practitioners are "cure-oriented." Cancer specialists talk of cures when urging patients and families to initiate noxious chemotherapy treatment. Their urgings are not wholly specious, as experimental data show substantial increases in long-term survival rates with many intensive chemotherapy regimens. But the cancer specialist and layperson may assign quite different meanings to the term *cure*. To the specialist, cure may mean freedom from disease for 5 or perhaps 7 to 10 years. For the layperson, cure may mean freedom from disease for a lifetime.

Verbal messages are not the only and perhaps not the most important type of social communication. Observations of other ill people and the way the well treat the ill can shape representations, coping, and the linkage of the illness to the self. Such influences may have greater impact than direct verbal communication.

Two examples come to mind. Ringler (1981) found that breast-cancer patients who observed a relative or close friend die of cancer were more distressed and viewed cancer as far more devastating than did women who lacked such first-hand observation. Images of physical decimation of another human being locked their own self-systems to the disease representation in a vivid and threatening manner. The second example is the not infrequent complaint of our cancer patients that family and friends are intruding on their autonomy. In an effort to be helpful, they take on tasks well within the patient's competency. By blocking coping in areas where the patient could readily succeed, they not only frustrate the individual's need to regulate his or her everyday life but force the individual to act as though cancer pervaded all of his or her activities and competencies.

Both of the above patterns describe how nonverbal interpersonal communication (observation of others and efforts of well persons to support and be helpful to the ill) can work against the patient's efforts to encapsulate a life-threatening chronic disease. But both observations of other ill persons and social support can assist as well as interfere with the patient's efforts to develop a rational encapsulation of the disease. Adams and Lindemann (1974) published two case examples of young men suffering from spinal injuries; one was successfully rehabilitated and the other was not. The individual who was rehabilitated accepted the injury and turned his energies to life problems within his competency: he abandoned that part of the self associated with outstanding athletic performance and developed his intellectual competency, becoming a high school history teacher. The other case provides a contrasting picture of someone who became a "living disability and depression," returning to and living at home, withdrawing from others and sustaining the false hope of eventual recovery. Unsuccessful efforts at total rejection of the debilitating injury resulted in total disability and self-destruction.

Adams and Lindemann point to one especially significant difference between these two young men: their social environments responded in vastly different ways to the fact of the injury. The parents and friends of the successful coper provided an environment of support for the individual's redefinition of himself. The parents and friends of the unsuccessful coper supported the young man's false hope for cure, were dejected by his injury, and rejected his self-redefinition. The cognitive or information differences between the two environments are clear, one discouraging and the other encouraging the creation of a larger sphere of self-value and competency, but we would like to emphasize the emotional or affective differences. The positive affective environment provided by family and friends for the young man who succeeded in redefining himself provided him with the freedom to accept injury, to stand off cognitively and observe the realities of his physical, intellectual, and psychological self, and to experience positive emotion in relation to new self-values and new self-competencies. The family and parents of the young man who failed to adapt supported his illusions, did not permit him to observe himself, and denied him positive affect to new self-values and new competencies.

Private Experience

The individual's concrete experience with his body is the final source of information shaping the illness representation and linking the illness to the self-system. There are many factors that could be discussed in this area, but we will focus on just two: the role of changes in energy level and emotional state and the role of diurnal rhythms in sustaining the sense of wholeness and integrity of the self.

We believe that the onset of depression and the depletion of energy can function to establish a connection between illness and the self. Evidence for this is available in studies of chronic pain and illness behavior; depressed persons appear more likely to develop long-lasting syndromes of pain and illness behavior such as dependency, irritability, and focusing on symptoms (see Wooley, Blackwell, & Winget, 1978). Depression and the depletion of energy undercut coping, and active coping is important for solving nearly all problems. Hence the depletion of energy resulting either from the debilitating effects of illness or from the onset of depression in response to the threat of illness provides concrete, subjective evidence that the disease is invading all provinces of the self-system, including its values and perceived problems and opportunities. Being prepared for the appearance of depressed feelings, and being ready to accept a passive coping role for the short term may prove critical in avoiding this particular cause of generalization of the illness to the self-system.

We also suspect that diurnal rhythms play a critical role in keeping alive the ability to encapsulate or isolate an illness to specific components of the self. For most people, as the day goes on energy is depleted, competency declines, the symptoms (pain and distress) of illness worsen, and moods change. The morning typically sees new energy, more favorable mood, and reduced pain and distress. These changes in feeling can serve as sources of information about one's condition. The positive changes provide hope and define a segment of the day and self which can be focused on nonillness problems, thus allowing cognitive efforts to encapsulate the illness and prevent it from consuming the self-system. Depressive disorders that disrupt this rhythm will permit the illness to engulf the self.

Our discussion has barely scratched the surface of the ways in which concrete body experiences and the experience of emotions can affect whether a chronic illness is represented as an encapsulated entity in the self or whether this same illness overwhelms the self, causing psychological deficits and disability. Prior experience with chronic disease, success in rehabilitation, and the response of the social environment to acute illness episodes (for example, the degree to which the individual is not only cared for but excused from efforts to rehabilitate) can influence reactions to the concrete experiences of chronic illnesses. This is a rich area for study and a potentially important one for identification of at-risk persons and for the development of interventions.

Conclusion: The Self as a Determinant of Regulation

We wish to make clear that the linkage of self to illness-regulatory mechanisms—to representations of illness and coping—is shaped from within the cognitive system. Thus, the organization of the self, how it relates to the environment and to its own emotional reactions, is critical in determining whether the illness is integrated with or remains alien to the self, and whether the links of illness to self take on the characteristics of a total, encapsualted, or at-risk model.

The aspect of self we wish to emphasize is its hierarchical differentiation. At the most abstract, or top, end of this sytem is the overall self-worth or esteem associated to self. Very close to it are the values like warmth and lovingness, commitment to scientific ideals, or family integrity, that define areas for self-worth. This hierarchical organization plays an important role in determining whether illness is associated with the total self or encapsulated in specific areas. A well-differentiated self-system with components well instantiated in concrete, everyday experiences is more likely to succeed in isolating illness impact to specific functions and contents.

Below the most abstract levels of the self-system are two more specific and concrete layers. The most concrete involves the representation of the perceived (seen, kinesthetically felt, heard, and thought of) self in specific problem-solving situations. At this level the self is experienced as producing acts to cope with and regulate problems and to cope with and regulate emotional experiences. This is the level of specific coping tactics, specific criteria, and the experience of specific outcome appraisals. It is in this nitty gritty level of processing that we experience success and failure.

A crucial aspect of this everyday concrete experience is the way the outcome experiences are attributed to and influence the processing system. Does the success and failure confirm or disconfirm the adequacy of specific coping tactics, and adequacy of the representation of the problem, the reasonableness of the criteria for apprisal, the adequacy of self-worth, the adequacy of self-competency, and the value and competency of the individual's social, medical, and institutional support systems?

When new problems are experienced, when coping fails to produce expected outcomes, and when discrepancies exist between abstract and concrete problem definitions, moment-by-moment regulatory processes are disrupted; they are in a state of "positive feedback." Positive feedback means that outcomes are not appraised as meeting goals, that the gap between present and anticipated state is increasing rather than decreasing. These are the occasions when both the problem-specific system and the self-system are most likely to undergo change. If coping efforts continually fail to close the gap and the individual struggles more and more intensely with his problem, the feedback implies failure in coping, lack of self-competency, and destruction or domination of the self by the illness if its threat is sufficiently large.

Moments of disregulation or positive feedback (Schwartz, 1979) are crucial for re-evaluating coping tactics, representations, appraisal criteria, and self-systems, but it is not clear which of these elements will bear the brunt of change. In the previous section we reviewed the cultural, interpersonal–communicative, and subjective factors that can constrain or direct feedback. In this section we suggest that the hierarchical differentiation of the self-system also contributes to this feedback process. We believe there is an intermediate level to the self-system that is extremely important in affecting the feedback process. For lack of a better term, we have called it a level of strategies for relating oneself to specific problem situations. Strategies are well learned sets or readinesses for relating self to moment-by-moment problem solving. They are especially important during moments of crisis or positive feedback. How is the self viewed in relation to the problem? Does the individual view him- or herself as a problem solver, as having to observe, collect evidence, appraise outcomes, and accept good tactics and reject poor ones? Does the individual see him- or herself as constructing a view of the problem situation, as correcting this view with new information, and as acting as best one can with currently available data? Does the individual expect, observe, tolerate, and adjust to his or her own subjective emotional reactions or does he or she ignore and attempt to override, deny, or distort these feelings?

Generalized strategies are brought to bear in specific situations and connect self-values to tactics and direct the readout from appraisals. Whether the traditional vocabulary of cognitive styles and defenses will describe and make sense of this material is not yet clear. We suspect, however, that a somewhat different vocabulary will be needed as control theory is expanded to deal with the long- as well as the short-term aspects of adapting to chronic illness.

References

Adams, J. E., & Lindemann, E. Coping with long term disability. In G. V. Coelho, D. A. Hamburg, & J. E. Adams (Eds.), *Coping and adaptation*. New York: Basic Books, 1974.

Baumann, L. *Psychological and physiological correlates of blood pressure and predicted blood pressure*. Master's thesis in progress, University of Wisconsin—Madison, 1982.

Broadbent, D. E. The hidden preattentive process. *American Psychologist*, 1977, 32, 109–118.

Carver, C. S., & Scheier, M. F. Self-focusing effects of dispositional self-consciousness, mirror presence, and audience presence. *Journal of Personality and Social Psychology*, 1978, 36, 324–332.

Carver, C. S., & Scheier, M. F. *Attention and self-regulation: A control-theory approach to human behavior*. New York: Springer-Verlag, 1981.

Epstein, S. The self-concept: Or, a theory of a theory. *American Psychologist*, 1973, 28, 404–416.

Glynne, K., Hirschman, R., & Leventhal, H. *Smoking in school children*. Manuscript in preparation, University of Wisconsin—Madison, 1982.

Gutmann, M. C., Pollock, M. L., Schmidt, D. H., & Dudek, S. *Symptom monitoring and attribution by cardiac patients*. Paper presented at the annual meeting of the American Federation for Clinical Research, 1981.

Herzlich, C. *Health and illness: A social psychological analysis*. New York: Academic Press, 1973.

Johnson, J. E. Stress reduction through sensation information. In I. C. Sarason & C. D. Spielberger (Eds.), *Stress and anxiety* (Vol. 2). Washington: Hemisphere, 1975.

Johnson, J. E., & Leventhal, H. Effects of accurate expectations and behavioral instructions on reactions during a noxious medical examination. *Journal of Personality and Social Psychology*, 1974, *29*, 710–718.

Johnson, J. E., Rice, V. H., Fuller, S. S., & Endress, M. P. Sensory information, instruction in a coping strategy, and recovery from surgery. *Research in Nursing and Health*, 1978, *1*, 4–17.

Kelly, G. A. *The psychology of personal constructs* (Vols. 1 & 2). New York: Norton, 1955.

Lazarus, R. *Psychological stress and the coping process*. New York: McGraw-Hill, 1966.

Leventhal, E., Shacham, S., Boothe, L., & Leventhal, H. *The role of attention in distress control during childbirth*. Unpublished manuscript, University of Wisconsin—Madison, 1981.

Leventhal, H. Findings and theory in the study of fear communications. In L. Berkowitz (Ed.), *Advances in experimental social psychology* (Vol. 5). New York: Academic Press, 1970.

Leventhal, H. The consequences of depersonalization during illness and treatment. In J. Howard & A. Strauss (Eds.), *Humanizing health care*. New York: Wiley, 1975.

Leventhal, H., & Everhart, D. Emotion, pain, and physical illness. In C. Izard (Ed.), *Emotions and psychopathology*. New York: Plenum Press, 1979.

Leventhal, H., Nerenz, D. R., & Steele, D. Disease representations and coping with health threats. In A. Baum & J. Singer (Eds.), *Handbook of psychology and health*. Hillsdale, N.J.: Erlbaum, 1983.

Linz, D., Penrod, S., & Leventhal, H. *Lay persons' conceptions of illness*. Unpublished manuscript, University of Wisconsin—Madison, 1981.

Melzack, R. *The puzzle of pain*. New York: Basic Books, 1973.

Meyer, D. L. *The effects of patients' representations of·high blood pressure on behavior in treatment*. Unpublished doctoral dissertation, University of Wisconsin—Madison, 1981.

Meyer, D. L., Leventhal, H., & Gutmann, M. Symptoms in hypertension: How patients evaluate and treat them. *New England Journal of Medicine*, in press.

Miller, G. A., Galanter, E., & Pribram, K. H. *Plans and the structure of behavior*. New York: Henry Holt, 1960.

Mosbach, P. *Factors associated with delay in seeking care for mental health problems*. Unpublished master's thesis, University of Wisconsin—Madison, 1982.

Neisser, U. *Cognitive psychology*. New York: Appleton-Century-Crofts, 1967.

Nerenz, D. R. *Control of emotional distress in cancer chemotherapy*. Unpublished doctoral dissertation, University of Wisconsin—Madison, 1979.

Nisbett, R. E., & Ross, L. *Human inference: Strategies and shortcomings of social judgment*. Englewood Cliffs, N.J.: Prentice-Hall, 1980.

Powers, W. T. *Behavior: The control of perception*. Chicago:.Aldine, 1973.

Ringler, K. E. *Processes of coping with cancer chemotherapy*. Unpublished doctoral dissertation, University of Wisconsin—Madison, 1981.

Rogers, R. W. Cognitive and physiological processes in fear appeals and attitude change: A revised theory of protection motivation. In J. Cacioppo and R. Petty (Eds.), *Social psychophysiology*. New York: Guilford Press, 1982.

Safer, M. A., Tharps, Q., Jackson, T., & Leventhal, H. Determinants of three stages of delay in seeking care at a medical clinic. *Medical Care*, 1979, *17*, 11–29.

Schwartz, G. The brain as a health care system. In G. C. Stone, F. Cohen, & N. E. Adler (Eds.), *Health psychology: A handbook*. San Francisco: Jossey-Bass, 1979.

Shiffrin, R. M., & Schneider, W. Controlled and automatic human information processing: II. Perceptual learning, automatic attending, and a general theory. *Psychological Review*, 1977, *84*, 127–190.

Suchman, E. A. Stages of illness and medical care. *Journal of Health and Social Behavior*, 1965, 6, 114.
von Bertalanffy, L. *General systems theory*. New York: Braziller, 1968.
Wooley, S. C., Blackwell, B., & Winget, C. A learning theory model of chronic illness behavior: Theory, treatment, and research. *Psychosomatic Medicine*, 1978, *40*, 379–401.
Zimmerman, R., Linz, D., Leventhal, H., & Penrod, S. *The effects of blood pressure information on perception of symptoms*. Manuscript in preparation, University of Wisconsin—Madison, 1982.

3

Methodological Issues in Research on Coping with Chronic Disease

DAVID WATSON
PHILIP C. KENDALL

All interest in disease and death is only another expression of interest in life.
THOMAS MANN

Introduction

There has been a proliferation of research concerning the psychological consequences of chronic disease since the 1970s. This research has assumed an increasingly important position in medical psychology and behavioral medicine. And, happily, it appears to have increased in quality as well as in quantity.

However, many problems remain—problems that hamper the interpretation of results and diminish the overall utility and impact of much of the research. It should be noted that many of the practices and procedures we criticize are not, strictly speaking, "wrong," but instead represent less-than-optimal approaches to research design and data analysis. Thus, many of our recommendations pertain to ways of extracting the *most* information from a study and from a particular set of data. Our suggestions will center on the following major points: (*a*) *coping* is a multifaceted concept that cannot be fully assessed by a single measure, but requires several diverse assessment measures; (*b*) the dependent variables included in a study should be carefully selected and should be of demonstrable reliability and validity; (c) correlational and multivariate analyses are necessary to explicate the relationships among the variables; and (d) long-term longitudinal designs provide the clearest view of the process of psychological adaptation to chronic disease.

The present chapter is divided into four main sections. The first section contains a discussion of the major issues in the formulation of a research design. The second section is devoted to the specific problem of assessment and provides general guidelines for the inclusion of measures in a study. The third section discusses some major issues that should be considered in the data analysis, and the final section presents conclusions and suggestions for further research.

Most of the research that will be discussed can be classified into one of two categories:

1. *Coping studies* that investigate the impact of the chronic disease on the individual (e.g., by comparing the mean personality characteristics of a patient group with those of an appropriate control group). This type of research seeks to answer the question "How well or how poorly are these patients coping?"
2. *Outcome studies* that evaluate the effectiveness of a particular intervention in ameliorating the negative impact of the disease. This type of research attempts to answer the question "Does the intervention enhance the patients' coping?"

The issues involved in the two types of research noted above are often somewhat different and, thus, will be discussed separately at various points in the review.

Research Design Issues

SAMPLE CHARACTERISTICS: COPING STUDIES

One of the first problems facing an investigator is that of specifying the exact nature of the population to be studied. As pointed out by several authors (Bradley, Prokop, Gentry, Van der Heide, & Prieto, 1981; Fordyce, 1976; Hardyck & Moos, 1966; Meyerowitz, 1970), chronic disease patient groups often are mistakenly viewed as single, homogeneous populations. In fact, they typically are heterogeneous groups that may include individuals differing greatly with respect to demographic characteristics such as vocational and social problems, psychopathology, and etiology, severity, and duration of disease. Moreover, patient group characteristics generally will not be randomly distributed across clinic and hospital sites. For example, teaching hospital clinics often will treat the most severely affected or most difficult patients, or those with special complicating problems. Roberts and Reinhardt (1980) studied a sample of chronic pain patients seen at a university teaching hospital clinic and noted that "patients referred to the clinic for evaluation are almost always particularly difficult chronic pain patients not deemed suitable for referral to or treatment in other local programs (p. 152)." Similarly, Chapman, Sola, and Bonica (1979) found more somatic complaints and depression in a university teaching hospital sample of chronic pain patients than in a chronic pain sample seen in private practice.

The implication is that samples of patients seen at a single site may not constitute a representative sample of a total chronic disease population; hence, results based solely on one such sample cannot be used to characterize the entire patient population. Unfortunately, however, most coping studies use "samples of convenience" obtained at a single site.

Nonetheless, it is not necessary to study the total patient population. An investigator might only be interested, for example, in tension headache or severe rheumatoid arthritis patients. Whatever the target group, however, it is absolutely necessary to obtain a representative sample of that population. If, as is very often the case, an investigator is interested in describing the psychological characteristics of a general patient group, then it often will be necessary to obtain patients from a variety of clinic sites.

Constructing a sample from multiple sites also may be desirable when an investigator is interested in conducting correlational research, because correlations will necessarily be low when the variance of one or more variables is attenuated. For example, Fordyce and his associates (Fordyce, Brena, Holcomb, DeLateur, & Loeser, 1978) found little relationship between pain descriptions and Minnesota Multiphasic Personality Inventory (MMPI) scores, while other researchers (Leavitt & Garron, 1979; McCreary, Turner, & Dawson, 1981) have reported substantial relationships between pain ratings and scores on the MMPI. McCreary et al. (1981) suggest that the discrepant results of Fordyce et al. may be due to the fact that the latter group's sample (pain patients referred to a university hospital pain clinic) produced more homogeneous MMPI scores than did their sample (patients seen at a university hospital orthopedic clinic).

Differences in patient selection also may contribute to dissimilarities among the samples used in different studies. Goldstein (1981), for example, has noted that some studies of the psychological characteristics of hypertensive patients have used only essential (i.e., of unknown etiology) hypertensives, whereas others have included patients whose problems are of endocrine or renal origin. Similarly, some chronic pain investigators have used only low back patients, and others have included those suffering from headache or other pain. Investigations that use very different samples can produce very different results.

Dissimilar samples also may reflect differences in diagnostic criteria or simply diagnostic error. Pickering (1968), for example, has pointed out that some experimenters have used a blood pressure as low as 120/80 mm Hg to define hypertension, whereas others have established a criterion as high as 180/110 mm Hg. Goldstein (1981) has noted that hypertensive patients have been selected on the basis of only systolic or diastolic blood pressure levels as well as on various combinations of the two. Creer (1979) has argued that, due to diagnostic error, many patients have been included in asthma research who actually have suffered from other respiratory disorders (see Creer, Chapter 12).

Clearly, investigators must give careful consideration to the specific populations of interest and to the question of whether or not their patient samples are truly representative of those populations. Investigators also should consider patient selection and diagnostic criteria more carefully than have many previous researchers. In addition, investigators should report in greater detail the characteristics of their samples, the sites at which they are obtained, and the criteria used for diagnosis and selection.

SAMPLE CHARACTERISTICS: OUTCOME STUDIES

The samples used in outcome research generally will not be representative of the overall patient populations, if for no other reason than that the studied patients will tend to be those who are not coping well.[1] The extent of a sample's deviation from its population norm will depend on several factors such as the goal of the intervention (e.g., chronic pain treatment programs designed as last resorts for patients who have not been helped by previous medical or psychological interventions will include patients who are very atypical) and the cost of treatment (e.g., inpatient chronic pain programs usually try to screen out those patients who are not likely to be helped and thus tend to produce atypical samples). Adequate reporting of the sample characteristics as well as inclusion or exclusion criteria will enable other health care professionals to determine exactly what kinds of patients were helped by the intervention.

The prediction of which patients will be helped by the psychosocial intervention under investigation is an important part of any outcome research.

[1]However, Sobel and Worden (1979) have pointed out that many psychosocial interventions have been indiscriminately applied to entire groups of medical patients, including those manifesting no coping problems.

Prediction efforts benefit from some form of correlation analysis (whether through a chi square, simple correlation, multiple regression, or another procedure); it therefore is important for an investigator to anticipate (e.g., through pilot testing) the distributions of potentially important predictor variables within the sample. If any such variables have little variance or a highly skewed distribution, an investigator may wish to broaden the composition of the sample through changes in selection or diagnostic criteria. For example, several studies have found that high scores on the Hypochondriasis (Hs) scale of the MMPI are associated with poor outcomes following a variety of medical treatments to relieve chronic pain (e.g., Blumetti & Modesti, 1976; McCreary, Turner, & Dawson, 1979; Phillips, 1964; Wiltse & Rocchio, 1975). The Hs scale might also prove to be an important predictor of success in operant pain treatment approaches. However, the Hs scores of pain patients seen in some inpatient programs tend to be very high (see, for example, Reinhardt, 1979); the attenuated variance in these samples limits the scale's potential ability to predict successful outcomes. Correlations corrected for attenuation would be desirable in such cases (Guilford & Fruchter, 1973).[2]

RELIABILITY OF DIAGNOSIS

Patients often are selected for inclusion in a study and/or assigned to a particular treatment group on the basis of a medical diagnosis. Medical diagnoses usually are seen as objective, reliable, and valid judgments that require little analysis or comment. In fact, the reliability and validity of medical diagnoses can be questioned (Feinstein, 1977). For example, a number of studies have compared the average MMPI scale scores of patients with functional pain (i.e., pain with no demonstrable physical etiology) with those of patients whose pain has a clear organic basis. Although some studies (e.g., Calsyn, Louks, & Freeman, 1976; Louks, Freeman, & Calsyn, 1978; McCreary, Turner, & Dawson, 1977) have found substantial differences between the two groups, others have not (e.g., Carr, Brownsberger, & Rutherford, 1966; Cox, Chapman, & Black, 1978; Fordyce et al., 1978; Lair & Trapp, 1962). Of all these studies, only the Fordyce et al. investigation included a measure of the extent to which different physicians had made the same diagnosis. Six physicians were asked to place 100 pain patients on an organic–functional continuum; it was reported that the average interphysician correlation was only .59. This interrater reliability coefficient was far too

[2]For a discussion of factors that affect the value of a correlation coefficient, see Nunnally, 1978, pp. 138–146; Guilford and Fruchter, 1973, pp. 324–334.

low to have permitted any important decisions regarding individual cases. Of course, it is certainly possible that physicians used in some of the other studies were able to make more reliable and meaningful judgments about the etiology of patients' pain experiences; this might explain the inconsistency of the results across studies. However, reliability of diagnosis cannot be assumed, and the burden of proof lies with those who claim that such judgments can be reliably and meaningfully rendered.

Hypertension research also is plagued with questionable diagnoses. Smith (1977) and Goldstein (1981) have noted that a single blood pressure reading can easily lead to the misclassification of individual patients. Nonetheless, there appears to be no general consensus regarding the number of measurements necessary to obtain a stable value (see Goldstein, 1981); in fact, studies have varied widely in the number of blood pressure readings taken. This issue deserves more thought and investigation (see Coates, Perry, Killen, & Slinkard, 1981).

General reviews of medical diagnoses (e.g., Feinstein, 1977; Koran, 1975) indicate that reliability should not be assumed in most cases, but rather should be measured and reported. Diagnostic reliability can be demonstrated, for example, by obtaining two or more independent judgments for each patient and calculating an interrater reliability coefficient (for a recent discussion of interrater reliability, see Mitchell, 1979). For unstable measures, such as blood pressure readings, the best approach is to obtain a number of readings from each subject. These individual measurements then can be summed to form an aggregate measure, the internal consistency of which can be assessed using Cronbach's (1951) coefficient alpha. If the reliability of this aggregate score is too low, more measurements should be taken (Nunnally, 1978, pp. 245–246 discusses satisfactory levels of reliability in basic research and in applied settings).

CONTROL GROUPS: COPING STUDIES

Much of the early research concerning the psychological characteristics of patients with chronic disease was based upon subjective data, obtained through interviews and other clinical contact, and was conducted without benefit of control groups. It is now recognized that meaningful scientific research requires objective data and control group comparisons.

However, it is not clear which individuals constitute the most appropriate control subjects. Many studies, for example, have used scale norms (e.g., MMPI *T* scores) derived from a normal (control) population. Other studies (e.g., Moos & Solomon, 1965) have used patients' siblings or other relatives to control for a variety of demographic and environmental characteristics.

Many researchers have judged normal controls to be inappropriate, and instead have turned to individuals suffering from physical problems other than those suffered by the patients of interest. Thus, some investigators (e.g., Bond & Pearson, 1969) have used a general medical patient sample to control for factors such as hospitalization and physical symptomatology, and others (e.g., Cleveland, Reitman, & Brewer, 1965; Ostfeld & Lebovitz, 1959; Spergel, Ehrlich, & Glass, 1978) have used other chronic disease groups to control for the effects of chronic disease per se.

Some researchers have attempted to make appropriate comparisons by using two or more control groups. For example, Spergel et al. (1978) compared the MMPI scores of rheumatoid arthritics with those of patients with gastric ulcers, multiple sclerosis, low back pain, and pulmonary disease. Hardyck and Moos (1966) studied the MMPI responses of two chronic disease groups (rheumatoid arthritics and hypertensives) and two control groups (relatives of the arthritics and normals). Ward (1971) compared the Maudsley Personality Inventory (MPI; Eysenck, 1959) scores of rheumatoid arthritics with those of surgery patients and neurotics. Dattore, Shontz, and Coyne (1980) compared the premorbid MMPI scores of cancer patients to those of an aggregate control group that was constructed from equal numbers of normals, schizophrenics, essential hypertensives, patients with gastrointestinal ulcers, and those with benign neoplasms.

It is obvious that the use of different types of control groups can lead to very different conclusions regarding the psychological characteristics of a patient group. Hardyck and Moos (1966), for example, found that their two control groups were as different from one another as each was from either of the two chronic disease groups. Bond and Pearson (1969) compared the MPI Neuroticism scores of cervical cancer patients with those of a medical patient sample and a housewife normative sample. The cancer patients appeared quite normal when compared to the housewives (their mean score of 10.64 was very close to the normative mean of 10.52); however, their Neuroticism scores were significantly *lower* than those of the medical patients. This cancer patient sample thus may be viewed as either normal or defensive, depending upon the control group used to make the comparison.

The importance of the control sample is perhaps most strikingly illustrated in the study conducted by Dattore et al. (1980). As noted previously, the authors compared scores on 17 MMPI scales produced by a group of cancer patients to those of an aggregate control sample. An interesting aspect of the study is that the MMPIs were collected at least 1 year before the initial diagnoses had been made (i.e., when the subjects were not experiencing any significant medical or psychiatric difficulty). Any differences between the groups thus reflected differences in premorbid personality functioning. Analyses showed that the cancer patients had significantly lower scores than did the control subjects on the Depression (D), Repression–Sensitization $(R–S;$ Byrne, 1961), and Denial of Symptoms $(Dn;$ Little & Fisher, 1958) scales. It was concluded that the cancer patients showed relatively greater premorbid repressive tendencies, particularly with regard to depressive affect. This interpretation is consistent with Bahnson and Bahnson's (1964) "psychophysiological complementarity" theory of cancer, which holds that repression is a primary feature of the premorbid cancer personality. The interpretation offered by Dattore et al. (1980) assumes, of course, that the control patients represented a fairly normal sample; thus, the cancer patients reported lower than normal levels of maladjustment. An alternative interpretation might be that the cancer patients were essentially normal premorbidly, and that the control patients (recall that this sample included schizophrenics, essential hypertensives, and patients with gastrointestinal ulcers) reported greater than normal maladjustment. It would be possible to choose between these two explanations if the authors had reported the actual T scores for the two groups; in the absence of such information the latter interpretation seems more plausible.

Finding the appropriate control groups for comparison is a major problem that is not easily resolved. However, with some tests and with certain populations it is clear that normals do not represent an adequate control sample. Consider, for example, the most widely used instrument in research of this type, the MMPI. Studies with this test invariably find that chronic disease patients have elevated mean scores on the "neurotic triad": the Hs, D, and Hysteria (Hy) scales. Such elevations have been found, for example, among multiple sclerotics (Baldwin, 1952; Bourestom & Howard, 1965; Lanyon, 1968), rheumatoid arthritics (Bourestom & Howard, 1965; Moos & Solomon, 1964; Nalven & O'Brien, 1964; Spergel et al., 1978), ulcer patients (Lanyon, 1968; Sullivan & Welsh, 1952), spinal cord injured patients (Bourestom & Howard, 1965; Taylor, 1970), persons with pulmonary disease (Lanyon, 1968), and chronic pain patients (Cox et al., 1978; Freeman, Calsyn, & Louks, 1976; Lanyon, 1968; Phillips, 1964; Sternbach, Wolf, Murphy, & Akeson, 1973; Strassberg, Reimherr, Ward, Russell, & Cole, 1981; Watson, 1982b). The pervasiveness of this finding has led Spergel et al. (1978) to suggest that there may be a "chronic disease personality" characterized by somatic overconcern, depression, and repression that is common to all of the patient groups noted above.

However, many investigators (e.g., Baldwin, 1952; Kendall, Edinger, & Eberly, 1978; Meyerson, 1957; Nalven & O'Brien, 1964, 1968; Taylor, 1970; Watson, 1982b) have pointed out that it is inappropriate to describe patients with chronic diseases on the basis of norms that are derived from normal populations. The neurotic triad scales of the MMPI contain many items referring to specific physical problems as well as more general health-related items such as "I am about as able to work as I ever was"; "I am in just as good physical health as most of my friends"; and "During the past few years I have been well most of the time." It is important to remember that these items were included in the neurotic triad scales because patients diagnosed as hypochondriacal, depressed, or hysterical endorsed them more frequently than did normals. However, a patient with chronic disease who admits to having poor physical health and many pains is not necessarily hypochondriacal or depressed!

The problem outlined above is not confined solely to the MMPI. The MPI Neuroticism scale and its successor, the Eysenck Personality Inventory (EPI; Eysenck & Eysenck, 1964) Neuroticism scale are other measures frequently used in chronic disease research. Hill (1971) has noted that the EPI Neuroticism scale includes several questions referring to somatic problems, including "Are you troubled by aches and pains?" and "Do you worry about your health?" Hill (1971) and Levy (1981) have pointed out that many depression and extraversion scales include items that may reflect impaired mobility subsequent to a chronic physical problem. Other investigators (Goldstein, 1981; Suess & Chai, 1981) have argued that the test scores of hypertensives and asthmatics can be greatly affected by medications, the effects of which may persist after the cessation of usage. Levy (1981) has delineated several artifactual variables (fatigue and low motivation, as well as sensory and motor deficits) that may present a distorted picture of the psychological status of geriatric patients. As noted by Meyerson (1957), Taylor (1970), and Kendall et al. (1978), the problem is essentially one of validity generalization—that is, do test scores have the same psychological implications for patients with chronic diseases that they have for relatively healthy individuals? Validity generalization should not be assumed, but instead needs to be demonstrated for each patient group.

By now the limitations of a coping study that compares mean characteristics of patient and control samples should be clear. The use of atypical samples, inappropriate and/or poorly understood control groups, or tests of unknown or questionable validity in the patient population can undermine meaningful interpretations of the results.

CONTROL GROUPS: OUTCOME STUDIES

Confounding Effects

Comparison groups in outcome studies are necessary to control for a number of different types of confounding effects (see Kendall & Norton-Ford, 1982). First, there is *spontaneous remission*, or what might be called *time effects*. That is, patients' coping levels may change simply with the passage of time. For example, cancer patients may experience a marked increase in emotional distress or vocational and marital problems with the initial diagnosis of the disease. As time passes, however, many patients return nearly to premorbid levels of functioning as they adjust to the disease. Any intervention designed to help these patients obviously must be evaluated against the effects of time. A no-treatment control group (e.g., Andrasik & Holroyd, 1980; Kendall, Williams, Pechacek, Graham, Shisslak, & Herzoff, 1979) is sufficient for this purpose as long as the patients are randomly assigned to the groups. Nonetheless, time effects will not be controlled if the groups differ on variables other than the assignment to treatment conditions. For example, Roberts and Reinhardt (1980) compared the adjustment of patients who had completed an inpatient pain treatment program (after posttreatment intervals ranging from 1 to 8 years) with that of patients who either had been rejected for treatment or had refused to enter the program. Reasons for patient rejection included unwillingness to return to work, a complicating medical problem, pending litigation, a primary chemical dependency problem, and severe mental disorder. There is no good reason to believe that patients who had been rejected for treatment or who had refused to enter the program would have exhibited changes over time similar to those that patients in the intervention group would have shown in the absence of treatment.

Comparison groups also must be used in order to control for *placebo effects*. These effects are nonspecific changes that result from the process of being treated per se, rather than from aspects specific to the treatment. The factors that produce placebo effects are very interesting in their own right (see Bootzin & Lick, 1979; Jospe, 1978; Prokop & Bradley, 1981b), but are a great nuisance in outcome research.

Sources of Placebo Effects

There are two main sources of placebo effects. First, there are patients' expectations of benefits. It frequently has been shown that many patients will exhibit some improvement simply because they expect to get better. For example, Brena and his colleagues (Brena, Wolf, Chapman, & Hammonds, 1980) examined 20 chronic low back pain patients who received 12 lumbar sympathetic injections. Each patient received six injections of the drug bupivacaine and six saline injections. The drug and placebo injections led to significant and equivalent reductions in the patients' subjective pain ratings. Another illustration of expectancy effects can be seen in a study conducted by Andrasik and Holroyd (1980). These authors studied 39 tension headache sufferers in an investigation of the effects of EMG biofeedback on frontal muscle tension. Subjects were assigned to either one of three biofeedback groups or to a no-treatment control group. Subjects in the treatment groups received several sessions of biofeedback training designed to produce decreased, stable, or increased levels of frontal muscle tension. However, all three groups were led to believe that they were learning to reduce muscle tension levels. Analysis of EMG data indicated that all three treatment groups were appropriately affected by the feedback—for example, the tension-increase group exhibited an increase in muscle tension levels. Nonetheless, following treatment all three biofeedback groups had significantly lower levels of self-reported headache pain than did the no-treatment control group; there were no significant differences among the three biofeedback groups. It is clear that frontal muscle tension reduction per se was not a factor in reducing patients' headache pain, and that patients' expectations that biofeedback would benefit them partially mediated patients' pain rating changes.

The second source of placebo effects is the nonspecific increase in attention and interpersonal interaction provided to patients by most psychosocial interventions. For example, Lucas (1976) investigated the effectiveness of various preoperative interventions in facilitating the recovery of heart surgery patients. The patients were divided into four groups: (a) patients who were trained to actively focus on plans for recovery and future life; (b) patients who merely were asked to think about recovery and future plans; (c) patients who only were given increased attention commensurate with that provided to patients in the former two groups; and (d) patients who received no treatment. The results indicated that the first three groups showed significantly better recoveries than did the no-treatment controls, but that they did not differ significantly among themselves. Thus, increased attention alone produced significant improvements in patients' postsurgery recovery.

It is generally believed that most placebo effects are short-lived, and that they will have largely dissipated at a long-term follow-up assessment (e.g., Fordyce & Steger, 1979). This might imply that the inclusion of a follow-up assessment reduces or eliminates the need for an appropriate control group. However, there appear to be no good data to support this belief (Roberts, 1981).

Placebo control groups are both a scientific and practical necessity. They are a scientific necessity because without adequate controls it is possible to determine the efficacy of an intervention but it is not possible to specify what factors contributed to the outcome. In other words, one may be able to determine that a treatment worked, but without the use of placebo control groups one cannot say *why* or *how* it worked. Failure to use adequate controls is thus inimical to the basic scientific goal of *understanding*—that is, of ascertaining why and how events occur.

Placebo control groups are a practical necessity because scarce treatment resources are wasted when they are used in ways that do not benefit the patient population. Interventions designed for patients with chronic disease are frequently lengthy and very expensive, and require extensive use of staff and other hospital-based resources. Inpatient chronic pain treatment programs, for example, typically require 3–8 weeks of hospitalization and cost several thousand dollars per patient (Fordyce & Steger, 1979; Roberts, 1981; Turk & Genest, 1979). The cost effectiveness of these interventions can be increased through the isolation and elimination of ineffective programs and procedures.

Placebo Control Procedures

Several characteristics of an adequate placebo control procedure can be noted. First, assignment of patients to treatment and control groups must be completely random so that the control group patients are as nearly identical to the treatment group patients as possible. This point may seem too obvious to mention, but it can be more difficult to achieve subject randomization in practice than is commonly supposed. For example, one method frequently used to eliminate bias in group composition is to alternate assignment to the groups—for example, odd-numbered admissions are placed in the primary intervention group and even-numbered admissions are assigned to a control condition. Kraemer (1981), however, has argued that staff members or investigators often consciously or unconsciously gerrymander assignment order, thereby biasing the samples. She has noted that "even the risk of such bias is good reason to avoid this procedure [p. 313]." A technique that is superior to alternate assignment is the randomization procedure developed by Efron (1971). The procedure requires (*a*) the first patient to enter the study and (*b*) any patient who enters when the group sizes are equal to be randomly assigned to one of the groups. When group sizes are unequal, an entering patient has a one-in-three chance of being put into the larger group, and a two-in-three chance of being placed into the smaller group. The most crucial aspect of this procedure is that there never is sure knowledge of group assignment, and yet there remains a constant pressure to equalize the group sizes (see Kraemer, 1981).

The second attribute of a proper placebo control intervention is that it must be similar to the primary intervention in terms of credibility to the patients and in the generation of patients' expectations for success (Kendall & Norton-Ford, 1982). That is, the patients in the primary intervention and placebo control groups must view their respective treatments as being equally likely to help them. Many studies have used control groups that do not satisfy this criterion. For example, several researchers (e.g., Alexander & Smith, 1979; Andrasik & Holroyd, 1980; Beaty & Haynes, 1979; Miller &

Dworkin, 1977; Shapiro & Surwit, 1976) have questioned the credibility of the false feedback procedures (in which feedback is manipulated by the experimenter) that have been widely used as attention placebo treatments in biofeedback studies. Whether or not the placebo effects associated with any treatment intervention actually have been controlled can be directly assessed by requiring patients in the primary intervention and placebo control groups to rate the credibility of their respective treatments and their expectations for treatment success (see Andrasik & Holroyd, 1980; Borkovec, 1972; Borkovec & Nau, 1972; Prokop & Bradley, 1981b).

The credibility of any control treatment also can be assessed by comparing the attrition rates (the percentage of patients in a group who drop out of treatment during the study) within the primary intervention and placebo control groups. If a control group has a relatively higher attrition rate, the credibility of the placebo control treatment can be seriously questioned. It therefore is desirable to report the attrition rates for each treatment group included in a study.[3]

The third attribute of a proper placebo control intervention is that it should provide patients with as much interaction with the treatment staff as that provided to patients in the primary intervention group. This can be easily arranged by scheduling comparable amounts of staff contact with each patient, regardless of group assignment.

Finally, many interventions that are used with chronic disease patients are multidisciplinary and include a wide variety of specific treatment elements (see Fordyce & Steger, 1979; Gordon, Friedenbergs, Diller, Hibbard, Wolf, Levine, Lipkins, Ezrachi, & Lucido, 1980; Turk & Genest, 1979; Ziesat, 1981). A single program may include patient education, behavior modification, physical therapy, withdrawal from addictive drugs, occupational and marital counseling, and psychotherapy. It is important to tease out the separate effect of each component so that factors contributing to treatment success can be isolated and ineffectual procedures can be eliminated. Such a dismantling study (Kazdin & Wilson, 1978) can be performed using a factorial design in which groups of patients are provided the intervention with one of the component procedures removed. A factorial design minimizes the ethical problems raised by the withholding of treatment from control group patients, which have been partially responsible for the lack of no-treatment control groups in many areas of outcome research. Furthermore, 'Ziesat (1981) has noted that clinics treating large numbers of patients can investigate the separate effects of several treatment facets within the same dismantling study.

[3]It is also important to compare treatment drop-outs from "remainers" across all relevant variables. These comparisons are necessary to establish whether or not the remainer group is representative of the original sample (Kendall & Norton-Ford, 1982).

LONGITUDINAL RESEARCH DESIGNS: COPING STUDIES

We already have noted some of the limitations of the typical coping study in which the mean responses of a chronic patient group are compared with those of one or more control samples. In this section we consider other problems with this research approach and discuss the benefits of using predictive, longitudinal designs in coping studies.

As was discussed in "Sample Characteristics: Coping Studies" and "Control Groups: Coping Studies," one basic problem with the majority of coping studies is that the obtained group differences may reflect methodological artifacts (e.g., atypical patient samples, inappropriate comparison groups, uncontrolled drug effects, or the use of tests that contain many items regarding chronic physical problems and/or impaired mobility) rather than true psychological differences. Moreover, even if the results may be assumed to reflect meaningful between-group differences, they often are open to a variety of interpretations. Most importantly, *if patients are assessed only once it is impossible to separate out premorbid personality differences from psychological changes resulting from the chronic physical problem.* The interpretative problem is particularly acute when psychophysiologic (e.g., asthma, hypertension, ulcers) or somatization (e.g., chronic benign pain) processes are thought to have a role in the development of some patients' symptoms.

Some investigators have vainly sought to circumvent this problem by comparing the test scores of patients who have suffered from the disease for varying lengths of time (e.g., Shadish, Hickman, & Arrick, 1981; Sternbach et al., 1973; Ward, 1971). For example, Sternbach et al. (1973) found that patients with chronic benign pain (lasting 6 months or longer) had higher scores on the neurotic triad scales of the MMPI than did patients with acute pain (lasting less than 6 months). This study was based upon the assumption that "acute patients are those who will, with the passage of time, become chronic patients [Sternbach, 1974, p. 16]." If this assumption were valid, then the Sternbach et al. results would indicate that pain patients' elevations on the neurotic triad scales are at least partially due to the chronicity of their physical problems.

However, it is unreasonable to assume that patients sampled at different points of the disease process represent samples drawn from the same population. In the case of some diseases (e.g., cancer, coronary heart disease), it is reasonable to believe that psychological factors (such as the adaptive use of denial; see Krantz, 1980; Krantz & Deckel, Chapter 4) are related to patient survival. Thus, patients assessed at a relatively late point in the course of a disease will be a selected subset, and will necessarily have higher mean scores on the survival-related factors than will patients assessed soon after disease onset. For other diseases (e.g., chronic benign pain), it is reasonable to believe that poor coping ability is related to the continuation of physical symptoms. For example, several studies (Blumetti & Modesti, 1976; McCreary *et al.*, 1979; Phillips, 1964; Wiltse & Rocchio, 1975) have shown that high neurotic triad scores among back pain patients are associated with poor outcomes following medical or psychological treatments. This suggests that acute pain patients with low neurotic triad scores are less likely than those with high scores to become chronically disabled. Given this selection factor, the neurotic triad scores of patients with chronic pain will necessarily tend to be higher than those of patients with acute pain.

Because of selection factors such as these, it cannot be assumed that patients measured at different points in the disease process are sampled from the same population. This pseudolongitudinal design therefore should not be used. Instead, investigations of psychological changes resulting from a chronic disease must employ a longitudinal design in which the same patients are studied on two or more occasions (see, for example, Crown & Crown, 1973). Obviously, it is best to perform the initial assessment as early in the disease process as is possible. Premorbid vocational status and other important demographic information usually can be obtained from the patient and, in some settings (e.g., Veterans Administration hospitals), one may have access to premorbid scores on intelligence and personality measures. Barring this, it is desirable to minimize the time span between disease onset and the collection of psychological data.

Longitudinal designs allow for another important benefit in addition to those previously described: they permit predictive analyses. For example, those patient characteristics that are associated with an early return to premorbid vocational status or other indicators of positive treatment outcome can be assessed. Unfortunately, many coping studies have employed only one measurement of patient attributes and have reported only mean group differences. Thus, they have tended to create what Fordyce has called "the illusion of homogeneity [1976, p. 141]"—the belief that each of the patients individually manifests the group's mean characteristics. For example, many investigators using the MMPI have mistakenly interpreted a mean group profile as if it were an individual profile (e.g., Bourestom & Howard, 1965; Spergel *et al.*, 1978; Sternbach, 1974; Sternbach *et al.*, 1973). Butcher and Tellegen (1978), however, have pointed out that personality correlates established for individuals cannot be applied to group MMPI profiles. They note that "it may actually be the case that *no* individual in the group has the code type corresponding to the group mean score [p. 626]."

A better approach to coping studies is to identify those individuals who are coping poorly and who are most in need of an ameliorative intervention (Sobel & Worden, 1979). This strategy permits more efficient use of scarce treatment resources. A predictive longitudinal approach is particularly useful here. Patients can be assessed at disease onset and at subsequent points in the disease process. Patient characteristics at disease onset that are related to long-term coping ability then can be identified. For example, Sobel and Worden (1979) found that the MMPI scores of newly diagnosed cancer patients were highly related to several indices of coping ability (e.g., mood disturbance, an inventory of psychosocial problems) that were assessed several months later. Additional efforts toward the identification of variables that predict coping ability among patient groups with various chronic diseases would permit early preventive interventions with those patients who were most likely to face long-term adjustment problems.

It must be emphasized that predictive longitudinal designs, although possibly quite useful, cannot be used to establish cause-and-effect relationships. Even if one were to find, for example, that premorbid *Hs* scores were highly predictive of long-term disability caused by chronic pain, it could not be concluded that disability is caused by hypochondriacal or other neurotic tendencies of the patients. Shontz (1970) has noted: "If a third factor (say, malnutrition) produces, first, personality changes and only later produces bodily disease, longitudinal tests would show predictive validity for personality tests and still fail to reveal the true cause of the illness [p. 60]."

PREDICTIVE DESIGNS IN OUTCOME RESEARCH

Perhaps the most typical design used in outcome research involves the assessment of two groups at pre- and posttreatment. The mean scores of the groups then are compared at each assessment point, and the pre- to posttreatment differences in each group are evaluated for significance (i.e., factorial designs using analyses of variance). We will now consider two additions to this basic design that greatly increase its utility.

First, predictive analyses are an extremely important aspect of outcome studies. Several writers (e.g., Bradley *et al.*, 1981; Kendall & Norton-Ford, 1982; Turk & Genest, 1979) have pointed out that, in addition to evaluating whether or not an intervention is effective, it is important for investigators to determine what kinds of patients are most likely to be helped or not helped by that intervention. With this information, programs can admit those patients who are most likely to show improvement. The information also can be used to design modifications of existing programs, or to develop new interventions for improving the care of patients who are not being helped by current treatment regimens. The ultimate goal of this predictive approach is the development of an actuarial system in which each patient is referred to that intervention program most likely to benefit him or her.

A major design problem with many previous prediction studies is that all patients were not given the same treatment (e.g., Blumetti & Modesti, 1976; McCreary et al., 1979; Strassberg et al., 1981; Waring, Weisz, & Bailey, 1976). For example, Strassberg et al. (1981) entered chronic pain patients' MMPI scores in a regression analysis in order to predict their responses to diverse treatments (e.g., nerve block, transcutaneous electrical stimulation) provided in an anesthesiology clinic. However, there is no reason to believe that the same variables will predict successful outcomes across all the treatments. Each treatment modality should therefore be individually examined through its own regression analysis.

Another design problem with many published predictive studies is the failure to perform long-term follow-up assessments of treatment success (Bradley et al., 1981; Fordyce & Steger, 1979; Prokop & Bradley, 1981b; Roberts, 1981). An intervention that produces long-lasting benefits obviously is to be preferred over one that does not; indeed, one can question the utility of an intervention that does not maintain its benefits months after treatment. Thus, the addition of a long-term follow-up assessment represents the second addition to the design of outcome studies that enhances their utility.

The lack of follow-up assessment in chronic disease research is particularly distressing because there is every reason to suspect that treatment effects may not endure in many patient groups. Environmental events (such as operant reinforcement of physical complaints and/or disability) or personality characteristics (such as those found in persons with disorders featuring a psychophysiologic or somatization component) associated with various chronic disorders may not be permanently affected by treatment interventions and in time may undo patient gains. Gordon et al. (1980), for example, found significant differences at posttreatment between their intervention and control groups; however, these differences virtually disappeared at a 3-month follow-up assessment (primarily because the control patients showed improved coping relative to intervention patients at follow-up).

CONCLUSION

Because many critical decisions will necessarily depend upon the general goals of the study, basic aspects of research (e.g., the population of interest, the questions to be investigated, the analyses to be performed) must be clearly formulated long before data are collected. For example, complex factorial and predictive designs require much larger sample sizes than simple group mean comparisons. We have outlined a basic predictive, longitudinal design that we feel provides clear answers to important research questions. We now turn to a discussion of some general considerations of the measures to be included in a study.

Assessment

RELIABILITY OF MEASURES

Adequate reliability of assessment measures is essential. Nunnally (1978) has defined reliability as follows:

> Reliability concerns the extent to which measurements are *repeatable*—when different persons make the measurements, on different occasions, with supposedly alternative instruments for measuring the same thing and when there are small variations in circumstances for making measurements that are not intended to influence results. In other words, measurements are intended to be *stable* over a variety of conditions in which essentially the same results should be obtained [p. 191].

As this definition suggests, reliability can be calculated in a number of ways. We already have mentioned the interrater and internal consistency reliability coefficients (see "Reliability of Diagnosis"). The former is obtained by correlating independent ratings of the same phenomena, and the latter is based on the average correlation among the component items of an aggregate measure. Another important index of reliability is the stability or test–retest coefficient, or the correlation between scores on the same measure obtained at different times.

It is unfortunate that a great many researchers in the chronic disease literature have not fully considered the reliability of their instruments. We have already noted, for example, that the reliabilities of medical and other criterion diagnoses (e.g., organic versus functional pain) generally are not assessed and reported. When the reliabilities of such diagnoses have been reported they often have been only moderate (e.g., Feinstein, 1977; Fordyce et al., 1978; Koran, 1975; Prokop & Bradley, 1981b). The interrater reliability of any diagnosis can be determined easily by having several judges independently provide a diagnosis for each patient. An interrater reliability coefficient then can be calculated. If the reliability of the diagnosis is low, retraining of diagnosticians or providing a more precise definition of the disorder may be required. Also, a low reliability coefficient can be increased by summing the individual ratings to form a composite measure. As a general rule, reliability increases as the number of component measurements in an aggregate measure increases (e.g., Horowitz, Inouye, & Siegelman, 1979; Strahan, 1980).

Similar points can be made about other types of ratings. For example, most of the studies investigating factors related to treatment success (e.g., Blumetti & Modesti, 1976; Else & Hastings, 1981; Wilfling, Klonoff, & Kokan, 1973; Wiltse & Rocchio, 1975) have used as the criterion variable simple ratings of treatment outcome made by the treating physician or another staff member (e.g., Else and Hastings had a nurse rate the recovery of their heart surgery patients as "good," "psychiatric," or "catastrophic"). There is no good reason to believe that the reliabilities of such ratings are very high. This fact is especially disturbing since the unreliability of a variable tends to limit its validity. That is, the random "noise" of measurement error tends to obscure lawful and systematic relationships between the variable of interest and other measures. The use of an unreliable criterion in a predictive study therefore is self-defeating.

It also has been pointed out (e.g., Bradley et al., 1981) that the reliability of behavioral measures (e.g., observer recordings of the number of pain behaviors emitted by patients during a given period) needs to be more carefully considered. Fordyce (1976) and Sternbach (1974) have noted that careful training of raters is an important step toward obtaining reliable behavioral assessments. In addition, Bradley et al. (1981) have advocated periodic "reliability checks" to correct "drift" (Kent & Foster, 1977) and other possible sources of unreliability in the behavioral ratings.

Many studies in the chronic disease literature have individually examined numerous variables by performing a separate analysis (e.g., t test) for each variable (see Bradley et al., 1981; Cox & Chapman, 1976; Prokop & Bradley, 1981b). An extreme example of this can be seen in a study conducted by Roberts and Reinhardt (1980) who compared their chronic pain groups on 164 and 213 variables at base-line and follow-up assessments, respectively. Several basic problems with a multiple t tests approach to data analysis can be noted. First, individual variables generally will be less reliable than will aggregate measures achieved by combining individual variables. With a sufficient sample size, aggregate measures can be easily developed by correlating all single variables and submitting them to a factor analysis (e.g., Strassberg et al., 1981; Trabin, 1981). A factor score can be calculated for each factor, and this score can then be treated as any other variable (Gorsuch, 1974). Second, if individual variables are significantly correlated with one another then the t tests performed on them will not be independent; the interpretation of these t tests will be relatively complicated. Third, as the number of t tests performed increases, so does the number of significant relationships to be expected by chance. For example, Roberts and Reinhardt (1980) reported that 11 of their 164 base-line group comparisons were significant. Given the extremely large number of significance tests that were performed, several significant relationships would be expected by chance alone and the few significant findings should not be interpreted as reflecting real group differences. Fourth, the use of numerous variables and analyses tends to obfuscate, rather than to enlighten. It is much easier to interpret results obtained on a small number of well-understood variables than it is to understand the meaning of a large number of individual t tests or other analyses. Finally, as the number of analyses increases, it becomes easier for a truly interesting and important relationship to become lost in a sea of variables. To return to the Roberts and Reinhardt example, the 11 significant findings included differences on the Hs, D, and Ego Strength (Es) scales of MMPI. Chronic pain patients who participated in treatment had lower Hs and D scores, and higher Es scores, than did the patients who declined to participate. These interesting differences suggest that the patients who volunteered for the study generally had fewer somatic complaints, were less depressed, and were coping better than were those who did not volunteer. However, because of the 153 nonsignificant t tests, these differences cannot be interpreted.

As noted above, the benefits to be gained from the use of a relatively small number of highly reliable measures are very substantial. However, it must be emphasized that only variables that are significantly related to one another should be combined to form an aggregate measure. If unrelated variables are combined, the resulting composite will *not* be reliable. For this reason, before any measures are combined their relationships should be assessed through correlational and/or factor analysis, and the reliability of the composite should be reported. This procedure frequently has not been followed. For example, some chronic pain outcome studies (e.g., Malec, Cayner, Harvey, & Timming, 1981; Maruta, Swanson, & Swenson, 1979; Roberts & Reinhardt, 1980) have used a composite index as a criterion for treatment success or failure. To be classified as a treatment "success" in the Maruta *et al.* (1979) study, a patient had to show moderate or marked improvement in each of three categories: improved attitude, reduced use of pain-related medications, and better physical functioning. No data were provided to indicate that these individual criteria were significantly related to one another, or that the resulting composite had adequate internal consistency. It could not be assumed that the individual categories were related, because studies in the chronic disease literature frequently have found that outcome criteria are not highly associated with one another. The failure to demonstrate the reliability of the composite was particularly unfortunate in the Maruta *et al.* (1979) study, as these authors were interested in identifying factors associated with treatment success; in fact, they developed a scale designed to differentiate between patients with successful versus unsuccessful outcomes. As previously stated, however, it is self-defeating to attempt to predict an unreliable criterion.

VALIDITY OF MEASURES

Questions of validity are questions of what may properly be inferred from a test score; validity refers to the appropriateness of inferences from test scores or other forms of assessment. The many types of validity questions can, for convenience, be reduced to two: (a) What can be inferred about what is being measured by the test? (b) What can be inferred about other behavior [American Psychological Association, 1974, p. 25]?

We already have touched on the topic of validity in our discussion of the appropriateness of using the MMPI and other tests (e.g., of neuroticism and extraversion) in chronic disease populations (see "Control Groups: Coping Studies"). The use of these tests with chronic disease patients was questioned because they include many items reflecting persistently poor physical health and reduced mobility. The nature of these items and their relationship to the special life problems of people who have a chronic disease mean that it is likely test scores of chronic disease patients require inferences that are different from those required of the scores produced by physically normal patients (Kendall *et al.*, 1978). Other factors, including uncontrolled drug effects, also can affect the validity of test scores in some patient groups such as hypertensives and chronically ill geriatric patients (e.g., Goldstein, 1981; Levy, 1981). Clearly, the validity of even very well-established and widely used measures should be re-evaluated in light of the special circumstances of specific patient populations. Let us consider some issues in the validity of specific types of measures, beginning with the MMPI.

MMPI

The MMPI has been used very extensively in the chronic disease literature. This test has been shown to have a variety of important uses, for example, as a predictor of treatment outcome (Blumetti & Modesti, 1976; McCreary *et al.*, 1979; Strassberg *et al.*, 1981; Wiltse & Rocchio, 1975) and as a predictor of early return to normal employment among orthopedic patients (Phillips, 1964). However, the test has been used inappropriately in revised, shortened forms and for purposes to which other measures are better suited. For example, many researchers have used one of the several short-form versions of the MMPI such as the Midi–Mult (Dean, 1972) and the Faschingbauer Abbreviated MMPI (Faschingbauer, 1974). These short forms are very attractive to researchers because of the difficulties involved in persuading chronically ill patients to complete either the full 566-item version or the 399-item Form R (Bradley *et al.*, 1981). Although scale scores on the short forms have been shown to be strongly correlated with those on the full test, it has been repeatedly found (Fillenbaum & Pfeiffer, 1976; Hedlund, Won Cho, & Powell, 1975; Hoffman & Butcher, 1975) that there is little congruence between the code types produced by the short forms and those obtained with the full test. While the abbreviated versions of the MMPI may have some useful applications, they should *not*, in general, be viewed as valid substitutes for the 566- or 399-item versions (Butcher, Kendall, & Hoffman, 1980; Butcher & Tellegen, 1978).

It also is recommended that *K*-corrected scale scores not be used in chronic disease research, since *K*'s "suppressor" function has not been well validated in these patient populations (see Butcher & Tellegen, 1978). Scale *K* instead should be used as a separate measure; multiple regression or some other type of multivariate analysis may be used to examine *K*'s possible role as a suppressor.

In addition, it should be emphasized that the MMPI was designed as a measure of psychopathology rather than normal range personality. Nonetheless, the test frequently has been used as a measure of normal personality characteristics. Other inventories that have been specifically designed to assess normal range personality attributes, such as the California Psychological Inventory (CPI; Gough, 1957), the Personality Research Form (PRF; Jackson, 1967), and the Differential Personality Questionnaire (DPQ; Tellegen, 1980) are much better instruments than the MMPI for the study of nonpathological personality characteristics.

Finally, content homogeneous MMPI scales, such as factor or cluster scales (e.g., Block, 1965; Wiggins, 1969), are superior to the basic clinical scales for many research purposes. The clinical scales were constructed from items differentiating a relevant chinical group from normals; thus, the logic of their development means they are for the most part quite heterogeneous in their content and internal structure. For example, *Hy* consists of two basic types of items: (*a*) the admission of various problems (e.g., specific somatic complaints, dissatisfaction, and malaise) and denial of good health and (*b*) the general denial of psychological and emotional problems and of interpersonal anxiety. Scores on these two sets of items have been found to be moderately *negatively* correlated with one another in most subject groups (e.g., chronic pain patients; Watson, 1982b). Relative to the homogeneous content scales noted previously, the heterogeneous MMPI clinical scales are undesirable for use in predictive analyses (either as a predictor or as a criterion) or correlational research because of their low internal consistency reliability coefficients (see "Reliability of Diagnosis"; "Reliability of Measures"; Anastasi, 1976). In addition, it is difficult to interpret changes (e.g., after treatment, as in Roberts & Reinhardt, 1980; Sternbach & Timmermans, 1975) on the heterogeneous clinical scales, as the changes may be confined to any one of the component clusters (Butcher & Tellegen, 1978). Investigators are thus advised to consider carefully the appropriateness of the basic clinical scales for their particular research needs.[4]

Self Reports

Patient self-reports have been used to study a variety of constructs other than those measured by the standardized psychological inventories, including pain intensity, mood, psychosocial problems, physical functioning, and effects of treatment. Investigators of contingency management treatment programs have questioned the general validity of self-report measures, noting that they may be susceptible to a number of response biases, and often do not correlate significantly with other types of variables (Fordyce & Steger, 1979). Fordyce and his associates (Fordyce, Fowler, Lehmann, De-Lateur, Sand, & Trieschmann, 1973) found that, although observable outcome variables (activity tolerance, uptime, medication use) indicated substantial improvement, patient self-ratings of discomfort and pain-related interference with daily activities tended to remain constant over the course of the treatment.

However, self-report measures retain an important place in research because there are no good alternatives for assessing certain types of constructs. For example, although verbal report may be distorted, there is no more direct method for measuring pain as it is subjectively experienced by the patient. Similarly, a patient's current mood can be assessed most directly by verbal self-report. Pain and mood are important constructs, even if they do not correlate significantly with other variables, as they provide the most direct access to the patient's view of his or her current situation. Moreover, it is unwise to assume that self-reports will not demonstrate any predictive value. For example, posttreatment pain ratings may prove to be significantly related to the maintenance of observable treatment gains (e.g., increases in activity tolerance and uptime) between the termination of treatment and follow-up.

The use of self-reports to measure constructs other than subjective experiences does pose serious problems. For example, chronic pain patients frequently are asked to self-monitor and record behaviors such as uptime and drug use (e.g., Fordyce et al., 1973). Sternbach (1974) has argued that patients can be relied upon to provide fairly accurate behavioral records since they expect that the data will help the staff provide more effective treatment. This belief is supported by the results of Fordyce et al. (1973)

---

[4]It is noteworthy that Hs, which has shown considerable promise as a predictor, is one of the most homogeneous of the clinical scales.

who obtained a correlation of .82 between staff observations and patients' ratings of uptime. However, Kremer, Block, and Gaylor (1981) reported very different findings in their intensive investigation of four chronic pain patients. At the end of each hour patients recorded whether or not they had been "up" (i.e., standing or walking), and whether or not they had interacted with at least one other person. A Physical Activity Index was constructed for each patient by dividing the number of "up" hours by the total number of hours; similarly, a Social Activity Index was created by dividing the number of social interaction hours by the total number of hours. These indices were compared with similar measures constructed from unobtrusive staff observations. Analyses showed that three of the four patients significantly underreported their physical activity. Furthermore, one of the patients reported a marked decrease in physical activity over the course of hospitalization, whereas the staff observed a significant increase. Another patient underreported her social activity as well as physical activity.

It should be noted that several investigators (e.g., Bradley et al., 1981; Nelson, 1977) have argued that self-monitoring of activity may itself affect behavior. This notion raises the possibility that behavior changes attributed to an intervention may in part result simply from patients monitoring their own behavior. Self-monitoring effects (see also Ciminero, Nelson, & Lipinski, 1977) clearly deserve further investigation.

Given the evidence reported above, it is recommended that unless the validity of patient self-reports of observable behaviors can be demonstrated, the self-reports should be used only in conjunction with corroborating measures. Examples of such corroborating measures include unobtrusive spouse or staff ratings (e.g., Kremer et al., 1981; Nelson, 1977); low cost, automated uptime instruments (e.g., Cairns & Pasino, 1977; Sanders, 1980); precise, objective, measures of range-of-motion and current physical capability (Gottlieb, Strite, Koller, Madorsky, Hockersmith, Kleeman, & Wagner, 1977; Newman, Seres, Yospe, & Garlington, 1978; Pope, Rosen, Wilder, & Frymoyer, 1980; Trabin, 1981); and exercise tolerance (Fordyce et al., 1973).

The validity of retrospective self-report data is even more questionable than that of self-reports of observable behaviors. For example, Fordyce et al. (1973) asked chronic benign pain patients "to rate on a ten-point scale the amount of pain they remembered themselves as having had at the time of admission and discharge from the program and at the time of completing the follow-up questionnaire [p. 406]." The patients were similarly instructed to remember the extent to which pain had interferred with their activities at admission and discharge, and to rate the current level of interference. The authors reported that there were significant differences between admission and discharge scores on both measures. These results may suggest that the patients felt that they had benefited in some way from the treatment program, but they do not indicate that the patients actually experienced decreased pain or interference with their daily activities at discharge. In the absence of any validation data, reliance on the patients' memories is a very poor substitute for actual longitudinal data.

Subjective Measures

Finally, it must be strongly emphasized that data obtained from interviews, projective techniques, ratings, or any other subjective measure must be obtained by someone who is blind to the study's hypotheses and to the patients' group membership (Jospe, 1978; Prokop & Bradley, 1981b). The possibility of experimenter bias is so great that any subjective data that have not been obtained blindly (e.g., Forester, Kornfeld, & Fleiss, 1978; Gordon et al., 1980) cannot be considered valid. For further discussions of validity and other assessment issues with a number of specific chronic disease groups, the reader is referred to the volume edited by Prokop and Bradley (1981a, especially Chapters 3–9 and 25).

ASSESSMENT OF COPING

In addition to the previously noted psychometric difficulties associated with rating and behavioral assessment data, chronic disease researchers also must confront the issue of appropriately measuring the construct of *coping* with disease. A review of the literature suggests that researchers often have evaluated coping in a limited fashion. Freeman and his associates (Freeman, Calsyn, Sherrard, & Paige, 1980) for example, used ratings of vocational rehabilitation as the measure of adjustment in renal dialysis patients. Similarly, Krantz (1980) noted that vocational adjustment and patient morale generally have been used to assess recovery from heart attack. Indeed, many outcome studies have used a single "success of treatment" criterion measure. In many cases (Abram, Anderson, & Maitra-D'Cruze, 1981; Blumetti & Modesti, 1976; Else & Hastings, 1981; Wilfling et al., 1973; Wiltse & Rocchio, 1975), the measure simply has been a staff member's subjective rating of treatment success, whereas in others (Malec et al., 1981; Maruta et al., 1979; Roberts & Reinhardt, 1980) several apparently unrelated individual criteria have been combined to form a composite measure of dubious reliability. Some investigators (e.g., McCreary et al., 1979; Sobel & Worden, 1979) merely have used a number of self-report outcome measures to assess coping.

If an investigator is interested solely in a patient group's adjustment in a particular area (e.g., vocational rehabilitation), then it is entirely appropriate to restrict the assessment of coping to that area. However, if an investigator is interested in coping in a broader sense, then it seems inappropriate to restrict assessment to one, or a few, limited areas of adjustment. Chronic physical problems affect a broad range of areas in a patient's life (e.g., physical activity, mood, drug use, vocational status, marital satisfaction), and also affect the lives of others (e.g., spouses, children, parents, siblings, friends).

If changes in these diverse areas were highly related to one another, then it would be sufficient to assess coping by measuring one or two types of variables. However, it has been frequently reported that various facets of coping are not highly interrelated. For example, several studies have found that patient self-report variables were not affected by a treatment intervention, despite the fact that gains were exhibited on other variables. Thus, Gruen (1975) found that myocardial infarction patients who received a psychological support intervention spent significantly fewer days in intensive care and under intensive observation than did control subjects; however, self-reported anxiety levels of the patient groups did not differ from one another (see also Fordyce et al., 1973).

Conversely, other investigations have shown that some treatments (especially those with a strong placebo element) affect self-report measures, but not other types of variables. Brena et al. (1980) found that sympathetic nerve block injections did not affect electromyographic (EMG) or physical activity levels, but did lead to a significant reduction in subjective pain ratings. Similarly, Berk, Moore, and Resnick (1977) and Murphy (1976) reported that acupuncture significantly reduced verbal reports of pain, but did not affect range-of-motion measures.

Other evidence indicating that many commonly used measures of coping are unrelated to one another is found in a study by Trabin (1981). Trabin factor-analyzed the posttreatment scores of chronic pain patients on 17 outcome variables: subjective pain level, 3 range-of-motion measures, and the 13 basic MMPI scales. Four factors were found. The first was a general *negative affect* or *emotional distress* dimension that included the first 8 MMPI clinical scales. Next was a *physical functioning* factor that comprised the three range-of-motion measures. The third dimension appeared to be a *complaining* factor; subjective pain level and the MMPI *F* scale showed positive loadings while the *L* and *K* scales had negative loadings on the factor. The fourth factor was an *extraversion* or *positive affect* dimension that was defined by the *Ma* (positive loading) and *Si* (negative loading) scales.

The consistent finding that different coping measures are unrelated to one another has led several writers (e.g., Freeman et al., 1980; Ziesat, 1981) to conclude that future research must include several types of coping measures. We strongly concur with this view. Although appropriate measures will vary with the goals of the study and the patient group being investigated, as a general rule researchers would profit from a consideration of the following types of measures:

1. *Patient self-ratings of pain and discomfort*. There are many diverse approaches to the measurement of the sensory, affective, and cognitive–evaluative dimensions of pain (see Bradley *et al.*, 1981; Frederiksen, Lynd, & Ross, 1978; Sternbach, 1974; Trabin, 1981).

2. *Patient self-ratings of mood*. Recent research has consistently indicated that two broad dimensions underlie self-ratings of transient mood (e.g., Russell, 1980; Zevon & Tellegen, 1982; Watson, 1982a). We recommend that investigators assess both positive affect and negative affect (see Hall, 1977; Zevon & Tellegen, 1982).

3. *Physical activity*. Objective measures of uptime (Fordyce *et al.*, 1973), range of motion (Trabin, 1981), and/or functional ability (Granger & Greer, 1976; Jette, 1980) may be used to assess patients' physical activity.

4. *Use of the health care system*. Assessments may include variables such as number of hospitalizations, number of surgeries, number of physicians seen, and number of days spent in the hospital (e.g., Roberts & Reinhardt, 1980; Strassberg *et al.*, 1981). These may be especially important variables because of the high costs with which they are associated. Thus, interventions that reduce health care system use could prove to be very cost effective (see Item 9).

5. *Vocational rehabilitation*. This variable has been used primarily in the recent literature. Freeman *et al.* (1980), for example, rated the vocational readjustment of their renal dialysis patients as good (full employment), fair (part-time work), or poor (not working). Another approach involves the assessment of whether or not the patients have fully returned to their premorbid vocational status (e.g., full employment, part-time work, homemaking; see Roberts & Reinhardt, 1980). Vocational rehabilitation is an important variable because of the high costs associated with disability and worker's compensation benefits. Interventions that help persons return to work should be highly cost effective (see Item 9).

6. *Family and social life*. Measures of marital satisfaction (e.g., Jacobson, Waldron, & Moore, 1980; Locke & Wallace, 1959; Wills, Weiss, & Patterson, 1974), family environment (e.g., Moos & Moos, 1976), sexual functioning (e.g., Roberts & Reinhardt, 1980), and social activity (e.g., Kremer *et al.*, 1981) are all appropriate for the assessment of the family and social life.

7. *Medication use*. This variable could be assessed, for example, as the number of hypnosedative medications needed to fall asleep and/or the number of drugs used in a specific category (e.g., muscle relaxants, analgesics, tranquilizers and sedatives, narcotics; Roberts & Reinhardt, 1980).

8. *Measures of cognitive functioning*. These measures assess the internal

experience of the patient (e.g., the thought pattern of a pain patient exposed to a variety of stimuli, noxious or otherwise). Cognitive variables may be found to mediate observable patterns of coping behavior. In the study of anxiety, for instance, individuals reporting high levels of anxiety were found to have internal dialogues that were in conflict, whereas less anxious subjects were shown to have less conflicted internal dialogues; both groups had positive thoughts, but the less anxious group had fewer negative counterthoughts (Kendall & Hollon, 1981). Investigation of cognitive functioning of patients with chronic pain, specifically their internal dialogues and the corresponding ways in which they view the world, is a fruitful direction for future research.

9. *Cost effectiveness.* Unfortunately, this highly important dependent variable is very seldom assessed (our informal survey suggests that less than 1% of studies in the chronic disease literature report cost effectiveness data). As noted above, cost effectiveness can be measured by estimating pre- to posttreatment changes in costs associated with hospitalizations, medical and surgical procedures, staff time, medication use, disability and worker compensation payments, and other disease-related variables; the monetary savings produced by treatment then can be compared to the costs of treatment. It is our belief that many of the interventions that have been developed for patients with chronic diseases will prove to be highly cost effective. Research that uses cost effectiveness variables therefore should serve to increase public and private support for these and similar intervention programs.

10. *Assessment of coping in the patient's social environment.* There is no good reason to assume that a chronic disease affects only the patient. Family members, close friends, and others in the patient's social environment experience stress and disruptions of their lives, and in some cases (e.g., the parents of children with leukemia), family members may have as great a need for psychosocial support as do the patients. Thus, assessment in coping and outcome studies may be extended to include family members and others who may have been affected by the disease. Measures of the mood and marital satisfaction of the patient's family members as well as assessment of the general family environment can provide very useful information about the coping levels of family members and others affected by the patient's disease.

11. *Important predictor variables.* Investigators may attempt to anticipate and to include variables, such as level of knowledge concerning the disease, that might be related to one or more facets of patients' posttreatment coping (Kendall & Watson, 1981). In addition, Bradley et al. (1981) suggest that investigators try to identify those patients who are likely to drop out during the course of a study (e.g., Gordon et al., 1980). As well as being of considerable interest in its own right, any nonrandom attrition will alter

the characteristics (and hence the representativeness) of the final patient sample. Thus, it is both interesting and important to know which patients are likely to drop out during treatment or decline to participate in a follow-up assessment.

Researchers might also consider employing different *levels* of assessment as a means of completely explicating treatment outcome. Two such levels of assessment have been noted (Kendall, Pellegrini, & Urbain, 1981). The *specifying* level of assessment consists of behaviors, affects, and other specific aspects of coping that have been changed by the treatment intervention. This level of assessment includes measures such as those listed. The *general impact* level of assessment comprises measures of general and pervasive changes in the patients' overall levels of coping. Measures of general impact include, for example, overall ratings of improved coping made by the patients, their spouses, and health care professionals.

Finally, we must emphasize very strongly that, while we are advocating the use of widely diverse measures, we also feel that the total number of variables should be kept to a minimum. Overinclusion of variables has several disadvantages. Overtaxing the patience and motivation of the subjects, for example, may affect the overall quality of the data. We also have seen that data analysis and interpretation become more difficult as the number of measures increases. Moreover, valuable data-analytic procedures such as multiple regression and factor analysis require more subjects as the number of variables increases. The total number of variables can be kept acceptably low by eliminating unreliable, invalid, or redundant measures (see "Reliability of Measures" and "Validity of Measures"). Our view on this issue has been well expressed by Kraemer (1981):

> Finally, and very important, one should eliminate redundant response measures. It is a peculiar response to difficult problems of measurement that when one distrusts any one measure, one might believe that separate use of 5 to 10 such untrustworthy measures will clarify the situation. In general, the issues can only be further confused. From any such redundant set, one should discard any measures of questionable validity, and that are distinctly lower than others in reliability, and combine the remaining measures, if any, to step up reliability. The basic principle is that one has the best chance at solidly hitting a target by aiming carefully and taking one's best shot, not by spraying buckshot wildly in the general direction of the target [p. 317].

Data Analysis

CORRELATIONAL ANALYSES

We have recommended that investigators use simple or multivariate correlational analyses in two important ways. First, correlational analyses can

be used to reduce and simplify complex data sets by identifying and grouping highly related variables. Second, they can be employed to predict important criterion measures. We now consider some general issues pertaining to
correlational research.

The first issue is the requirement of much larger sample sizes for correlational research than for purely experimental studies. Large sample sizes are
needed because correlational research can be used not only to determine
whether or not a relationship exists between two variables, but also to estimate the *strength* of that relationship. As sample size decreases, the confidence interval of the correlation coefficient increases; thus, relatively large
samples are required to produce estimates of relationship strength that
closely approximate the true population relationship. For example, Butcher
and Tellegen (1978) point out that with a very small sample of 19 subjects
and a correlation coefficient of .50, the 95% confidence interval ranges
from .06 to .78. Hence, a sample of 19 subjects does not allow an investigator to retain confidence concerning the strength and importance of the relationship.

Large sample sizes are especially important in multivariate correlational
analyses, such as multiple regression and factor analysis. Because of their
large confidence intervals, individual correlation coefficients produced by
small samples will be highly unstable. Hence, multivariate analyses that are
based upon many such correlations will tend to produce very different results from sample to sample.

Clearly, in correlational research, an investigator should strive to obtain
samples that are as large as possible. It is impossible, however, to specify
exactly what constitutes an acceptable sample size. As a general rule of
thumb, it is preferable to have a sample size of at least 100 subjects in any
correlational analysis; multivariate procedures ideally should have a sample
size of several hundred (e.g., Comrey, 1978; Nunnally, 1978). Comrey
(1978), for example, recommends a minimum sample size of 200 for factor
analysis, and notes that adding subjects will improve the clarity of results
until stability in structure is reached at approximately 2000 subjects.

Nonetheless, it must be emphasized that these general guidelines represent *ideal* conditions. It can be very difficult to obtain samples in applied
settings that meet the standards set by psychometrics textbooks. A researcher must balance the costs (e.g., unstable covariance matrices) and
benefits (e.g., data reduction) associated with employing correlational analyses under less-than-optimal conditions.

An additional consideration in multivariate correlational research is that of
the ratio of subjects to variables. Multivariate techniques such as multiple
regression and factor analysis are designed to maximize or to minimize some
mathematical function. In multiple regression, for example, weights are

assigned to each predictor in such a way as to maximize the multiple correlation between the predictors and the criterion. Similarly, a principal factor analysis extracts as a first factor the dimension that accounts for the maximum possible variance among the variables. As a result, these procedures will capitalize greatly on chance sampling errors (i.e., sample correlations that are higher than the true population correlation). It therefore is important to minimize the influence of sampling error when using these techniques. The best way to minimize sampling error is to have a large number of subjects for each variable employed in the analysis. Most writers advise that at least 5 (Comrey, 1978; Gorsuch, 1974) or 10 (Nunnally, 1978) subjects be used for each variable included in a factor analysis. Similarly, it generally is recommended (e.g., Nunnally, 1978) that at least a 10:1 subject-to-predictor ratio be employed in multiple regression analyses. It is also important to attempt to cross-validate the results of any multivariate analysis on a new sample of subjects; cross-validation is critical when the initial analysis is based upon a small sample or a low variable-to-subject ratio (i.e., when sampling error tends to be quite large). For a discussion of cross-validation in multivariate correlational analyses, see Guilford and Fruchter (1973, Chapter 18); Nunnally (1978, Chapter 5); and Schmidt, Coyle, and Rauschenberger (1977). The need for large sample sizes and the cross-validation of results is not intended to discourage researchers from employing correlational analyses. These requirements are necessary in order to demonstrate the strength of the relationship among the variables of interest and the real-world significance of one's findings.

It should be noted that a great deal of research that appears to use an experimental design is actually correlational research. Such research often employs t tests to determine the relationship between two continuous variables, one of which has been dichotomized (e.g., the division of a particular patient group's scores on an MMPI scale by means of a median split). For example, Hardyck and Moos (1966) divided their sample of hypertensives into "high complainers" and "low complainers" by performing a median split of the patients' scores on a complaint scale. These two groups then were compared (using t tests) on a number of MMPI scales. Since these analyses were designed solely to uncover relationships between complaining and MMPI scale scores, the research clearly was correlational in nature. Three basic problems with the dichotomization of a continuous variable can be noted. First, dichotomization leads to a substantial loss of (a) information (Nunnally, 1978, Chapter 4) and (b) reliability (Kraemer, 1981). Furthermore, the procedure does not allow for (c) the estimation of the magnitude of the relationship between the two variables. As noted previously, the use of a correlational analysis with a large sample size may provide a fairly precise estimate of the magnitude of the relationship among variables.

Finally, it is important to comment on the reporting of correlational analyses, particularly with regard to factor analytic investigations. The few studies in the chronic disease literature that have performed factor analyses generally have not reported them in sufficient detail. For example, Strassberg *et al.* (1981) simply noted that "subjects' responses to these 11 items were factor analyzed, yielding two theoretically and empirically independent factors [p. 222]." Similarly, Gordon *et al.* (1980) reported only that a factor analysis was performed, and that it "confirmed" the results of an earlier analysis. Stating that a factor analysis has been performed does not provide other investigators with a clear idea of the procedures that have been used, nor does it give them sufficient information to replicate the analysis. A discussion of each of the following is essential for an adequate reporting of a factor analysis: (*a*) the method used to extract the factors (e.g., principal factor, image, centroid); (*b*) the technique used for the community estimates (e.g., 1.00, squared multiple correlations, highest off-diagonal correlation), and whether or not an iterative procedure was used; (*c*) how the number of factors was determined (e.g., the Kaiser–Guttman criterion, the scree test); (*d*) the method of factor rotation (e.g., Varimax, Promax) and the rationale for its use; and (*e*) the criterion used to define variables with significant loadings on a factor (e.g., all variables with factor loadings greater than .30 or less than −.30). Other information, such as the original correlation matrix, the unrotated and rotated factor loading matrices, and the factor correlation matrix (if an oblique rotation has been used) might also be made available to readers by indicating their availability in a footnote.

ANALYSIS OF REPEATED MEASURES

We previously have recommended that coping studies use longitudinal designs in which a patient group is studied at several points in time (see "Longitudinal Research Designs: Coping Studies"). We now consider a critical issue of data analysis that often arises when the same subjects are assessed on the same variables on more than one occasion: the use of change scores.

Change scores have considerable intuitive appeal and thus have been extensively employed. Cronbach and Furby (1970) have listed four principal ways in which change scores have been used; two uses appear especially relevant to the chronic disease literature. First, change scores have been used as dependent variables in outcome studies to test whether or not two treatments (or one treatment and a no-treatment control) have had an equally large effect on a particular measure. Second, they have been employed as criterion variables in analyses designed to predict what patients would be most helped by a particular treatment.

There are three problems inherent in the use of change scores. First, change scores tend to be very unreliable. The measurement error present in each of the component assessments is compounded in the change score. Second, floor or ceiling effects tend to produce a spurious negative correlation between initial score level and the extent of change. For example, patients reporting little or no drug use at pretreatment cannot show as much improvement as those patients who report high pretreatment drug use. The third problem is that regression to the mean also can be expected to produce a spurious relationship between initial score level and change. That is, patients who have extreme initial scores on most variables (e.g., state anxiety) can be expected to produce scores that are closer to the population mean on subsequent assessments (Hays, 1973, pp. 626–627).

If one is interested in comparing the effects of two treatments (or one treatment versus no treatment), then posttreatment scores on the variables can be used as dependent measures (Cronbach & Furby, 1970; Mintz, Luborsky, & Christoph, 1979). If patients are assigned to treatment groups in a random or stratified-random manner, and if the correlation between pre- and posttreatment scores is moderately high (e.g., .40 or greater; see Elashoff, 1969), then analysis of covariance can be used to control for individual differences at pretreatment. If the correlation between pre- and posttreatment scores is not high, then a randomized blocks procedure (i.e., assigning patients to the groups on the basis of their pretreatment score) may be preferable to an analysis of covariance. However, when patients are *not* randomly assigned to treatment groups, it is likely that the groups will differ on a number of pretreatment variables and analysis of covariance cannot be used to eliminate the confounding. As Lord (1967) noted, "there simply is no logical or statistical procedure that can be counted on to make proper allowances for uncontrolled preexisting differences between groups [p. 305]."

When one is interested in identifying variables associated with treatment success, multiple regression can be used to calculate residual gain scores (see, for example, Cronbach & Furby, 1970; Mintz *et al.*, 1979). This procedure partials out the part of the posttreatment score on a variable that can be predicted by the pretreatment score. A residual gain score is produced that can then be correlated with other pretreatment variables.

LINEAR VERSUS CONFIGURAL PREDICTION

Several investigators have identified distinct subgroups within their patient samples. For example, Sternbach *et al.* (1973) constructed four separate pain patient subgroups using the patients' MMPI profiles. Similarly, Bradley, Prokop, Margolis, and Gentry (1978) and Prokop, Bradley, Margolis, and Gentry (1980) replicated several low back pain and multiple pain patient subgroups through a cluster analysis of their MMPI profiles. It has been argued (e.g., Prokop & Bradley, 1981b) that such subgroups are likely to have important correlates and thus will prove useful in predictive analyses. For example, patient subgroups might show differential response to treatment.

A potential advantage of this technique over other approaches is that it employs certain configural relationships among the predictors that may facilitate prediction. For example, an *Hs–D–Hy* MMPI code type might be a better predictor of poor treatment outcome than would any of the scales used either individually or in a linear combination. However, the subgroup technique has some potential disadvantages. One problem is that even with a very large initial sample, many of the subgroups will be rather small. For example, one of the subgroups in the Prokop *et al.* (1980) study included only five patients (these were drawn from a sample of patients seen over a 2-year period), and one of Sternbach *et al.*'s (1973) subgroups comprised only six patients. Predictive analyses require large sample sizes and it may be difficult to obtain adequate samples for a great many subgroups. If this is the case, then the potential benefits of the subgroup technique will be diminished.

There is some evidence that linear predictions using entire samples are as adequate as configural approaches. Several studies (Gianetti, Johnson, Klingler, & Williams, 1978; Goldberg, 1965, 1969; see also Butcher & Tellegen, 1978) have shown, for example, that a simple linear combination of MMPI scales discriminates psychotics from neurotics better than such highly configural methods as the Meehl–Dahlstrom rules (Meehl & Dahlstrom, 1960). Moreover, an investigator may determine whether a particular configural relaionship will enhance prediction through a linear predictive technique (e.g., multiple regression) by adding specific configural relationships to the regression equation as separate predictors.[5] Butcher and Tellegen (1978) note:

> even non-linear relations may emerge from systematic [linear] analyses provided the search is guided by a certain degree of theorizing permitting a focus on a smaller set of possible configurations, thus reducing the probability of drowning a few actual configural relations in a sea of unreplicable chance relationships. The reason is that without some theoretical constraints the number of configural patterns that would have to be considered in an exhaustive search easily becomes extremely and unmanageably large, thus requiring unattainably large sample sizes to minimize the occurrence of chance patterns [p. 625]

[5]For a discussion of how a systematic search for nonlinear relationships might be undertaken, see Tellegen, Kamp, and Watson (1982).

Conclusions and Recommendations

Our discussion of the design, assessment, and data analysis issues in research on coping with chronic disease has attempted to focus on those problems and research strategies that appear to be of general interest across a wide variety of patient groups. In doing so, we have tried to point out essential aspects of high quality research, at the same time recognizing the practical limitations faced by many investigators. For example, it was stressed that valuable multivariate techniques should ideally be used with very large sample sizes, but also it was noted that these analyses may still prove useful, even when the conditions established by textbook writers are not strictly met.

Our major recommendations can be summarized as follows:

1. *Long-term, longitudinal designs have merit.* An investigator interested in how a chronic disease affects patients' coping should obtain an initial assessment as soon after disease onset as possible. In addition, any premorbid information (e.g., personality and vocational characteristics) that can be collected would be especially valuable. Follow-up assessments then can be made at periodic intervals. An investigator interested in how a particular psychosocial intervention affects patients' coping should obtain periodic follow-up assessments as long after the cessation of treatment as research resources will allow.

2. *Predictive analyses can be employed to complement simple mean comparisons.* For example, in addition to examining how well a patient group is coping, it is also important to determine what patient characteristics at disease onset are highly related to later coping level. Early intervention programs then could be designed for patients who are likely to experience later coping problems. Similarly, in addition to investigating whether or not a given intervention significantly improves a patient group's coping ability, it is also important to identify patients who are most likely to be helped by the treatment. Thus, alternative interventions can be developed for those patients who are not likely to be helped by the current treatment program.

3. *Appropriate control groups must be used.* Outcome studies require comparison groups that control for the passage of time and placebo effects (as well as other factors associated with particular investigations). A factorial design, in which each treatment group is given a slightly different combination of treatment facets, can be employed to identify those aspects of the intervention that contribute to treatment success.

4. *Coping is a multifaceted concept that cannot be assessed through a single measure or a single type of measure.* Rather, a wide variety of mea-

sures should be used to assess the many aspects of coping. These measures might include patient self-ratings of pain, discomfort, and mood; objective measures of physical activity and medication use; variables indicating use of the health care system (e.g., number of hospitalizations); and general family environment, vocational adjustment, marital satisfaction, and sexual functioning.

5. *Assessment should include only reliable and valid measures.* The reliability and validity of the assessment measures must be determined and reported unless they already have been reasonably established. Reliability can be increased by combining related variables into aggregate measures. Factor analysis can be used to identify related variables.

6. *Although a variety of measures is valued, the total number of variables should not overtax the subjects.* Use of multivariate correlational techniques as well as interpretation of results is made easier as the number of dependent measures is reduced. Furthermore, the use of a relatively small number of nonredundant measures reduces strain on the patients.

References

Abram, S. E., Anderson, R. A., & Maitra-D'Cruze, A. M. Factors predicting short-term outcome of nerve blocks in the management of chronic pain. *Pain*, 1981, *10*, 323–330.

Alexander, A. B., & Smith, D. D. Clinical applications of electromyographic biofeedback. In R. J. Gatchel & K. P. Price (Eds.), *Clinical applications of biofeedback: Appraisal and status.* New York: Pergamon Press, 1979.

American Psychological Association. *Standards for educational and psychological tests.* Washington, D.C.: Author, 1974.

Anastasi, A. *Psychological testing* (4th ed.). New York: Macmillan, 1976.

Andrasik, F., & Holroyd, K. A. A test of specific and nonspecific effects in the biofeedback treatment of tension headache. *Journal of Consulting and Clinical Psychology*, 1980, *48*, 575–586.

Bahnson, C. B., & Bahnson, M. B. Denial and repression of primitive impulses and of disturbing emotions in patients with malignant neoplasms. In D. M. Kissen & L. L. LeShan (Eds.), *Psychosomatic aspects of neoplastic disease.* Philadelphia: Lippincott, 1964.

Baldwin, M. J. A clinico-experimental investigation into the psychological aspects of multiple sclerosis. *Journal of Nervous and Mental Disease*, 1952, *115*, 299–342.

Beaty, E. T., & Haynes, S. N. Behavioral intervention with muscle-contraction headache: A review. *Psychosomatic Medicine*, 1979, *41*, 165–180.

Berk, S. N., Moore, M. E., & Resnick, J. H. Psychosocial factors as mediators of acupuncture therapy. *Journal of Clinical and Consulting Psychology*, 1977, *45*, 612–619.

Block, J. *The challenge of response sets: Unconfounding meaning, acquiescence and social desirability in the MMPI.* New York: Appleton-Century-Crofts, 1965.

Blumetti, A. E., & Modesti, L. M. Psychological predictors of success or failure of surgical intervention for intractable back pain. In J. J. Bonica & D. Albe-Fessard (Eds.), *Advances in pain research and therapy* (Vol. 1). New York: Raven Press, 1976.

Bond, M. R., & Pearson, I. B. Psychological aspects of pain in women with advanced cancer of the cervix. *Journal of Psychosomatic Research,* 1969, *13,* 13–19.

Bootzin, R. R., & Lick, J. R. Expectancies in therapy research: Interpretive artifact or mediating mechanism? *Journal of Consulting and Clinical Psychology,* 1979, *47,* 852–855.

Borkovec, T. D. Effects of expectancy on the outcome of systematic desensitization and implosive treatments for analogue anxiety. *Behavior Therapy,* 1972, *3,* 29–40.

Borkovec, T. D., & Nau, S. D. Credibility of analogue therapy rationales. *Journal of Behavior Therapy and Experimental Psychiatry,* 1972, *3,* 257–260.

Bourestom, N. C., & Howard, M. T. Personality characteristics of three disability groups. *Archives of Physical Medicine and Rehabilitation,* 1965, *46,* 626–632.

Bradley, L. A., Prokop, C. K., Gentry, W. D., Van der Heide, L. H., & Prieto, E. J. Assessment of chronic pain. In C. K. Prokop & L. A. Bradley (Eds.), *Medical psychology: Contributions to behavioral medicine.* New York: Academic Press, 1981.

Bradley, L. A., Prokop, C. K., Margolis, R., & Gentry, W. D. Multivariate analyses of the MMPI profiles of low back pain patients. *Journal of Behavioral Medicine,* 1978, *1,* 253–272.

Brena, S. G., Wolf, S. L., Chapman, S. L., & Hammonds, W. D. Chronic back pain: Electromyographic, motion and behavioral assessments following sympathetic nerve blocks and placebos. *Pain,* 1980, *8,* 1–10.

Butcher, J. N., Kendall, P. C., & Hoffman, N. MMPI short forms: Caution. *Journal of Consulting and Clinical Psychology,* 1980, *48,* 275–278.

Butcher, J. N., & Tellegen, A. Common methodological problems in MMPI research. *Journal of Consulting and Clinical Psychology,* 1978, *46,* 620–628.

Byrne, D. The Repression–Sensitization scale: Rationale, reliability, and validity. *Journal of Personality,* 1961, *29,* 334–349.

Cairns, D., & Pasino, J. A. Comparison of verbal reinforcement and feedback in the operant treatment of disability due to chronic low back pain. *Behavior Therapy,* 1977, *8,* 621–630.

Calsyn, D. A., Louks, J., & Freeman, C. W. The use of the MMPI with chronic low back pain patients with a mixed diagnosis. *Journal of Clinical Psychology,* 1976, *32,* 532–536.

Chapman, C. R., Sola, A. E., & Bonica, J. J. Illness behavior and depression compared in pain center and private practice patients. *Pain,* 1979, *6,* 1–7.

Ciminero, A. R., Nelson, R. O., & Lipinski, D. P. Self-monitoring procedures. In A. R. Ciminero, K. S. Calhoun, & H. E. Adams (Eds.), *Handbook of behavioral assessment.* New York: Wiley, 1977.

Cleveland, S. E., Reitman, E. E., & Brewer, E. J., Jr. Psychological factors in juvenile rheumatoid arthritis. *Arthritis and Rheumatism,* 1965, *8,* 1152–1158.

Coates, T. J., Perry, C., Killen, J., & Slinkard, L. A. Primary prevention of cardiovascular disease in children and adolescents. In C. K. Prokop & L. A. Bradley (Eds.), *Medical psychology: Contributions to behavioral medicine.* New York: Academic Press, 1981.

Comrey, A. L. Common methodological problems in factor analytic studies. *Journal of Consulting and Clinical Psychology,* 1978, *46,* 648–659.

Cox, G. B., & Chapman, C. R. Multivariate analysis of pain data. In J. J. Bonica & D. Albe-Fessard (Eds.), *Advances in pain research and therapy* (Vol. 1). New York: Raven Press, 1976.

Cox, G. B., Chapman, C. R., & Black, R. G. The MMPI and chronic pain: The diagnosis of psychogenic pain. *Journal of Behavioral Medicine,* 1978, *1,* 437–443.

Creer, T. L. *Asthma therapy: A behavioral health care system for respiratory disorders.* New York: Springer, 1979.

Cronbach, L. J. Coefficient alpha and the internal structure of tests. *Psychometrika,* 1951, *16,* 297–334.

Cronbach, L. J., & Furby, L. How should we measure "change"—or should we? *Psychological Bulletin,* 1970, *74,* 68–80.

Crown, S., & Crown, J. M. Personality in early rheumatoid disease. *Journal of Psychosomatic Research,* 1973, *17,* 189–196.

Dattore, P. J., Shontz, F. C., & Coyne, L. Premorbid personality differentiation of cancer and noncancer groups: A test of the hypothesis of cancer proneness. *Journal of Consulting and Clinical Psychology,* 1980, *48,* 388–394.

Dean, E. F. A lengthened Mini: The Midi–Mult. *Journal of Clinical Psychology,* 1972, *28,* 68–71.

Efron, B. Forcing a sequential experiment to be balanced. *Biometrika,* 1971, *58,* 403–417.

Elashoff, J. D. Analysis of covariance: A delicate instrument. *American Educational Research Journal,* 1969, *6,* 383–402.

Else, B. A., & Hastings, J. E. The relationship of the conceptual level analogy test to outcome following open heart surgery. *Comprehensive Psychiatry,* 1981, *22,* 326–333.

Eysenck, H. J. *Manual of the Maudsley Personality Inventory.* London: University of London Press, 1959.

Eysenck, H. J., & Eysenck, S. G. B. *Manual of the Eysenck Personality Inventory.* London: University of London Press, 1964.

Faschingbauer, T. R. A 166 item short-form of the MMPI: The FAM. *Journal of Consulting and Clinical Psychology,* 1974, *42,* 645–655.

Feinstein, A. R. A critical overview of diagnosis in psychiatry. In V. M. Rakoff, H. C. Stancer, & H. B. Kedward (Eds.), *Psychiatric diagnosis.* New York: Brunner/Mazel, 1977.

Fillenbaum, G. G., & Pfeiffer, E. The Mini–Mult: A cautionary note. *Journal of Consulting and Clinical Psychology,* 1976, *44,* 698–703.

Fordyce, W. E. *Behavioral methods for chronic pain and illness.* St. Louis, Mo.: C. V. Mosby, 1976.

Fordyce, W. E., Brena, S. F., Holcomb, R. F., DeLateur, B. J., & Loeser, J. C. Relationship of patient semantic pain descriptions to physician diagnostic judgments, activity level measures and MMPI. *Pain,* 1978, *5,* 293–303.

Fordyce, W. E., Fowler, R. S., Lehmann, J. F., DeLateur, B., Sand, P., & Trieschmann, R. B. Operant conditioning in the treatment of chronic pain. *Archives of Physical Medicine and Rehabilitation,* 1973, *54,* 399–408.

Fordyce, W. E., & Steger, J. C. Chronic pain. In O. F. Pomerleau & J. P. Brady (Eds.), *Behavioral medicine: Theory and practice.* Baltimore: Williams & Wilkins, 1979.

Forester, B. M., Kornfeld, D. S., & Fleiss, J. Psychiatric aspects of radiotherapy. *American Journal of Psychiatry,* 1978, *135,* 960–963.

Frederiksen, L. W., Lynd, R. S., & Ross, J. Methodology in measurement of pain. *Behavior Therapy,* 1978, *9,* 486–488.

Freeman, C. W., Calsyn, D. A., & Louks, J. The use of the MMPI with low back pain patients. *Journal of Clinical Psychology,* 1976, *32,* 294–298.

Freeman, C. W., Calsyn, D. A., Sherrard, D. J., & Paige, A. B. Psychological assessment of renal dialysis patients using standard psychometric techniques. *Journal of Consulting and Clinical Psychology,* 1980, *48,* 537–539.

Gianetti, R. A., Johnson, J. H., Klingler, D. E., & Williams, T. A. Comparison of linear and configural MMPI diagnostic methods with an uncontaminated criterion. *Journal of Consulting and Clinical Psychology,* 1978, *46,* 1046–1052.

Goldberg, L. R. Diagnosticians vs. diagnostic signs: The diagnosis of psychosis vs. neurosis from the MMPI. *Psychological Monographs,* 1965, *79*(9, Whole No. 602).

Goldberg, L. R. The search for configural relationships in personality assessment: The diagnosis of psychosis vs. neurosis from the MMPI. *Multivariate Behavioral Research*, 1969, *4*, 523–536.

Goldstein, I. B. Assessment of hypertension. In C. K. Prokop & L. A. Bradley (Eds.), *Medical psychology: Contributions to behavioral medicine.* New York: Academic Press, 1981.

Gordon, W. A., Freidenbergs, I., Diller, L., Hibbard, M., Wolf, C., Levine, L., Lipkins, R., Ezrachi, O., & Lucido, D. Efficacy of psychosocial intervention with cancer patients. *Journal of Consulting and Clinical Psychology*, 1980, *48*, 743–759.

Gorsuch, R. L. *Factor analysis*. Philadelphia: W. B. Saunders, 1974.

Gottlieb, H., Strite, L., Koller, R., Madorsky, A., Hockersmith, V., Kleeman, M., & Wagner, J. Comprehensive rehabilitation of patients having chronic low back pain. *Archives of Physical Medicine and Rehabilitation*, 1977, *58*, 101–107.

Gough, H. G. *Manual for the California Psychological Inventory*. Palo Alto, Ca.: Consulting Psychologists Press, 1957.

Granger, C. V., & Greer, D. S. Functional status measurement and medical rehabilitation outcomes. *Archives of Physical Medicine and Rehabilitation*, 1976, *57*, 103–108.

Gruen, W. Effects of brief psychotherapy during the hospitalization period on the recovery process in heart attacks. *Journal of Consulting and Clinical Psychology*, 1975, *43*, 223–232.

Guilford, J. P., & Fruchter, B. *Fundamental statistics in psychology and education* (5th ed.). New York: McGraw-Hill, 1973.

Hall, C. A. *Differential relationships of pleasure and distress with depression and anxiety over a past, present and future time framework.* Unpublished doctoral dissertation, University of Minnesota, 1977.

Hardyck, C. D., & Moos, R. H. Sampling problems in studies of psychosomatic disorders: Difficulties in determining personality correlates. *Journal of Psychosomatic Research*, 1966, *10*, 171–182.

Hays, W. L. *Statistics for the social sciences* (2nd ed.). New York: Holt, Rinehart & Winston, 1973.

Hedlund, J. L., Won Cho, D., & Powell, B. J. Use of MMPI short forms with psychiatric patients. *Journal of Consulting and Clinical Psychology*, 1975, *43*, 924.

Hill, O. W. Personality and rheumatoid arthritis. *British Medical Journal*, 1971, *2*, 588.

Hoffman, N. G., & Butcher, J. N. Clinical limitations of three MMPI short forms. *Journal of Consulting and Clinical Psychology*, 1975, *43*, 32–39.

Horowitz, L. M., Inouye, D., & Siegelman, E. Y. On averaging judges' ratings to increase their correlations with an external criterion. *Journal of Consulting and Clinical Psychology*, 1979, *47*, 453–458.

Jackson, D. N. *Personality Research Form manual*. Goshen, N.Y.: Research Psychologists Press, 1967.

Jacobson, N. S., Waldron, H., & Moore, D. Toward a behavioral profile of marital distress. *Journal of Consulting and Clinical Psychology*, 1980, *48*, 696–703.

Jette, A. M. Functional status index: Reliability of a chronic disease evaluation instrument. *Archives of Physical Medicine and Rehabilitation*, 1980, *61*, 395–401.

Jospe, M. *The placebo effect in healing*. Lexington, Mass.: D. C. Heath, 1978.

Kazdin, A. E., & Wilson, G. T. *Evaluation of behavior therapy*. Cambridge, Mass.: Ballinger, 1978.

Kendall, P. C., Edinger, J., & Eberly, C. Taylor's MMPI correction factor for spinal cord injury: Empirical endorsement. *Journal of Consulting and Clinical Psychology*, 1978, *46*, 370–371.

Kendall, P. C., & Hollon, S. D. Assessing self-referent speech: Methods in the measurement of self-statements. In P. C. Kendall & S. D. Hollon (Eds.), *Assessment strategies for cognitive–behavioral interventions*. New York: Academic Press, 1981.

Kendall, P. C., & Norton-Ford, J. D. Therapy outcome research methods. In P. C. Kendall & J. N. Butcher (Eds.), *Handbook of research methods in clinical psychology*. New York: Wiley, 1982.

Kendall, P. C., Pellegrini, D. S., & Urbain, E. S. Approaches to assessment for cognitive–behavioral interventions with children. In P. C. Kendall & S. D. Hollon (Eds.), *Assessment strategies for cognitive–behavioral interventions*. New York: Academic Press, 1981.

Kendall, P. C., & Watson, D. Psychological preparation for stressful medical procedures. In C. K. Prokop & L. A. Bradley (Eds.), *Medical psychology: Contributions to behavioral medicine*. New York: Academic Press, 1981.

Kendall, P. C., Williams, L., Pechacek, T. F., Graham, L. E., Shisslak, C., & Herzoff, N. Cognitive–behavioral and patient education interventions in cardiac catheterization procedures: The Palo Alto medical psychology project. *Journal of Consulting and Clinical Psychology*, 1979, *47*, 49–58.

Kent, R. N., & Foster, S. L. Direct observational procedures: Methodological issues in naturalistic settings. In A. R. Ciminero, K. S. Calhoun, & H. E. Adams (Eds.), *Handbook of behavioral assessment*. New York: Wiley, 1977.

Koran, L. M. The reliability of clinical methods, data, and judgments: Part I. *New England Journal of Medicine*, 1975, *293*, 642–646.

Kraemer, H. C. Coping strategies in psychiatric clinical research. *Journal of Consulting and Clinical Psychology*, 1981, *49*, 309–319.

Krantz, D. S. Cognitive processes and recovery from heart attack: A review and theoretical analysis. *Journal of Human Stress*, 1980, *6*, 27–38.

Kremer, E. G., Block, A., & Gaylor, M. S. Behavioral approaches to treatment of chronic pain: The inaccuracy of patient self-report measures. *Archives of Physical Medicine and Rehabilitation*, 1981, *62*, 188–191.

Lair, C., & Trapp, E. The differential diagnostic value of the MMPI with somatically disturbed patients. *Journal of Clinical Psychology*, 1962, *18*, 146–147.

Lanyon, R. I. *An handbook of MMPI group profiles*. Minneapolis: University of Minnesota Press, 1968.

Leavitt, F., & Garron, D. C. Psychological disturbance and pain report differences in both organic and non-organic low back pain patients. *Pain*, 1979, *7*, 187–196.

Levy, S. M. The psychosocial assessment of the chronically ill geriatric patient. In C. K. Prokop & L. A. Bradley (Eds.), *Medical psychology: Contributions to behavioral medicine*. New York: Academic Press, 1981.

Little, K. B., & Fisher, J. Two new experimental scales of the MMPI. *Journal of Consulting Psychology*, 1958, *22*, 305–306.

Locke, H. J., & Wallace, K. M. Short marital adjustment and prediction tests: Their reliability and validity. *Marriage and Family Living*, 1959, *21*, 251–255.

Lord, F. M. A paradox in the interpretation of group comparisons. *Psychological Bulletin*, 1967, *68*, 304–305.

Louks, J. L., Freeman, C. W., & Calsyn, D. A. Personality organization as an aspect of back pain in a medical setting. *Journal of Personality Assessment*, 1978, *42*, 152–158.

Lucas, R. H. The affective and medical effects of different preoperative interventions with heart surgery patients (Doctoral dissertation, University of Houston, 1975). *Dissertation Abstracts International*, 1976, *36*, 5763B.

Malec, J., Cayner, J. J., Harvey, R. F., & Timming, R. C. Pain management: Long-term follow-up of an inpatient program. *Archives of Physical Medicine and Rehabilitation*, 1981, *62*, 369–372.

Maruta, T., Swanson, D. W., & Swenson, W. M. Chronic pain: Which patients may a pain-management program help? *Pain*, 1979, *7*, 321–329.

McCreary, C. P., Turner, J., & Dawson, E. Differences between functional and organic low back pain patients. *Pain*, 1977, *4*, 73–78.

McCreary, C. P., Turner, J., & Dawson, E. The MMPI as a predictor of response to conservative treatment for low back pain. *Journal of Clinical Psychology*, 1979, *35*, 278–284.

McCreary, C. P., Turner, J., & Dawson, E. Principal dimensions of the pain experience and psychological disturbance in chronic low back pain patients. *Pain*, 1981, *11*, 85–92.

Mechl, P. E., & Dahlstrom, W. G. Objective configural rules for discriminating psychotic from neurotic MMPI profiles. *Journal of Consulting Psychology*, 1960, *24*, 375–387.

Meyerowitz, S. Psychosocial factors in the etiology of somatic disease. *Annals of Internal Medicine*, 1970, *72*, 753–754.

Meyerson, L. Special disabilities. *Annual Review of Psychology*, 1957, *8*, 437–457.

Miller, N. E., & Dworkin, B. R. Critical issues in therapeutic applications of biofeedback. In G. E. Schwartz & J. Beatty (Eds.), *Biofeedback: Theory and research*. New York: Academic Press, 1977.

Mintz, J., Luborsky, L., & Christoph, P. Measuring the outcome of psychotherapy: Findings of the Penn Psychotherapy Project. *Journal of Consulting and Clinical Psychology*, 1979, *47*, 319–334.

Mitchell, S. K. Interobserver agreement, reliability, and generalizability of data collected in observational studies. *Psychological Bulletin*, 1979, *86*, 376–390.

Moos, R. H., & Moos, B. S. A typology of family social environments. *Family Process*, 1976, *15*, 357–371.

Moos, R. H., & Solomon, G. F. MMPI response patterns in patients with rheumatoid arthritis. *Journal of Psychosomatic Research*, 1964, *8*, 17–28.

Moos, R. H., & Solomon, G. F. Personality correlates of the degree of incapacity of patients with physical disease. *Journal of Chronic Diseases*, 1965, *18*, 1019–1038.

Murphy, T. M. Subjective and objective follow-up assessment of acupuncture therapy without suggestion in 100 chronic pain patients. In J. J. Bonica & D. Albe-Fessard (Eds.), *Advances in pain research and therapy* (Vol. 1). New York: Raven Press, 1976.

Nalven, F. B., & O'Brien, J. F. Personality patterns of rheumatoid arthritis patients. *Arthritis and Rheumatism*, 1964, *7*, 18–28.

Nalven, F. B., & O'Brien, J. F. On the use of the MMPI with rheumatoid arthritic patients. *Journal of Clinical Psychology*, 1968, *24*, 70.

Nelson, R. O. Methodological issues in assessment via self-monitoring. In J. D. Cone & R. P. Hawkins (Eds.), *Behavioral assessment: New directions in clinical psychology*. New York: Brunner/Mazel, 1977.

Newman, R., Seres, J., Yospe, L., & Garlington, B. Multidisciplinary treatment of chronic pain: Long-term follow-up of low-back pain patients. *Pain*, 1978, *4*, 283–292.

Nunnally, J. C. *Psychometric theory* (2nd ed.). New York: McGraw-Hill, 1978.

Ostfeld, A. M., & Lebovitz, B. Z. Personality factors and pressor mechanisms in renal and essential hypertension. *Archives of Internal Medicine*, 1959, *104*, 43–52.

Phillips, E. L. Some psychological characteristics associated with orthpaedic complaints. *Current Practices in Orthopedic Surgery*, 1964, *2*, 165–176.

Pickering, G. *High blood pressure*. London: J. & A. Churchill, 1968.

Pope, M. H., Rosen, J. C., Wilder, D. G., & Frymoyer, J. W. The relationship between biomechanical and psychological factors in patients with low-back pain. *Spine*, 1980, *5*, 173–177.

Prokop, C. K., & Bradley, L. A. (Eds.). *Medical psychology: Contributions to behavioral medicine*. New York: Academic Press, 1981. (a)

Prokop, C. K., & Bradley, L. A. Methodological issues in medical psychology and behavioral medicine research. In C. K. Prokop & L. A. Bradley (Eds.), *Medical psychology: Contributions to behavioral medicine*. New York: Academic Press, 1981. (b)

Prokop, C. K., Bradley, L. A., Margolis, R., & Gentry, W. D. Multivariate analyses of the MMPI profiles of multiple pain patients. *Journal of Personality Assessment*, 1980, *44*, 246–252.

Reinhardt, L. *A long-term follow-up study of chronic pain patients treated with a behaviorally oriented inpatient pain treatment program*. Unpublished doctoral dissertation, University of Minnesota, 1979.

Roberts, A. H. The behavioral treatment of pain. In J. M. Ferguson & C. B. Taylor (Eds.), *A comprehensive handbook of behavioral medicine* (Vol. 2). Jamaica, N.Y.: Spectrum, 1981.

Roberts, A. H., & Reinhardt, L. The behavioral management of chronic pain: Long-term follow-up with comparison groups. *Pain*, 1980, *8*, 151–162.

Russell, J. A. A circumplex model of affect. *Journal of Personality and Social Psychology*, 1980, *39*, 1161–1178.

Sanders, S. H. Toward a practical instrument system for the automatic measurement of "uptime" in chronic pain patients. *Pain*, 1980, *9*, 103–109.

Schmidt, N., Coyle, B. S., & Rauschenberger, J. A Monte Carlo evaluation of three formula estimates of cross-validated multiple correlation. *Psychological Bulletin*, 1977, *84*, 751–758.

Shadish, W. R., Hickman, E., & Arrick, M. C. Psychological problems of spinal cord injury patients: Emotional distress as a function of time and locus of control. *Journal of Consulting and Clinical Psychology*, 1981, *49*, 297.

Shapiro, C., & Surwit, R. S. Learned control of physiological function and disease. In H. Leitenberg (Ed.), *Handbook of behavior modification and behavior therapy*. Englewood Cliffs, N.J.: Prentice-Hall, 1976.

Shontz, F. C. Physical disability and personality: Theory and recent research. *Psychological Aspects of Disability*, 1970, *17*, 51–69.

Smith, W. M. Epidemiology of hypertension. *Medical Clinics of North America*, 1977, *61*, 467–486.

Sobel, H. J., & Worden, J. W. The MMPI as a predictor of psychosocial adaptation to cancer. *Journal of Consulting and Clinical Psychology*, 1979, *47*, 716–724.

Spergel, P., Ehrlich, G. E., & Glass, D. The rheumatoid arthritic personality: A psychodiagnostic myth. *Psychosomatics*, 1978, *19*, 79–86.

Sternbach, R. A. *Pain patients: Traits and treatment*. New York: Academic Press, 1974.

Sternbach, R. A., & Timmermans, G. Personality changes associated with reduction of pain. *Pain*, 1975, *1*, 171–179.

Sternbach, R. A., Wolf, S. R., Murphy, R. S., & Akeson, W. H. Traits of pain patients: The low-back "loser." *Psychosomatics*, 1973, *14*, 226–229.

Strahan, R. F. More on averaging judges' ratings: Determining the most reliable composite. *Journal of Consulting and Clinical Psychology*, 1980, *48*, 587–589.

Strassberg, D. S., Reimherr, F., Ward, M., Russell, S., & Cole, A. The MMPI and chronic pain. *Journal of Consulting and Clinical Psychology*, 1981, *49*, 220–226.

Suess, W. M., & Chai, H. Neuropsychological correlates of asthma: Brain damage or drug effects? *Journal of Consulting and Clinical Psychology*, 1981, *49*, 135–136.

Sullivan, P. L., & Welsh, G. S. A technique for objective configural analysis of MMPI profiles. *Journal of Consulting Psychology*, 1952, *16*, 383–388.

Taylor, G. P. Moderator-variable effects on personality-test-item endorsements of physically disabled patients. *Journal of Consulting and Clinical Psychology*, 1970, *35*, 183–188.

Tellegen, A. *The Differential Personality Questionnaire*. University of Minnesota, 1980.

Tellegen, A., Kamp, J., & Watson, D. Recognizing individual differences in predictive structure. *Psychological Review*, 1982, *89*, 95–105.

Trabin, T. *Evaluation and prediction of pain management program outcomes for chronic low back pain patients*. Unpublished doctoral dissertation, University of Minnesota, 1981.

Turk, D. C., & Genest, M. Regulation of pain: The application of cognitive and behavioral techniques for prevention and mediation. In P. C. Kendall & S. D. Hollon (Eds.), *Cognitive–behavioral interventions: Theory, research and procedures.* New York: Academic Press, 1979.

Ward, D. J. Rheumatoid arthritis and personality: A controlled study. *British Medical Journal,* 1971, *2,* 297–299.

Waring, E. M., Weisz, G. M., & Bailey, S. I. Predictive factors in the treatment of low back pain by surgical intervention. In J. J. Bonica & D. Albe-Fessard (Eds.), *Advances in pain research and therapy* (Vol. 1). New York: Raven Press, 1976.

Watson, D. *A cross-cultural study of the structure of mood.* Unpublished doctoral dissertation, University of Minnesota, 1982. (a)

Watson, D. Neurotic tendencies among chronic pain patients: An MMPI item analysis. *Pain,* 1982, *14,* 365–385. (b)

Wiggins, J. Content dimensions in the MMPI. In J. N. Butcher (Ed.), *MMPI: Research developments and clinical applications.* New York: McGraw-Hill, 1969.

Wilfling, F. J., Klonoff, H., & Kokan, P. Psychological, demographic and orthopedic factors associated with prediction of outcome of spinal fusion. *Clinical Orthopedics,* 1973, *90,* 153–160.

Wills, T. A., Weiss, R. L., & Patterson, G. R. A behavioral analysis of the determinants of marital satisfaction. *Journal of Consulting and Clinical Psychology,* 1974, *42,* 802–811.

Wiltse, L. L., & Rocchio, P. D. Preoperative psychological tests as predictors of success of chemonucleolysis in treatment of the low back syndrome. *Journal of Bone and Joint Surgery,* 1975, *57A,* 478–483.

Zevon, M. A., & Tellegen, A. The structure of mood change: An idiographic/nomothetic analysis. *Journal of Personality and Social Psychology,* 1982, *43,* 111–122.

Ziesat, H. A., Jr. Behavioral approaches to the treatment of chronic pain. In C. K. Prokop & L. A. Bradley (Eds.), *Medical psychology: Contributions to behavioral medicine.* New York: Academic Press, 1981.

PART II

Coping with Specific Illnesses
and Their Treatments

4

Coping with Coronary Heart Disease and Stroke*

DAVID S. KRANTZ
A. WALLACE DECKEL

Introduction

Diseases of the heart and the cerebral vasculature rank first and third as major causes of death and disability in the United States (U.S. Department of Health, Education, and Welfare, 1979). Although these disorders result in different physical impairments, they are similar in regard to risk factors, sudden onset, and the threat of recurrence. This chapter focuses on the overlapping constellation of psychological responses that are associated with coronary heart and cerebrovascular diseases.

During the past 20 years, numerous studies have been published on the psychosocial aspects of rehabilitation following myocardial infarction (MI) or heart attack. Considerably fewer investigations have examined the psychological aspects of a cerebrovascular accident or stroke, the other major symptomatic and disabling cardiovascular disease. Recovery from an MI or a stroke is more than just a medical problem. Complex and demanding social, vocational, and psychological adjustments are often required of patients and their families. Progress in medical treatment has increased the percentage of individuals surviving acute episodes of these disorders (Feigenson, McDowell, Meese, McCarthy, & Greenberg, 1977; Garrity, 1975; Lawrence

*Preparation of this chapter was assisted by Uniformed Services University of the Health Sciences Grant C07214. Portions of this chapter relating to heart attack were adapted from an article by D. S. Krantz (1980).

ISBN 0-12-144450-3

& Christie, 1979). However, many of the nonmedical problems resulting from
the onset of symptomatic cardiovascular disease remain as severe as the
primary illness itself (Croog & Levine, 1977; Croog, Levine, & Lurie, 1968;
Doehrman, 1977; Espmark, 1973).

Biomedical and psychological variables interact at many levels in the recovery process, and a growing body of data indicates that important recovery
outcomes may depend on the patient's interpretation of illness and the
success and failure of psychological coping mechanisms. The coping process
in stroke is further complicated by damaged cognitive capacity to monitor
and to deal with psychological adjustment to the disease (see Gordon and
Diller, Chapter 5). An understanding of coping mechanisms therefore may
suggest strategies for intervention and also provide insights into more general ways that psychosocial processes can influence health.

We begin this chapter by describing the nature of the physical disease
processes underlying MI and stroke. Next, we consider the social, vocational, and psychological impact of each disorder, and review various perspectives on coping with these diseases. In our discussion we also consider
psychological and behavioral intervention strategies for facilitating the recovery process.

Physical Disease Processes

Arteriosclerosis is thought to be the underlying structural disorder for most
cases of MI and for some cases of stroke. It is a symptomless condition
characterized by narrowing and deterioration of the arteries, including the
coronary arteries and blood vessels that nourish the brain. An excess accumulation of cholesterol and related lipids form a mound of tissue, or
plaque, on the inner wall of one or more of the arteries. The formation of
arteriosclerotic plaques may proceed undetected for years, affecting cardiac
and/or cerebral functioning only when the plaques cause a degree of
obstruction sufficient to diminish blood supply. Once this occurs, arteriosclerosis has evolved sufficiently to produce cardiovascular symptomatology.

Coronary heart disease (CHD) has several symptomatic or clinical manifestations. In one form of CHD, angina pectoris, occasional instances of
inadequate blood supply (ischemia) cause the individual to experience attacks of chest pain. Although ischemia per se does not cause permanent
tissue damage, angina is a painful condition that can lead to more serious
complications. A more severe and frequently fatal consequence of CHD is

MI, in which a prolonged state of ischemia results in death of a portion of the heart tissue. Other manifestations of CHD include congestive heart failure, conditions secondary to MI (e.g., ventricular failure, heart rupture), and disturbances of the conductive or beat-regulating portion of the heart, that is, the arrhythmias (Hurst, Logue, Schlant, & Wenger, 1978).

Some cases of stroke can result from an infarction—or a stoppage of the blood supply—to a localized, discrete area of the brain, causing death of the involved tissue. Although arteriosclerosis and/or hypertension are integral parts of this process, the sequence of events leading to stroke is somewhat different than that leading to heart disease. In one form of stroke, arteriosclerotic plaques directly damage the cerebral blood vessels, which then become capable of trapping blood clots (cerebral thrombi) or circulating substances or masses (e.g., dislodged pieces of plaque from distant blood vessels, collectively called cerebral emboli) that cause the infarction and subsequent brain lesion.

Stroke also can be caused by cerebral hemorrhage—a bleeding into the brain resulting from a rupture of a blood vessel. The extent of damage to nervous tissue caused by hemorrhage is considerable and represents a more immediate threat to life than stroke caused by infarction. Blood leaking into the brain from the hemorrhage compresses large areas of nervous tissue together within the rigid, bony skull and causes widespread and often fatal damage.

Dimensions of Recovery

A large number of predictor variables have been implicated and studied as possible determinants of postcardiovascular disease adjustment (Garrity and coauthors, 1976). These include physical variables (severity of disease, intensity of symptoms, physical activity, central nervous system damage), psychological processes (perceptions of illness, denial, locus of control), sociological and demographic characteristics (age, socioeconomic status, predisease work situation, money available for early retirement), and characteristics of the health care system (e.g., information received from physicians). Level of functioning (e.g., resumption of normal activities), vocational adjustment, and morale of the patient during recovery have been the most frequently studied outcome variables. One major problem with research on the recovery process has been the lack of standardized instruments for measuring outcome variables and their predictors. In addition, much of the research on the recovery process has been descriptive or correlational in nature and there has been a notable lack of prospective investigation. These facts have made it difficult to establish firm cause-and-effect relationships, and have made it difficult to predict effective rehabilitation interventions.

Despite extensive research, there is still no universally accepted definition of *recovery*. Some investigators define recovery in terms of physical health status and others in terms of behavioral outcomes such as return to work and vocational adjustment. There is some agreement in dividing the course of illness temporally into an acute (in-hospital) phase and a convalescent/recovery (posthospital) phase; however, there seems to be little consensus about how medical and psychosocial processes are interrelated at each stage. Given the diversity of recovery-related variables, we have chosen to discuss a limited number of variables and issues important in rehabilitation. These include cognitive and emotional disturbances and restoration of function in the work and home environments.

THE IMPACT OF ILLNESS ON WORK AND FAMILY

Myocardial Infarction

Some of the most significant barriers to recovery and rehabilitation of coronary patients are of a social and occupational nature. Three of the major concerns of the recovering heart patient after release from the hospital involve survival (fears of death and recurrence of disease), the effects of illness on ability to resume work activities, and the effects of illness on sexual functioning (Croog, 1983; Dillard, 1982). Reviews of the literature suggest that roughly 85% of patients are found to be reemployed 1 year after heart attack (Doehrman, 1977; Garrity, 1981). Delays or failures in returning to work occur more often among blue-collar workers, relatively less educated people, and patients with long-lasting depression or emotional distress. However, many individuals who resume employment reduce their levels of productivity, change jobs, or switch from full to part-time work schedules (Doehrman, 1977; Garrity, 1981). Physical variables such as severity of MI and number of previous MIs are related to patients' return to work. Nevertheless, medical status is by no means a sufficient predictor of occupational adjustment.

Data from several studies suggest that many, if not most, patients do not return to their previous levels of sexual activity after an MI. This is probably caused more by psychological and interpersonal concerns than by physiological factors (Doehrman, 1977). For example, in one study by Hellerstein and Freidman (1970), the five most common reasons given for diminished sexual activity were decreased desire, depression, anxiety, wife's decision, and fear of death. Much has been written about the role of the family in influencing the course of recovery and rehabilitation, with particular emphasis on how the wife can affect the way the husband copes with his disease (Croog, 1975; 1983). Some anecdotal and case reports have appeared on issues such as husband-and-wife conflict (Garrity, 1975) and spouse over-protectiveness (Wishnie, Hackett, & Cassem, 1971). However, there has been little systematic research on the patterns of interpersonal behaviors between husband and wife that are associated with good or poor adjustment to illness (Croog, 1975).

Stroke: Vocational Impact

Not surprisingly, the catastrophic changes that result from stroke also have been found to have a significant impact upon work and family. Stroke is often considered to be a disease afflicting persons beyond retirement age. However, stroke does affect all age groups, and medical developments that have lengthened survival expectancies have also increased the importance of research on vocational rehabilitation.

In one study of adjustment to stroke, Espmark (1973) found that the speed with which stroke patients returned to work primarily depended upon the extent of severity of the poststroke handicap. Most patients with a minimal to moderate degree of handicap returned to work within the first 3 months, whereas the more severely handicapped individuals took longer than 6 months to return. In a similar investigation, Weisbroth, Esibill, and Zuger (1971) reported an average length of time between onset of disability and return to work that was generally longer than was found in the Espmark (1973) study (approximately 18 months) and that was also, as one might expect, dependent on the location of the lesion in the brain.

Studies involving long-term vocational follow-up of stroke patients have produced somewhat inconsistent results. Several optimistic reports (e.g., Anderson, Anderson, & Kottke, 1977; Anderson & Kottke, 1978; Espmark, 1973) have suggested that there is a relatively high rate of return of stroke patients to active vocational functioning. These reports have concluded that, optimally, two-thirds of stroke patients can be expected to return to work of some kind. Moreover, one study concluded that adjustment to work among those able to resume activities was not significantly impaired by the extent of neurological handicap, although emotional problems secondary to the stroke were associated with poor occupational readjustment (Espmark, 1973).

The findings noted in the preceding discussion stand in constrast to several more pessimistic reports indicating that only a minority (certainly less than half) of stroke patients can be expected to resume work activity. For example, Powell, Diller, and Grynbaum (1976) reported on vocational readjustment in stroke patients from two hospitals with widely divergent patient populations: one hospital serviced a patient population that was low in socioeconomic status (SES) and the other serviced a middle- to high-SES population. It was found that few patients from either hospital were employed at a 2-year follow-up. Although the two populations contained equivalent proportions of unemployed patients, the impact of unemployment upon patients differed drastically as a function of social class. Higher SES stroke patients generally were very discouraged by their inability to work again; they felt that work had intrinsic value and meaning beyond income. In contrast, lower SES patients were less traumatized by the inability to work. They tended to report that their jobs had previously offered little satisfaction and did not feel that it was a personal failure to be unable to continue working. Thus, it is apparent that return to work by itself is not necessarily a useful parameter for evaluating quality of life in the recovering stroke patient.

In summary, there appears to be considerable disagreement concerning the consequences of stroke for vocational readjustment. This disagreement partially stems from major methodological differences among studies (e.g., some studies select only the highly favorable candidates for vocational rehabilitation, whereas others include all patients). Other causes for this lack of consensus include differences among studies in evaluating effects upon vocational readjustment of patient age and SES, side and extent of lesion, type of employment, and the meaning of the aforementioned variables for the affected individual.

Effects of the Family on Stroke Recovery

Although research indicates that there can be marked disruption of the interpersonal relationships among families of stroke victims (Aroskar & Dittmar, 1978; Lawrence & Christie, 1979), the effects of this disruption on the rehabilitation of the stroke patient are not well understood. It seems plausible that a supportive family structure would facilitate the recovery process; however, most studies do not support this hypothesis. For example, Hyman (1972) found trends suggesting that stroke victims' satisfaction with their families was negatively associated with functional improvement: the more content the patient was in his family setting, the poorer was the recovery from stroke. These data were explained by postulating that family cohesiveness generated overprotection of the patient and subsequently impaired the recovery process. Similar results were reported in a large and well-controlled study by Labi, Phillips, and Greshman (1980), who found that stroke survivors who lived alone were less likely than those who lived in a family to decrease outside socializations. A third corroborative study (Rogoff, Cooney, & Kutner, 1964) found that married hemiplegic persons showed less improvement than nonmarried hemiplegics, possibly as a result of the spouse's overprotection of the patient.

Findings in contrast to those described above also have been reported.

Anderson *et al.* (1977) demonstrated that living at home rather than in a nursing home correlated positively with patients' rehabilitation progress. Powell *et al.* (1976) found no differences between married and unmarried patients living alone with respect to performance in the rehabilitation program. Instead they reported that SES level was related to *both* marital status and the patient's disposition. Lower SES patients were less likely to be married and more likely to be institutionalized. Middle- to high-SES patients were more likely to be married and were more likely to return home.

The studies reviewed above suggest that the family may play a significant role in the rehabilitation process of the stroke patient. However, the small research literature does not presently allow general conclusions to be drawn about the nature of that role. It currently is not possible to predict with consistency the types of family setting that will foster or impede the rehabilitation process for the stroke-impaired individual.

COGNITIVE AND EMOTIONAL RESPONSES TO ILLNESS

The patient's psychological reactions to MI and stroke have been conceptualized in several ways by different investigators. One view (Cassem & Hackett, 1971) focuses on psychodynamic *defense mechanisms* and coping dispositions (particularly denial and depression) used in response to the acute stress of illness. In the case of CHD, other conceptual approaches have been offered as well. These include a *health-perception* perspective (Garrity, 1975) that emphasizes patients' attitudes and beliefs about their health status. These beliefs are thought to guide a series of conscious decisions that, in turn, lead to a variety of behaviors related to recovery. Alternatively, a third *control and predictability* model (Krantz, 1980) views the recovery process as a response to crisis and proposes that illness can induce feelings of helplessness. Therefore, particular aspects of illness will have a less negative impact to the extent that they are perceived (in the context of the illness situation) to be predictable and/or controllable. In the following discussion we describe psychological perspectives on recovery. We first consider approaches to coping with heart attack and then discuss the literature on stroke. In the presentation of each approach we also consider therapeutic interventions derived from that perspective.

Heart Attack Recovery: Psychological Perspectives

DEFENSE MECHANISMS AND COPING DISPOSITIONS

Denial

Cassem and Hackett (1971) have developed a model for the chronology of emotional reactions of the person who suffers an MI in which denial is implicated as the focal mechanism for the coronary patient. It is proposed that a patient feels heightened anxiety when first admitted to the coronary care unit (CCU). Denial is soon mobilized and the patient finds it difficult to believe that he or she has really had a heart attack. Subsequently, anxiety declines for a period, and the patient (a) often protests detention in the CCU, (b) insists on returning to normal activities, and (c) becomes difficult to manage. However, after several days the patient becomes more cognizant of the limitations of his or her true condition and experiences depression.

The Cassem and Hackett model implies that patients who use denial will experience less anxiety in the CCU than those who do not and, because of the presumed stress-reducing effects of denial, those who use the defense mechanism will show facilitated recovery. Therefore, Hackett and Cassem (1973) believe that deniers will have better survival records in the coronary care unit than nondeniers. In support of this model, several studies have found that patients who use denial tend to be less anxious in early phases of illness than those who do not (Froese, Hackett, Cassem, & Silverberg, 1974; Garrity et al., 1976). However, long-term follow-up studies examining the relationship between denial and longevity have not used sufficiently large samples to produce conclusive results regarding the Cassem and Hackett hypothesis. Paradoxically, the use of denial has been related in some studies to long-term resistance to compliance with medical regimens (Croog, Shapiro, & Levine, 1971; Garrity et al., 1976), as deniers have indicated less willingness to follow medical instructions than nondeniers. A recent report by Soloff (1980), however, did not find a relationship between denial and self-reported compliance.

In summary, patients' use of denial may make for better coping with the early stress of illness in the CCU. In the long term, however, patients may endanger their changes of recovery by ignoring medical recommendations that are important for satisfactory rehabilitation. The conflicting results relating denial to long-term outcomes suggest the need for further research on this question.

Greene, Moss, and Goldstein (1974) and Simon, Feinleib, and Thompson (1972) offer a view of denial that is somewhat different from that of Cassem and Hackett. They believe that denial of symptoms may appear even before hospitalization and cause delay in seeking help. Instead of viewing denial as an unconscious defense mechanism, Greene et al. and Simon et al. emphasize that patients may use denial as a (possibly conscious) instrumental cognitive coping strategy. These investigators report that many patients appreciate the seriousness of their symptoms but delay in seeking help because they cannot tolerate the helplessness that they perceive is entailed with illness and interruption of ongoing activities (Moss & Goldstein, 1970; Moss, Wynar, & Goldstein, 1969). Greene et al. (1974) present the argument that defense mechanisms among heart patients are developed in order to counter the perceived threat of helplessness that accompanies chronic illness. Although Hackett and Cassem have developed a questionnaire instrument to measure denial (Hackett & Cassem, 1974), defense mechanisms are notoriously difficult to measure operationally. This problem makes it difficult to test the denial hypothesis. Particularly with data gathered by face-to-face interviews, it is difficult to distinguish denial (as a defense mechanism) from inability or conscious unwillingness to discuss emotionally laden issues (Croog & Levine, 1977). For example, inconsistencies in data linking denial to recovery outcomes have been attributed to differences in patient willingness to admit troublesome feelings in brief interviews with strangers as opposed to in-depth interviews with trusted hospital staff (Doehrman, 1977).

To summarize, evidence for the efficacy of the Hackett and Cassem denial hypothesis is mixed, suggesting some benefits in the early stages of illness due to reduction of anxiety. However, some investigators (e.g., Moss *et al.*, 1969) have presented evidence implicating denial of symptoms as a source of delay in treatment and hospitalization. There is also the possibility, not yet thoroughly studied, that patients who persistently use denial may be less likely to comply with medical regimens than those who do not use denial. As a conceptualization of the recovery process, the Cassem and Hackett denial hypothesis seems to explain short-term in-hospital reactions best, but it is not sufficiently developed to account for long-term outcomes.

Depression

Depression is considered to be one of the most formidable problems in cardiac convalescence and rehabilitation (Hackett & Cassem, 1973). During the convalescence period patients must confront the realities of disability and deal directly with changes in life-style that are forced upon them. Moreover, after the period of hospitalization, a subset of patients are reluctant to resume normal activities or return to work—often to an extent not justified by their medical disability. One common reaction shown by this group of patients, termed *cardiac invalidism,* is characterized by excessive dependency, helplessness, and restriction of activity. This reaction may actually contribute toward worsening of medical status because of the physiological effects of deconditioning associated with physical inactivity (Wenger, 1973).

Other recent studies also have examined psychological characteristics of cardiac patients at various postinfarct time intervals. Pancheri and his co-workers (Pancheri, Bellaterra, Matteoli, Cristofari, Polizzi, & Puletti, 1978) administered a battery of psychological tests and interviews to patients in the CCU on the second and third day following infarction. Approximately 8 days later, upon release, the clinical condition of each patient was evaluated using medical parameters such as length of stay in the CCU and electrocardiographic and laboratory test data. Subjects were divided into two groups, labeled "improved" and "not improved," based on these clinical parameters. Results indicated that several psychological measures given earlier during the CCU stay distinguished the two groups. Patients categorized as "not improved" evidenced higher anxiety and heightened emotional reactions, including depression on several scales, as well as more work-related frustration. A difficulty in evaluating this study is that it is not entirely clear which medical variables distinguished the two groups in this study on admission. It should be noted, however, that patients in grave medical condition were excluded from the Pancheri *et al.* (1978) study sample.

Obier, MacPherson, and Haywood (1977) found evidence only partially supportive of the hypothesis that depression-related indices of coping ability may adversely affect survival outcomes. Measures of depression and pessimism were administered to patients while in the CCU and at 3, 6, and 12 months postinfarct. Out of a sample of 57 subjects, 12 died and 45 survived to participate in a final $2\frac{1}{2}$-year follow-up. Results indicated higher depression and pessimism in nonsurvivors at 3-, 6-, and 12-month periods. However, the groups did not differ on these measures during their stay in the CCU.

In a successful attempt to counter the effects of depression, Gruen (1975) subjected a random sample of cardiac patients to brief cognitively oriented psychotherapy designed to facilitate coping with illness. Data collected showed that treated patients, compared to a matched control group, had shorter stays in the hospital, were less likely to develop medical complications in the form of arrhythmias, showed fewer manifestations of depression or anxiety, and were more able to return to normal activities at a 4-month follow-up. The cognitive treatments consisted of reassurance and encouragement, and of strengthening the patients' positive beliefs and coping resources. These interventions, directed simultaneously at several psychological processes, demonstrate the efficacy of brief psychotherapy during the acute phase of illness.

To summarize, most research suggests that depression is associated with poorer post-MI outcomes. It is of course possible that patients who are in poorer physical condition merely report greater depression because of the physical or psychological impact of illness. However, there are enough prospective data to make it plausible that defense mechanisms such as denial reduce physiological stress responses, and that affective reactions such as depression increase stress during the acute phase of illness. Clearly, further intervention-oriented research is needed to examine the mechanisms whereby psychological defenses affect the recovery process (see Razin, 1982).

THE "HEALTH-PERCEPTION" APPROACH

As previously noted, a second perspective regarding the psychosocial aspects of cardiac rehabilitation assumes that patients' perceived health status is a central variable. This view is based on the notion that illness-related behaviors are products of a series of decisions based on the manner in which patients view their current health situations (Garrity *et al.*, 1976). Therefore, a patient's understanding of his/her clinical status is seen as equally important as actual physical status in determining behavioral outcomes. Mood and behavior in reaction to illness are seen as products of what people believe about the severity of their disorder, and, within the physical limitations imposed by disease, recovery-related variables are bound to health perceptions.

This view has received major impetus from research conducted by Garrity (1973a, 1973b, 1975) designed to explain why some MI patients return to work and recreational activities and achieve acceptable levels of morale although others do not. In this research, the study group consisted of male patients who had suffered an MI. Perceived health was measured by rating scales during the hospital stay and 6 months later. Self-reported morale and resumption of activities were also measured after a 6-month period. Results indicated that patients who perceived their health to be poor rated morale as lower and were less likely to have returned to work or to community involvement than patients who rated their health as relatively good. Health perceptions during and after hospitalization were related to one another, but perceived health status was only weakly related to clinical measures of physical health status. Therefore, perceptions of health had an independent relationship to measures of recovery and adjustment; controlling for the influence of physical health variables, health perceptions were related to recovery outcomes.

It should be noted that the conclusions of this research are limited by the fact that no attempt was made to manipulate or alter patients' health perceptions. Since this research was partly retrospective (patients were already ill when health self-ratings were initially made), it also is not clear to what extent reported poor health reflects rather than causes low morale. Self-reports of poor health may provide a justification for not returning to work and for withdrawal from outside involvements. Nevertheless, these findings highlight the importance of beliefs about the severity and nature of illness for the recovering heart-attack patient.

The health-perception model also suggests several interventions to improve self-assessed health status. Personnel involved in acute coronary care may be able to affect behavioral rehabilitation several months later by altering patient perceptions and fostering a belief (which is usually veridical) in the optimistic aspects of physical recovery (Garrity, 1975). Patient perceptions can be altered through instruction, education, and various nursing care and rehabilitation procedures. (See Rogers, Chapter 15, for further discussion of the role of nurses in changing patients' perceptions and behaviors.)

The health-perception model bears conceptual similarity to a more general health-belief model used to study participation in preventive health behavior (Kasl & Cobb, 1966; Rosenstock, 1966). Both models emphasize the decisions made by patients to reduce threats posed by illness. The health perception model proposes that many physical, psychosocial, and sociological predictors of post-MI adjustment may be mediated by patients' perceptions of personal health status (Garrity et al., 1976). This decisional model has the benefit of linking together many different predictor and outcome variables in cardiac rehabilitation, and also is intervention-oriented (although we know of no intervention studies to date that have been designed to test the model specifically).

A study by Soloff (1980) suggests that postcoronary mood disturbances (discussed in "Depression") may be related to patients' self-ratings of perceived quality of functioning. At a 3-month follow-up, total mood disturbance was (a) inversely related to perceptions of health status, and (b) a significant predictor of self-reported compliance and perceived quality of functioning. Thus, the interrelationships among patients' beliefs about their health, mood disturbances, and recovery outcomes warrant further investigation.

To summarize, research on the health-perception model has to date been confined to correlational studies designed to predict rehabilitation outcomes among cardiac patients. This model seems most applicable to behavioral outcomes of the rehabilitation process (e.g., return to work) rather than to psychophysiological outcomes (e.g., stress responses) that might affect recovery. The model suggests that clinical interventions that improve patients' perceived health will speed recovery, but the model has not been directly tested through intervention research.

CONTROL AND PREDICTABILITY MODEL

A third psychological approach toward understanding recovery from heart attack is based upon the fact that the onset of acute MI constitutes a stressful and potentially uncontrollable event of major proportions for most cardiac patients (Krantz & Schulz, 1980). In addition to physical discomfort and fear of death, patients are confronted with uncertainties about employment, family, and life-style activities. Restrictions of life-style and a certain degree of fear and uncertainty may persist for months or even years beyond the acute phase of illness. Extensive research with both humans and animals has suggested that two related psychological factors can mediate an organism's responses to stress: controllability and predictability. Perceived control may be defined as the felt ability to escape, avoid, and/or modify threatening stimuli (Averill, 1973; Seligman, 1975). Predictability represents the ability to anticipate a particular stimulus.

In general, the greater the perceived controllability of a stressor, the less harmful are its effects on the organism. The work of Seligman (1975), for example, suggests that a psychological state of helplessness results when individuals encounter aversive events about which they can do nothing—that is, events that involve a perceived noncontingency between responses and outcomes. A range of cognitive, emotional, and physiological disturbances have been attributed to this psychological state, including depressive affect and anxiety. Research also indicates that, within limits, increases in the ability to predict, anticipate, or understand an aversive stimulus often reduce distress (Averill, 1973; Seligman, 1975). It is important to note that perceived controllability and predictability (and their beneficial effects) are not solely determined by the objective arrangement of a particular situation. Therefore, changing a person's interpretation of a particular objective situation (e.g., by providing information) can lessen appraised threat (Johnson & Leventhal, 1974; Seligman, 1975).

Several investigators (Engel, 1968; Seligman, 1975) have proposed that severe feelings of helplessness may be a general precursor to physical disease.[1] The control and predictability conceptualization of heart-attack recovery (Krantz, 1980) hypothesizes that adverse reactions occurring after acute MI are mediated in part by feelings of helplessness induced by illness and potentially threatening hospital procedures. According to this view, certain cognitive appraisal processes should be linked predictively to recovery-related behavioral and physiological responses. Holding medical status constant, it would be expected that individuals who feel relatively more competent, less depressed, and less threatened (all reflections of perceived helplessness) during the acute phase of illness will fare better at later points in the recovery process. In addition, procedures which enhance the patient's behavioral control (providing choices, encouraging participation) or cognitive control

[1]The original "learned helplessness" model proposed by Seligman (1975) has been revised to take account of the types of attributions individuals make concerning outcomes (Abramson, Seligman, & Teasdale, 1978). This revised model, in turn, has been the subject of considerable recent research and debate. However, as the Seligman and the Abramson, Seligman, and Teasdale models are concerned largely with affective and behavioral aftereffects of uncontrollable events and not with physiological disease processes, the details of these models need not concern us here.

(providing information, increasing environmental predictability) should facilitate recovery from acute MI. However, in order for these various procedures to have the desired effect, they must be presented to individuals in a way that heightens their sense of personal control.

Evidence bearing on the control and predictability perspective is derived largely from two intervention studies with post-MI patients. These two studies were conceived independently of this conceptual perspective, but the operations employed in the research seem to represent variables suggested by the model.

Transfer from a Coronary Care Unit: Effects of
Increasing Predictability

When a patient is ready for transfer from a CCU to a general medical ward, adverse reactions are frequently observed accompanying the sudden disruption of the physician–patient and nurse–patient relationships in the CCU. Klein, Kliner, Zipes, Troyer, and Wallace (1968) undertook a study to examine patients' reactions to their transfer. Patients were observed for symptoms, changes in physical health status, and overt emotional responses. In addition, daily urine samples were collected and examined for catecholamine excretion (see Frankenhaeuser, 1971). Results indicated that of the first seven patients followed after transfer, five showed adverse emotional reactions to the transfer along with some form of cardiovascular complication. All five also exhibited an increase in catecholamine excretion coincident with or following departure from the CCU.

Although transfer was intended as a sign of recovery, the patients showing adverse reactions interpreted being moved as a sign of rejection by the staff, as these patients often were transferred abruptly without choice or warning. In addition, there was a great deal of uncertainty over who was to be the patient's physician in his/her new location because other changes in treatment programs between CCU and ward were often abrupt.

Accordingly, a number of alterations in the CCU and ward procedures were instituted, and a second group of seven patients was studied. These changes included having (a) the patients prepared in advance for transfer, (b) the same physician–nurse team follow each of the patients through the CCU stay and the transfer, and (c) the nurse visit the patients every day after transfer and provide information about illness as well as help them make adjustments and future plans. The results indicated that the second group of seven patients, in contrast to the first, evidenced no new cardiovascular complications or untoward emotional responses accompanying transfer and also showed a substantially lower incidence of elevated catecholamine excretion.

Unfortunately, conclusions regarding the Klein *et al.* (1968) study must be tempered by the fact that the two sets of patients differed in severity of illness, duration of CCU stay, and level of physical activity. Nevertheless, these data provide a dramatic demonstration of the impact that unpredictable and uncontrollable changes in hospital environment can have upon the recovering heart patient. They further suggest that instituting changes to increase environmental predictability can have profound medical and psychological effects.

Nursing Factors and Recovery

An implicit assumption made by practitioners of coronary treatment is that proper nursing and psychological care can reduce patient stress. A remarkable but rather complex study conducted by Cromwell and associates (Cromwell, Butterfield, Brayfield, & Curry, 1977) manipulated patient-care procedures that appear to represent, in part, mixtures of various types of personal control. Acute MI patients were randomly assigned to a factorial combination of three nursing care procedures. The first intervention, labeled *information*, involved systematically providing patients with different amounts of information concerning the causes, physiology, and treatment of heart attack. The second intervention, called *participation*, was manipulated by varying the extent to which subjects initiated and engaged in activities related to their own treatment. A third intervention, termed *diversion*, consisted of giving patients different degrees of access to television, reading materials, and visitors.

The major findings of the nursing-care study concerned length of patient hospitalization. A complex interaction among the three nursing-care factors was found such that if patients were given high information but low levels of diversion or participation, hospital stay tended to be long. High information with high participation or high diversion, in contrast, led to short stays in the hospital. The results, subject to limitations of the study described below, suggest that if an acutely ill MI patient is told about the severity of his or her condition, that patient also should be allowed to actively participate in treatment or at least be given some opportunity for diversion.

A second finding of the Cromwell *et al.* (1977) study was that an intermediate level of physical activity was optimal for a short CCU and hospital stay. Specifically, intermediate amounts of both participation and diversion (the two treatments associated with the most patient activity) were associated with short hospital stays; either high or low amounts of participation and diversion were associated with long stays in the hospital. As there was no indication that patients discharged early had less favorable medical outcomes than those discharged later, the economic and psychosocial benefits of the favorable treatment combinations are self-evident.

In terms of the control and predictability approach, several issues and questions are raised by the Cromwell *et al.* (1977) study. First, it appears that the effects of various treatments in an acute coronary care setting depend on their meaning to the patient, which, in turn, depends on the particular context in which the treatments are presented. This conclusion is reached by considering the interactive effects of the treatments and is reinforced by an additional pattern of results suggesting that hospital stress, as measured by several physiological indices, was minimized to the extent that subjects received treatments congruent with measured personality characteristics. Second, the operations used to vary participation and diversion seem to have confounded personal control with other factors; the results, therefore, are not amenable to simple conceptual interpretation. For example, although the high-participation treatment probably resulted in a heightened sense of patient control or responsibility for the outcome of illness, it differed from the low-participation treatment in amount of physical activity as well as personal control. Such physical activity could affect healing processes of the vascular system independent of its psychological concomitants (Wenger, 1973). The diversion treatment also confounded personal control with redirection of attention. For example, in addition to directing their attention away from fears and concerns connected with illness, high-diversion patients could control and regulate the amount of visitation they received (Schulz, 1976).

Aside from concerns about the efficacy of various types or combinations of nursing care interventions, the Cromwell *et al.* study raises questions as to how much participation and responsibility are optimal to facilitate recovery from MI. In some cases, patients may neither prefer nor expect responsibility for some medical decisions. Perceptions of excessive responsibility, choice, or information may not be beneficial to patients either psychologically or medically (Mills & Krantz, 1979). Moreover, recent research suggests that in health-care situations individuals differ in their receptiveness to self-care and information; indeed, preferences for self-care and information can be measured reliably and have consequences for health behavior (Krantz, Baum, & Wideman, 1980). The most favorable outcomes therefore may result from matching individual patients with particular treatment interventions (Auerbach, Martelli, & Mercuri, in press; Krantz *et al.*, 1980).

In health-care settings, the patient's role in treatment is a major variable that distinguishes between traditional medical model approaches and newer behavioral approaches to health care; unlike the former, the behavioral approaches encourage the patient to become an active participant in treatment (Krantz *et al.*, 1980; Linn & Lewis, 1979; Schulman, 1979). Common sense suggests that the most efficacious approach to patient participation in treatment would maximize patients' abilities to cope with stressful aspects of illness without leading them to develop unrealistic expectations or to make medical decisions beyond their realm of competence (Johnson & Leventhal, 1974; Mills & Krantz, 1979). A final consideration is derived from recent studies of personal control treatments in institutional settings (see Krantz & Schulz, 1980 for a complete review). Long-term positive effects require that subjects attribute enhanced control to stable factors that will persist over time.

Psychotherapeutic Effects of Physical Exercise

One type of participatory treatment that may be effective for the post-MI patient is physical exercise. An increasing body of data documents the effectiveness of regular, graduated programs of physical activity in the convalescence of cardiac patients (Naughton, Hellerstein, & Mohler, 1973). Yet, until recently little experimental attention had been paid to the psychological effects of exercise. Several studies (e.g., McPherson, Paivio, Yuhasz, Rechnitzer, Pickard, & Lefcoe, 1967; Naughton, Bruhn, & Lategola, 1968) indicate that participation in physical activity programs can lead to an increased sense of well-being and decreased anxiety and depression in postinfarction patients. Hackett and Cassem (1973) further consider physical exercise to be the most potent antidote for depression available to the cardiac patient, and they recommend an appropriate program of physical conditioning beginning while the patient is still in CCU. They propose that physical conditioning acts to counter depression by restoring self-esteem, sense of independence, and feelings of self-sufficiency and accomplishment—in short, it restores patients' feelings of control over relatively stable factors in their lives. This interpretation of the effects of exercise rehabilitation for the cardiac patient further links the concept of control to the depression that is an important difficulty encountered during the recovery process.

To sum up, the control and predictability model has served a heuristic function of highlighting the importance of perceived lack of control and helplessness as psychological barriers to the MI recovery process. By viewing the setting of MI as analogous to a stress or crisis situation, this approach suggests environmental interventions (such as heightening patients' choice and active participation) in order to aid patients in coping with the threat of illness. However, to date, the studies that support the control and predictability model of post-MI recovery are not specifically generated by this approach. Further experimental studies are needed to determine the precise treatment interventions that are effective in minimizing patients' perceived helplessness and in maximizing favorable recovery outcomes.

The three models of MI recovery described in the previous sections identify psychological variables that must be addressed by clinicians in order to maximize favorable recovery outcomes. An awareness of the importance of defense mechanisms, patients' self-perceived health, and perceived control over illness can suggest the kinds of cognitive and behavioral interventions that may help patients cope with the stress of MI. Razin (1982) has provided an extensive review of post-MI psychosocial interventions. He concludes, as we do, that further hypothesis-testing research is badly needed in this area.

Stroke Recovery: Psychological Variables

DEFENSE MECHANISMS AND AFFECTIVE RESPONSES

Denial

As in the case of acute MI, denial of disability also occurs soon after the onset of stroke (Cohen, 1979). Initially this defense may serve as an adaptive coping mechanism, preventing the individual from becoming overwhelmed by the significance of this disease (Bardach, 1973). Again, by its very nature denial can present a great obstacle to the recovery process, particularly when it leads to refusal to acknowledge paralysis or other functional limitations that occur following stroke. Because of its importance to the rehabilitation of the stroke patient, denial has proven to be a widely investigated psychological sequela of stroke.

Using a real/ideal self-image disparity score as their measure of denial, Levine and Zigler (1975) compared the incidence of denial in patients with stroke, lung cancer, and coronary disease, as well as in healthy controls. It was found that while all three patient groups employed denial to some extent, the use of denial was more common among stroke patients than among the other groups. It was suggested that cancer and heart disease do not threaten the sense of uniqueness, self, and psychological adequacy to the extent that brain injury does; therefore, stroke patients require more intense use of denial to preserve psychological integrity.

Whereas Levine and Zigler explained their results in psychodynamic terms, Nathanson, Bergman, and Gordon (1952) suggested an alternative view of the use of denial. They found that 28 of 76 stroke patients exhibited denial (measured by incomplete acknowledgement of disability) in direct relation to the degree of disorientation caused by the neuropathology. Of 48 patients who expressed seemingly complete awareness of their disability, further in-depth questioning revealed that their awareness was not always complete. In contrast to the psychodynamic interpretation offered previously, Nathanson *et al.* suggested that denial among stroke patients may represent in part a direct organic consequence of the stroke rather than solely the use of a psychological defense mechanism. (See Barth and Boll, 1981 for further discussion of this view of denial.)

In a replication of this finding, Ullman, Ashenhurst, Hurwitz, and Gruen (1960) examined the nature of the interplay between neurophysiological brain damage and motivational–psychological factors leading to denial. They selected for study (as did Nathanson *et al.*) only those patients who manifested no signs of denial of their disease during an initial medical interview. After subjecting these individuals to a more rigorous examination, it was found that approximately one-half exhibited various degrees of denial of their disease. Interestingly, most of these patients had right-sided paralysis (right hemiplegia) due to left-hemisphere brain damage. As a consequence of this damage, the stroke patients' sensory perceptions were altered. For example, various body parts, such as an arm or leg, no longer "felt" as if they belonged to the patients. The patients' denial of illness thus was a result of their acceptance of these altered physical changes as real; that is, they denied that certain body parts belonged to them because it did not feel as if those parts did belong.

The studies reviewed above do not permit teasing out the relative contributions made by psychological and neuropathological processes to poststroke denial. However, it appears relatively safe to conclude that both psychological denial (protecting the emotional integrity of the stroke patient) and sensory and perceptual deficits (resulting from tissue damage) need to be considered when denial presents itself as a significant obstacle to the rehabilitation of stroke patients. (See Barth and Boll, 1981 and Gordon and Diller, Chapter 5, for further discussions of denial and arousal– indifference problems among stroke patients and the treatment difficulties posed by these problems.)

Depression and Other Mood Disturbances

Many authors, particularly those writing from the perspective of their clinical experience, have reported the occurrence of reactive depression following stroke (Bardach, 1973; Charaton & Fisk, 1978; Cohen, 1979; Feldman & Schultz, 1975; Fisher, 1961; Mossman, 1976; Piskor & Paleos, 1968; Ripecky & Lazarus, 1980; Singler, 1975; Watzlawick & Coyne, 1980; Whithouse, 1963). The reasons postulated for this poststroke depression are many and include illness-induced disruptions in personality dynamics, the life-threatening nature of illness, increased dependence on others, and removal from normal social and work activities (Fisher, 1961). Given the emotional upheavals associated with the factors cited above, it is not surprising that persons may experience depression following a stroke.

Although the clinical literature contains many descriptions of poststroke depression, there is relatively little systematic research to support the clinical observations of depression. Of the studies that have been performed, few demonstrate that the incidence of depression is statistically greater for stroke patients than for either healthy control groups or patients with other disorders matched for extent of functional disability. Indeed, Espmark (1973), in an uncontrolled and retrospective report of symptoms occurring after the onset of stroke, found depression to occur relatively less frequently than general anxiety, fatigue, mood fluctuations, memory impairments, or irascibility. These results suggest that the frequency of emotional states such as those noted above may pose a greater management problem for the poststroke patient than previously recognized. Similarly, Weinstein and Friedland (1977) found that the frequency of mood changes (including depression) was no greater than the frequency of denial or disorientation in patients with few perceptual limitations resulting from brain damage. Conversely, in patients with brain damage leading to impaired perception of sensory stimuli, the frequency of marked mood changes was lower than that of disorientation and greater than that of denial or hallucinations. Because of the vagueness of the diagnostic categories and the ambiguity of the classification of mood changes, we can conclude only that the results suggest that diverse mood changes occur among acute stroke patients. (See Gordon and Diller, Chapter 5, for a discussion of the occurrence of depression among stroke patients with right hemisphere brain damage.)

A third study compared the frequency of depression in stroke patients to that of an orthopedically disabled patient population (Folstein, Maiberger, & McHugh, 1977). It was found that, relative to orthopedic patients, stroke victims more frequently experienced depression. Specifically, of 20 stroke patients, 45% were depressed, whereas only 1 of 10 orthopedic patients showed similar symptoms. While both patient samples were small and no statistical comparison was reported, the study suggested that the incidence of depression may be greater in stroke patients than in comparably dysfunctional nonstroke populations. However, the evidence for the greater frequency of depression among stroke patients must be regarded as quite weak.

In summary, it seems that depression occurs among poststroke patients. It should be noted that although the clinical literature heavily emphasizes the high frequency and intensity of depression following stroke, existing empirical research suggests that depression may occur less frequently than other emotional reactions such as emotional lability or irritability. Moreover, the relative contributions of psychological responses to illness versus organic factors in producing these mood alterations remain to be determined. Depression among stroke victims certainly has been identified and discussed to a greater extent than many other emotional changes. This emphasis upon depression in the literature suggests that it also has warranted relatively greater treatment efforts. Perhaps clinicians have emphasized depression because compared to other emotional states (e.g., anger, anxiety) it may have a greater impact on the observer and may tend to elicit a nurturing or "helpful" response. Alternatively, depression may be more disabling than other poststroke psychological sequelae and, therefore, may warrant relatively greater clinical attention.

Psychological Interventions in Stroke Recovery

Most therapeutic interventions for stroke are structured in one of three ways. The first approach maximizes intellectual and physical stimulation of the patient in a structured, predictable, and supportive environment (e.g., Cohen, 1979; Davidson, 1963; Feldman & Schultz, 1975; Jones, 1975; Stonnington, 1980). A second general approach, discussed by Gordon and Diller (Chapter 5), employs specific cognitive remediation programs. A third intervention strategy, of most relevance to the concerns of this chapter, applies conventional psychotherapies to enhance the patient's ability to cope with the psychological aftermath of stroke.

Although supportive counseling for stroke patients has been advocated by a number of authors (e.g., Carlson, 1980; Charaton & Fisk, 1978; Daylong, 1974; Fisher, 1961; Hungerford, 1972; Stonnington, 1980; Whithouse, 1963), group therapy is the most common psychotherapeutic intervention presently used to facilitate coping in the poststroke patient. Reports of subjectively rated improvement among stroke patients and their families after group participation are common (D'Affliti & Weitz, 1974; Manuel, 1979; Oradei & Waite, 1974; Piskor & Paleos, 1968; Singler, 1975; Smith, 1977; Watzlawick & Coyne, 1980). However, no controlled outcome studies have been published documenting the superiority of group therapy over no therapy or other therapy controls. In addition, it appears that the group therapies reported in the stroke rehabilitation literature have employed diverse procedures that have made it difficult to compare the therapies with one another. For example, frequency and duration of sessions have varied among studies (e.g., from daily to once per week), as has group membership (e.g., stroke patients only versus patients and family together). Furthermore, some studies have examined groups with open membership characterized by frequent patient entrances and terminations (D'Affliti & Weitz, 1974; Manuel, 1979; Singler, 1975), whereas others have used groups with fixed membership throughout the duration of therapy. In this regard, it has been suggested that the introduction of new group members be made infrequently (Singler, 1975) in order to permit the development of support among members and allow more time for discussion by members who had been in the group longer.

A novel and promising intervention for the treatment of poststroke psychosocial disorders was developed in England by Griffith (1975). A community-wide plan was created in which teams of lay volunteers made routine visits to 31 stroke patients. These visits were made to stimulate patients' desire to recover and to encourage patients to make optimal use of their intellectual strengths by engaging in numerous games and tasks. Patient outcome was assessed by the family, doctors, speech therapists, and volunteers. The physicians reported that the general attitude and morale of nearly all of the patients had improved. Similarly, 21 patients showed improvement in speech. The success and cost effectiveness of this program suggests that it may represent an ideal posthospital rehabilitation program: it employs community resources to provide patients with social and cognitive stimulation that would not be possible in other settings.

To summarize the literature on the psychological sequelae of stroke, denial and depression have been emphasized, with other cognitive or mood changes (e.g., anger, anxiety) receiving considerably less attention. An important question remaining in the stroke rehabilitation literature is the precise role of organic brain damage in generating poststroke affective and cognitive responses. Three principal types of psychological interventions for stroke have occupied the greatest attention in the stroke rehabilitation literature: (a) use of structured, stimulating environments; (b) cognitive remediation; and (c) group pychotherapies. Further systematic research is needed to evaluate the comparative efficacy of these various approaches for different types of stroke lesions.

Conclusion

The major focus of this chapter has been on the cognitive and emotional processes involved in recovery from MI and stroke. Because recovery involves the interaction of medical and psychological variables at many levels, an understanding of psychosocial influences on recovery require identification of the precise mechanisms linking cognitive and emotional processes to rehabilitation outcomes. In closing this chapter, it is appropriate to redirect attention to several of these possible mechanisms.

Broadly drawing from the MI recovery literature, it appears that during the acute phase of illness, cognitive processes can directly affect internal physiological states such as cardiac electrical and sympathetic nervous system activity (Gruen, 1975; Klein et al., 1968). Central to this mechanism is the concept of psychological stress, which refers to an internal state of the individual who perceives threats to physical and/or psychic well-being (Lazarus, 1966). Physiological (neural, endocrine, hormonal) components of the stress response presumably lead to cardiovascular complications that may impede the recovery process. For example, denial has an adaptive stress-reducing role in the acute phase of illness, and increasing the predictability of the hospital environment has a potentially beneficial effect (Hackett & Cassem, 1973; Klein *et al.*, 1968).

A second way that cognitive variables might be translated into physical health outcomes is by changing the individual's behavior in health-related areas (e.g., self-care, medical compliance). Thus, a more positive view of one's health is seen as leading to favorable mood and behavior in reaction to illness (Garrity, 1981) and consequently to more complete resumption of activities after heart attack.

In the case of recovery from stroke, further understanding and treatment of the maladaptive defense mechanisms of poststroke denial and depression depend on the ability to understand and integrate the psychosocial and organic effects of the disease. Clearly, the stroke patient has much about which to be depressed; however, poststroke depression is not entirely reactive in nature, but partially a result of the effects of tissue damage. Thus, further research may reveal that a pairing of psychotherapeutic and pharmacologic interventions may offer the most promise for treatment in this area.

This chapter has examined the impact of MI and stroke on work and family as well as patients' cognitive and emotional responses to illness. The aim has been to place emphasis on mechanisms linking psychological processes to physiological, behavioral, and cognitive–affective aspects of the recovery process. Several conceptual approaches to these problems were presented in an effort to understand these mechanisms. Because recovery from both MI and stroke involve the interaction of medical and psychological processes at many levels, any single conceptualization may not be sufficient to account for all the relevant variables. Nevertheless, an understanding of the complex relationships among recovery variables may suggest strategies for intervention and also provide insight into more general ways that psychological variables can influence health.

References

Abramson, L. Y., Seligman, M. E. P., & Teasdale, J. D. Learned helplessness in humans: Critique and reformulation. *Journal of Abnormal Psychology*, 1978, 87, 49–74.

Anderson, E., Anderson, T. P., & Kottke, F. J. Stroke rehabilitation: Maintenance of achieved gains. *Archives of Physical Medicine and Rehabilitation*, 1977, *58*, 345–352.

Anderson, T. P., & Kottke, F. J. Stroke rehabilitation: A reconsideration of some common attitudes. *Archives of Physical Medicine and Rehabilitation*, 1978, *59*, 175–181.

Aroskar, M. A., & Dittmar, S. S. Impact of a stroke on the family system. *Journal of the New York State Nurses Association*, 1978, *9*, 5–8.

Auerbach, S. M., Martelli, M. F., & Mercuri, L. G. Anxiety, information, interpersonal impacts, and adjustment to a stressful health care situation, *Journal of Personality and Social Psychology*, 1983, in press.

Averill, J. R. Personal control over aversive stimuli and its relationship to stress. *Psychological Bulletin*, 1973, *80*, 286–303.

Bardach, J. L. Psychological considerations in hemiplegia. In A. B. Cobb (Ed.), *Medical and psychological aspects of disability*. Springfield, Ill.: Thomas, 1973.

Barth, J. T., & Boll, T. J. Rehabilitation and treatment of central nervous system dysfunction: A behavioral medicine perspective. In C. K. Prokop & L. A. Bradley (Eds.), *Medical psychology: Contributions to behavioral medicine*. New York: Academic Press, 1981.

Carlson, C. E. Psychosocial aspects of neurologic disability. *Nursing Clinics of North America*, 1980, *15*, 309–320.

Cassem, N. H., & Hackett, T. P. Psychiatric consultation in a coronary care unit. *Annals of Internal Medicine*, 1971, *75*, 9–14.

Charaton, F. A., & Fisk, A. Mental and emotional results of stroke. *New York State Journal of Medicine*, 1978, *78*, 1403–1405.

Cohen, S. Rehabilitation of the stroke patient. *Maryland State Medical Journal*, 1979, *28*, 82–83.

Cromwell, R. L., Butterfield, E. C., Brayfield, F. M., & Curry, J. J. *Acute myocardial infarction: Reaction and recovery*. St. Louis, Mo.: C. V. Mosby, 1977.

Croog, S. H. Recovery and rehabilitation of coronary patients: Psychosocial aspects. In D. S. Krantz, A. Baum, & J. E. Singer (Eds.), *Handbook of psychology and health* (Vol. 3): *Cardiovascular disorders and behavior*. Hillsdale, N.J.: Erlbaum, 1983.

Croog, S. H. Problems of barriers in the rehabilitation of heart patients: Social and psychological aspects. *Cardiac Rehabilitation*, 1975, *6*, 27.

Croog, S. H., & Levine, S. *The heart patient recovers*. New York: Human Sciences Press, 1977.

Croog, S. H., Levine, S., & Lurie, Z. The heart patient and the recovery process: A review of directions of research on social and psychological factors. *Social Science and Medicine*, 1968, *2*, 111–164.

Croog, S. H., Shapiro, D. S., & Levine, S. Denial among male heart patients. *Psychosomatic Medicine*, 1971, *33*, 385–397.

D'Affliti, J. G., & Weitz, G. W. Rehabilitating the stroke patient through patient–family groups. *International Journal of Group Psychotherapy*, 1974, *24*, 323–332.

Davidson, R. The psychologic aspects of stroke. *Geriatrics*, 1963, *18*, 151.

Daylong, W. B. Beyond the wall of silence. *Journal of Pastoral Care*, 1974, *28*, 122–133.

Dillard, C. O. *The family viewpoint*. Presentation to Cardiac Seminar Program, *Heart Disease, Stress and Industry*, The President's Committee on Employment of the Handicapped, New York City, March 1982.

Doehrman, S. R. Psycho-social aspects of recovery from coronary heart disease: A review. *Social Science and Medicine*, 1977, *11*, 199–218.

Engel, G. L. A life setting conducive to illness: The giving-up–given-up complex. *Annals of Internal Medicine*, 1968, *69*, 293–300.

Espmark, S. Stroke before 50: A follow-up study of vocational and psychological adjustment. *Scandinavian Journal of Rehabilitation Medicine*, Supplement 2, 1973, 5, 1–107.

Feigenson, J. S., McDowell, F. H., Meese, P., McCarthy, M. L., & Greenberg, S. D. Factors influencing outcome and length of stay in a stroke rehabilitation unit. *Stroke*, 1977, 8, 651–656.

Feldman, J. L., & Schultz, M. E. Rehabilitation after stroke. *Cardiovascular Nursing*, 1975, 11, 29–34.

Fisher, S. H. Psychiatric considerations of cerebral vascular disease. *American Journal of Cardiology*, 1961, 7, 379–385.

Folstein, M. F., Maiberger, R., & McHugh, P. R. Mood disorders as specific complications of stroke. *Journal of Neurology, Neurosurgery, and Psychiatry*, 1977, 40, 1018–1020.

Frankenhaeuser, M. Behavior and circulating catecholamines. *Brain Research*, 1971, 31, 241–262.

Froese, A., Hackett, T. P., Cassem, N. H., & Silverberg, E. L. Trajectories of anxiety and depression in denying and nondenying acute myocardial infarction patients during hospitalization. *Journal of Psychosomatic Research*, 1974, 18, 413–420.

Garrity, T. F. Social involvement and activeness as predictors of morale six months after myocardial infarction. *Social Science and Medicine*, 1973, 7, 199–207. (a)

Garrity, T. F. Vocational adjustment after first myocardial infarction: Comparative assessment of several variables suggested in the literature. *Social Science and Medicine*, 1973, 7, 705–717. (b)

Garrity, T. F. Morbidity, mortality and rehabilitation. In W. D. Gentry & R. B. Williams, Jr. (Eds.), *Psychological aspects of myocardial infarction and coronary care*. St. Louis, Mo.: C. V. Mosby, 1975.

Garrity, T. F. Behavioral adjustment after myocardial infarction: A selective review of recent descriptive, correlational, and intervention research. In S. M. Weiss, J. A. Herd, & B. H. Fox (Eds.), *Perspectives on behavioral medicine*. New York: Academic Press, 1981.

Garrity, T. F., McGill, A., Becker, M., Blanchard, E., Crews, J., Cullen, J., Hackett, T., Taylor, J., & Valins, S. Report of the task group of cardiac rehabilitation. In S. M. Weiss (Ed.), *Proceedings of the National Heart and Lung Institute Working Conference on Health Behavior* (DHEW Publication No. 76-868). Washington, D.C.: U.S. Government Printing Office, 1976.

Greene, W. A., Moss, A. J., & Goldstein, S. Delay, denial, and death in coronary heart disease. In R. S. Eliot (Ed.), *Stress and the heart*. Mount Kisco, N.Y.: Futura, 1974.

Griffith, V. E. Volunteer scheme for dysphasia and allied problems in stroke patients. *British Medical Journal*, 1975, 3, 633–635.

Gruen, W. Effects of brief psychotherapy during the hospitalization period on the recovery process in heart attacks. *Journal of Consulting and Clinical Psychology*, 1975, 43, 232–233.

Hackett, T. P., & Cassem, N. H. Psychological adaptation to convalescence in myocardial infarction patients. In J. P. Naughton, H. K. Hellerstein, & I. C. Mohler (Eds.), *Exercise testing and exercise training in coronary heart disease*. New York: Academic Press, 1973.

Hackett, T. P., & Cassem, N. H. The impact of myocardial infarction. *Rhode Island Medical Journal*, 1974, 57, 327–331.

Hellerstein, H. K., & Freidman, E. H. Sexual activity and the post-coronary patient. *Archives of Internal Medicine*, 1970, 125, 987–999.

Hungerford, J. Psychological management of the stroke patient. *Australian Occupational Therapy Journal*, 1972, 19, 7–10.

Hurst, J. W., Logue, R. B., Schlant, R. C., Wenger, N. K. *The heart* (4th ed.). New York: McGraw-Hill, 1978.

Hyman, M. D. Social psychological determinants of patients' performance in stroke rehabilitation. *Archives of Physical Medicine and Rehabilitation*, 1972, *53*, 217–226.

Johnson, J. E., & Leventhal, H. Effects of accurate expectations and behavioral instructions on reactions during a noxious medical exam. *Journal of Personality and Social Psychology*, 1974, *29*, 710–718.

Jones, R. F. Stroke rehabilitation. Part I: General considerations. *Medical Journal of Australia*, 1975, *2*, 773–775.

Kasl, S. V., & Cobb, S. Health behavior, illness behavior, and sick role behavior. *Archives of Environmental Health*, 1966, *17*, 246–266.

Klein, R. F., Kliner, V. A., Zipes, D. P., Troyer, W. G., & Wallace, A. G. Transfer from a coronary care unit. *Archives of Internal Medicine*, 1968, *122*, 104–108.

Krantz, D. S. Cognitive processes and recovery from heart attack: A review and theoretical analysis. *Journal of Human Stress*, 1980, *6*, (3), 27–38.

Krantz, D. S., Baum, A., & Wideman, M. Assessment of preferences for self-treatment and information in health care. *Journal of Personality and Social Psychology*, 1980, *39*, 977–990.

Krantz, D. S., & Schulz, R. A model of life crisis, control, and health outcomes: Cardiac rehabilitation and relocation of the elderly. In A. Baum & J. E. Singer (Eds.), *Advances in environmental psychology* (Vol. 2). Hillsdale, N.J.: Erlbaum, 1980.

Labi, M. L., Phillips, T. F., & Greshman, G. E. Psychosocial disability in physically restored long-term stroke survivors. *Archives of Physical Medicine and Rehabilitation*, 1980, *61*, 561–565.

Lawrence, L., & Christie, D. Quality of life after stroke: A three year follow-up. *Age and Aging*, 1979, *8*, 167–172.

Lazarus, R. S. *Psychological stress and the coping process*. New York: McGraw Hill, 1966.

Levine, J., & Zigler, E. Denial and self-image in stroke, lung cancer, and heart disease patients. *Journal of Consulting and Clinical Psychology*, 1975, *43*, 751–757.

Linn, L. S., & Lewis, C. E. Attitudes toward self-care among practicing physicians. *Medical Care*, 1979, *17*, 183–190.

Manuel, M. Counseling: Doing it the family way. *Nursing Mirror*, 1979, *148*, 28–29.

McPherson, B. D., Paivio, A., Yuhasz, M. S., Rechnitzer, P. A., Pickard, H. A., & Lefcoe, N. M. Psychological effects of an exercise program for post-infarct and normal adult men. *Journal of Sports Medicine and Physical Fitness*, 1967, *7*, 95–102.

Mills, R. T., & Krantz, D. S. Information, choice, and reactions to stress: A field experiment in a blood bank with laboratory analogue. *Journal of Personality and Social Psychology*, 1979, *37*, 608–620.

Moss, A. J., & Goldstein, S. The pre-hospital phase of acute myocardial infarction. *Circulation*, 1970, *41*, 737–742.

Moss, A. J., Wynar, B., & Goldstein, S. Delay in hospitalization during the acute coronary period. *American Journal of Cardiology*, 1969, *24*, 659–673.

Mossman, P. L. *A problem oriented approach to stroke rehabilitation*. Springfield, Ill.: Thomas, 1976.

Nathanson, M., Bergman, P. S., & Gordon, G. G. Denial of illness: Its occurrence in one hundred consecutive cases of hemiplegia. *Archives of Neurology and Psychiatry*, 1952, *68*, 380–387.

Naughton, J. P., Bruhn, J. G., & Lategola, M. T. Effects of physical training on physiologic and behavioral characteristics of cardiac patients. *Archives of Physical Medicine and Rehabilitation*, 1968, *49*, 131–137.

Naughton, J. P., Hellerstein, H. K., & Mohler, I. C. (Eds.). *Exercise testing and exercise training in coronary heart disease*. New York: Academic Press, 1973.

Obier, K., MacPherson, M., & Haywood, J. L. Predictive value of psychosocial profiles following acute myocardial infarction. *Journal of the National Medical Association*, 1977, *69*, 59–61.

Oradei, D. M., & Waite, N. S. Group psychotherapy with stroke patients during the immediate recovery phase. *American Journal of Orthopsychiatry*, 1974, *44*, 386–395.

Pancheri, P., Bellaterra, M., Matteoli, S., Cristofari, M., Polizzi, C., & Puletti, M. Infarct as a stress agent: Life history and personality characteristics of improved versus not-improved patients after severe heart attack. *Journal of Human Stress*, 1978, *4*, 16–26.

Piskor, B. K., & Paleos, S. The group way to banish after-stroke blues. *American Journal of Nursing*, 1968, *68*, 1500–1503.

Powell, R. B., Diller, L. D., & Grynbaum, B. Rehabilitation performance and adjustment in stroke patients: A study of social class factors. *Genetic Psychology Monographs*, 1976, *93*, 287–352.

Razin, A. M. Psychosocial intervention in coronary artery disease: A review. *Psychosomatic Medicine*, 1982, *44*, 363–388.

Ripecky, J. A., & Lazarus, L. W. Family guide to the problems of the stroke patient. *Geriatrics*, 1980, *35*, 47–48.

Rogoff, J. B., Cooney, D. V., & Kutner, B. Hemiplegia: Study of home rehabilitation. *Journal of Chronic Diseases*, 1964, *17*, 539–550.

Rosenstock, I. M. Why people use health services. *Milbank Memorial Fund Quarterly*, 1966, *44*, 94–124.

Schulman, B. Active patient orientation and outcomes in hypertensive treatment: Application of a socio-organizational perspective. *Medical Care*, 1979, *17*, 267–280.

Schulz, R. The effects of control and predictability on the psychological and physical well-being of the institutionalized aged. *Journal of Personality and Social Psychology*, 1976, *33*, 563–573.

Seligman, M. E. P. *Helplessness*. San Francisco: W. H. Freeman, 1975.

Simon, A. B., Feinleib, M., & Thompson, H. K. Components of delay in the prehospital phase of acute myocardial infarction. *American Journal of Cardiology*, 1972, *30*, 476–482.

Singler, J. R. Group work with hospitalized stroke patients. *Social Casework*, 1975, *56*, 348–354.

Smith, C. W. Releasing pressure caps: Using TA with women whose husbands have had strokes. *Transactional Analysis Journal*, 1977, *7*, 55–57.

Soloff, P. H. Effects of denial on mood, compliance, and quality of functioning after cardiovascular rehabilitation. *General Hospital Psychiatry*, 1980, *2*, 134–140.

Stonnington, H. H. Rehabilitation in cerebrovascular diseases. *Primary Care*, 1980, *7*, 87–106.

Ullman, M., Ashenhurst, E. M., Hurwitz, L. J., & Gruen, A. Motivational and structural factors in the denial of hemiplegia. *Archives of Neurology*, 1960, *3*, 306–318.

U.S. Department of Health, Education and Welfare. *Healthy people: The surgeon general's report on health promotion and disease prevention* (U.S. Public Health Service Publication No. 79-55071). Washington, D.C.: U.S. Government Printing Office, 1979.

Watzlawick, P., & Coyne, J. C. Depression following stroke: Brief, problem-focused family treatment. *Family Process*, 1980, *19*, 13–18.

Wenger, N. K. Early ambulation after myocardial infarction: Grady Memorial Hospital Emory University School of Medicine. In J. P. Naughton, H. K. Hellerstein, & I. Mohler (Eds.), *Exercise testing and exercise training in coronary heart disease*. New York: Academic Press, 1973.

Weinstein, E. A., & Friedland, R. P. Behavioral disorders associated with hemi-inattention. *Advances in Neurology*, 1977, *18*, 51–62.

Weisboth, S., Esibill, N., & Zuger, R. Factors in the vocational success of hemiplegic patients. *Archives of Physical Medicine and Rehabilitation,* 1971, *52,* 441–446.

Whithouse, F. A. Stroke: Some psychosocial problems it causes. *American Journal of Nursing,* 1963, *63,* 81–87.

Wishnie, H. A., Hackett, T. P., & Cassem, N. H. Psychological hazards of convalescence following myocardial infarction. *Journal of the American Medical Association,* 1971, *215,* 1292–1296.

5

Stroke: Coping with a Cognitive Deficit*

WAYNE A. GORDON
LEONARD DILLER

Introduction

Stroke (cerebrovascular accident or CVA) is the third biggest killer in the United States, causing 10% of all deaths. Each year almost half a million Americans, about 1 in every 500, are hospitalized as a result of stroke. The mortality rate is 30% during the first 30 days post-CVA. The 70% who survive live an average of another 7 years—approximately 10% of their lives—with some degree of physical impairment. The direct cost of these 2.5 million survivors in medical bills and lost earnings has been estimated at $4 billion dollars per year (*Executive Summary*, 1979).

The patient who has suffered a stroke lives with a myriad of complex behavioral disturbances. The most common deficit is a motor impairment. Immediately after a stroke, the victim usually is unable to move the arm and leg on the side contralateral to the brain damage. Thus the person is no longer able to walk or dress without physical assistance from another adult or the use of an assistive device such as a wheelchair or a hand splint. The motor impairment interferes with most activities of daily living (ADL).

*The authors would like to thank Mary Hibbard, Susan Egelko, Martha Scotzin, and Anne Kinney for their assistance in the preparation of this manuscript. This work was supported in part by Grant No. NS 10236-10 from the National Institutes of Health and Grants G008003038, G008003039 and G008300039 from the National Institute of Handicapped Research, U.S. Department of Education to Leonard Diller.

COPING WITH
CHRONIC DISEASE

113

Medical rehabilitation lasts an average of 45 days and costs about $6,000–$8,000 (Feigenson, 1979); however, its benefits to the patient are great, cutting the mortality rate in half and doubling the improvement in motor strength (Truscott, Kretschmann, Toole, & Pajak, 1974). Almost 80% of rehabilitation recipients are discharged to their homes. On discharge, 85% are ambulatory (28% with no aids, 57% using a device); 51% are ADL independent, and 44% require supervision but no physical assistance (Feigenson, McCarthy, Meese, Feigenson, Greenberg, Rubin, & McDowell, 1977). In addition, the gains derived from rehabilitation are maintained following discharge (Anderson, Anderson, & Kottke, 1977).

The other impairments confronting the stroke victim depend upon the side of the brain that has been damaged. Those with left brain damage (LBD) manifest their motor impairment on the right side of their body and often have residual communication disorders, such as aphasia. Aphasic patients experience difficulty understanding others or expressing themselves verbally—orally, in writing, or both. The various types of nonlinguistic cognitive impairments associated with LBD are not as well studied as are the types of aphasia. This neglect is probably due to the difficulties of evaluating a cognitive disorder when verbal information processing is disrupted.

Those stroke victims with right brain damage (RBD) manifest their motor impairment on the left side of their body and often have a residual visual information processing (VIP) disorder. About 40% of RBD patients suffer from this disorder in its most severe form. Less severe forms afflict another 30%. Thus, only about 30% of RBD patients are free of a VIP impairment. Still other deficits are associated with RBD. For example, Heilman, Schwartz, and Watson (1978) studied seven RBDs with severe VIP difficulties and reported that they also suffer from a hypoarousal syndrome. Others have indicated that the behavior of RBD patients is characterized by an indifference reaction (Gainotti, 1972). Folstein, Maiberger, and McHugh (1977) reported that RBD patients manifest levels of depression higher than those of LBD patients. At present there are no empirical data based on the evaluation of a large sample of RBD patients that examine either the incidence or the interrelationship among these four deficits (VIP, arousal, indifference, and depression).

Most of this chapter concentrates on the disorders associated with RBD. This focus is not meant to belittle the communication disorders of LBD nor to deny that they present obstacles to which individuals must adapt. The disorders associated with LBD, however, together with their diagnosis and treatment, are well described in the literature (Goodglass & Kaplan, 1972; Kertesz & McCube, 1977). However, some issues pertinent to LBD are reviewed before the detailed discussion of RBD.

Disorders Associated with Left Brain Damage

APHASIA

That aphasia occurs following damage to the left hemisphere but not damage to the right hemisphere is not only of obvious clinical significance, but also of scientific interest. The possibility is raised that the nature of a language disturbance might reflect the locus and the extent of brain damage. This possibility has given rise to attempts to (a) develop taxonomies to describe the language disorders associated with aphasia (Bay, 1964; Geschwind, 1965; Kertesz, 1979; Luria, 1966), (b) search for neuroanatomic correlates of different types of language disorders (e.g., it has been demonstrated that the patient who cannot recognize words has a lesion in the left hemisphere that is not located in the same place as in the patient who cannot read or write), and (c) devise methods for evaluating the nature and severity of the language disturbance (Goodglass & Kaplan, 1972; Kertesz, 1980; Spreen & Risser, 1981). In addition, a growing body of literature has focused on factors pertinent to recovery of function, including demographic and etiologic variables as well as the type, severity, and duration of aphasia (M. T. Sarno, 1981). Studies on prognosis and the efficacy of treatment for aphasia have resulted in a sizable body of literature and produced equivocal results (Darley, 1972; M. T. Sarno, 1980, 1981a, 1981b). From a rehabilitation perspective, a frequently neglected clinical consideration is the possible discrepancy between patterns of recovery in test performance and patterns of recovery in functional communication (M. T. Sarno & Levita, 1979). This discrepancy suggests that the clinical concerns that gave rise to the majority of scientific studies in the field might be at variance with the clinical issues that enter into day-to-day management decisions (Diller & Gordon, 1981b).

Consideration of aphasia aside, three other points of inquiry are of interest. These are emotions, intelligence, and learning.

EMOTIONS

Since the early work of Goldstein (1948), who observed the "catastrophic reactions" in left brain damaged people, the relatively high incidence of anxiety and depression associated with aphasia has been noted by many observers. More recently a growing interest in the neurology of emotional behavior has led to more careful and quantified observations of patients with LBD (Benson, 1980). Although it is reasonable to infer that emotional disturbance is a direct consequence of language disturbance, Robinson (Robinson,

1979; Robinson & Benson, 1981; Robinson, Shoemaker, Schlumpf, Valk, & Bloom, 1975), using an animal model of hemispheric damage, argues for a neurologic basis. Aside from several reports on the psychotherapeutic approaches to the management of emotional problems of aphasia, there is little work designed to deal directly with the management of emotional disturbances in LBD patients. Family counseling, either on an individual basis or structured groups for family members, has been found to be helpful (J. Sarno & M. T. Sarno, 1979). J. Sarno (1981) has reviewed the emotional aspects of aphasia and their management.

INTELLIGENCE

Because language and thinking are so intimately connected (Gardner & Winner, 1981), the relationship between language disorders and intellect has been a source of concern to students in the field. Some have argued that aphasia has a direct impact on nonverbal cognition (Weisenburg & McBride, 1935); others have argued for the possibility that cognitive disorders exist independent of language disturbance (Weinstein & Teuber, 1957). There have been many studies of the incidence and nature of disturbances in thinking and perception in LBD. In our own setting (Diller & Weinberg, 1962), individuals with LBD have been shown to have two substrata of difficulties—one in processing information via the auditory as opposed to the visual mode, and the second in retaining and processing sequential information. Thus, LBDs have difficulty in holding on to information. Intellectual operations that require short-term storage of some information while other information is being processed are particularly vulnerable to memory loss.

LEARNING

Rehabilitation involves mastering skills to compensate for deficits in functional activities caused by LBD; therefore, understanding the learning process is an important consideration. A number of studies have indicated that LBDs have difficulty in learning new tasks and cannot shift when cues are changed (Diller & Weinberg, 1962). Studies have shown that memory can be improved by the use of visual imagery mnemonic techniques (Gasparrini & Satz, 1979) and that order of information can serve as a significant cueing device in accord with the problems in processing serial information that were previously noted (Leftoff, 1981).

The problem of retraining impaired cognitive functions in LBD is attracting increasing attention from neuropsychologists (Diller & Gordon, 1981b). Students of speech therapy have tried various approaches to treat the language problems of aphasia. Hundreds of specific techniques have been reported. In general, the treatment methods can be categorized into those that are essentially direct–structured–pedagogic and those that largely entail stimulation–facilitation (M. T. Sarno, 1981a). These two approaches reflect underlying views of the nature of aphasia and of whether aphasia reflects impaired access to language or a loss of language. Pedagogic approaches are based on a theory of aphasia as a language loss. Stimulation methods generally follow an impaired access theory. Behavior modification programs have been employed in the treatment of aphasics in the form of programmed instruction (Holland & Sonderman, 1974) and in order to stimulate patients' access to a lexicon rather than in the form of a lexicon itself (Seron, Deloche, Bastard, Chassin, & Hermand, 1979).

Disorders Associated with Right Brain Damage

It is clear that many different professional groups (speech pathologists, neurologists, psychologists) have made major contributions to our understanding of aphasia caused by LBD as well as to its diagnosis and treatment. However, a different situation exists with respect to RBD research. Although the specific disorders associated with RBD are well documented, there have been few attempts to draw together what is known about the diffuse impact of RBD or to conceptualize the nature of its disturbance in order to develop a taxonomy of deficits. In the absence of such information it has been impossible either to ensure systematic diagnosis or to devise approaches to treatment of RBD-related impairments. It is scarcely surprising, then, that there exists among those who work in rehabilitation settings a pervasive despair concerning remediation of the complex behavioral disorders associated with RBD. Identification of the impairments associated with RBD does have diagnostic value, because these deficits are viewed as the hallmarks of brain damage. It is crucial, therefore, to review the current knowledge of diagnosis and treatment of the major disorders associated with RBD: VIP, arousal, indifference, and depression.

VISUAL INFORMATION PROCESSING DISORDERS

A discussion of the problems caused by RBD might best be begun with a description of the ways VIP disorders may interfere with a patient's daily functioning during medical rehabilitation. For example, a patient might arrive late for appointments for any of several reasons directly related to a

VIP disorder: (a) inability to read whole words and to see the hands of a clock on the left side of the clock face; (b) place disorientation, manifested by the patient frequently becoming lost on the ward; and (c) inability to perceive distances veridically, resulting in the patient bumping into objects, walls, or doors. The hazardous wheelchair performance of RBDs has also been observed. In addition, Diller and Weinberg (1970) have found that RBD individuals with VIP problems are "accident prone." Finally, a patient with a VIP disorder may often feel that he or she is "going crazy" either because (a) what the patient reads has no meaning, since he or she can read only the last few words on a line or the last syllable of a word; or (b) the patient feels that he or she hears voices (i.e., the patient believes he or she has auditory hallucinations, because the person with whom the patient is conversing, if standing or sitting on the patient's imparied side, can be heard but not seen). Table 5.1 presents other clinical examples of behavioral problems caused by VIP disorders. Most of these difficulties are related to the patient's inability to see his or her environment. Medically these RBD patients are diagnosed as having homonymous hemianopsia or visual–spatial neglect. The behavioral translation of these diagnostic labels is that the patient is unable to scan

TABLE 5.1

Behavioral Manifestations of VIP Disorders Observed in RBD Patients
in a Rehabilitation Setting

  I. Grooming
     A. Men unshaven
     B. Women with makeup applied on one side only
 II. Time
     A. Difficulty reading time on a clock
     B. Difficulty estimating time
III. Academic skills
     A. Difficulty reading
     B. Difficulty copying
     C. Difficulty with written arithmetic
 IV. Rehabilitation activities
     A. Increased incidence of accidents
     B. Difficulty walking and dressing
     C. Bumping into a wall while moving in a wheelchair or walking with a cane
  V. Daily activities
     A. Difficulty shopping
     B. Difficulty making change
     C. Difficulty dialing a phone
     D. Difficulty watching TV or movie
 VI. Eating
     A. Ignoring food on the left side of a tray
     B. Ignoring items on the left side of a menu

his or her environment adequately and consequently misses or misperceives information on the impaired side. Thus, for example, if asked to read the words *education* or *exit*, the patient will read *ion* or *it*. Similarly the patient will recognize only a part of a face, be it familiar or unfamiliar. This difficulty in processing information is not limited to the visual sense; it just as frequently exists in the auditory and tactile senses. Unfortunately, RBD patients are usually unaware that the above-mentioned problems are related to their VIP difficulties. People with interpersonal problems usually have a source of social validation—that is, feedback that a problem exists—but this source of feedback is often lacking with VIP disorders. Patients have no way of knowing that what they are seeing is not veridical. Thus, the probability of denial is increased.

What can be done to help RBD patients with VIP disorders? Investigators in our laboratory have developed and evaluated a series of programs designed to ameliorate VIP problems associated with RBD. Although it is beyond the scope of this chapter to review this research in great detail, several comments about the training programs are of value here.[1]

The first and perhaps overriding goal of treatment is to make patients with VIP deficits aware of their errors without arousing a sense of failure and consequent abandonment of the task. It is important, therefore, to develop several simple demonstrations in which failure to scan the environment is made obvious to patients, that is, they are made aware of what is missed by failure to scan. Patients can be taught an external stimulus that is compelling or attractive enough to force turning the head toward the impaired side. For example, an array of money is placed on the table in front of a patient. The large bills are purposely put on the impaired side. The patient is asked to pick up all of the money on the table. Naturally, a large sum of money remains on the table after the patient says that he or she has completed the task. Having the patient turn his or her head to see all the money that was left on the table is one way to begin to teach the patient that a VIP problem exists and that this difficulty can be overcome by turning the head. In order to teach this skill in a more systematic fashion, a device called a scanning machine was developed (Weinberg, Diller, Gordon, Gerstman, Lieberman, Lakin, Hodges & Ezrachi, 1977). The scanning machine requires patients to point to a target as it moves on a track around the perimeter of a board (similar to taking aim at a moving target in a shooting gallery). In general, patients can track the stimulus when it is on the right side of their field of vision but they quickly lose it when it moves to the left side. Treatment

---

[1]The reader is referred to the following articles for a complete review of this work: Barth & Boll, 1981; Diller, 1976; Diller & Gordon, 1981a, 1981b; Diller & Weinberg, 1977; Weinberg, Diller, Gordon, Gerstman, Lieberman, Lakin, Hodges, & Ezrachi, 1977, 1979.

consists of teaching patients to turn their heads to the left so that the stimulus can be seen in the right visual field. Once patients grasp this method of tracking, they tend to turn their heads with decreasing resistance even when the speed stimulus increases. After some practice, it has been observed that patients make head movements that are less gross and overt and track stimuli smoothly. Once patients have been taught to track, they can be easily taught to transfer this skill from the scanning machine to paper and pencil tasks. Cancellation tasks have been developed for this purpose. Patients are presented sheets of paper with several lines of letters, numbers, or figures. The patients are asked to cancel (draw a line through) all of the target stimuli (e.g., each h, 8, or star that they see). Patients are told not to begin cancelling until they see a prominent visual marker or anchor at the far left side of the page. This marker is used to anchor the patient's performance, as it provides the patient with a place to begin scanning. As patients become more proficient at cancellation tasks, the anchor is gradually faded. Anchoring of this sort improves the performance of even the most severely impaired patients (Diller, Ben-Yishay, Gerstman, Goodkin, Gordon, & Weinberg, 1974). Patients also are encouraged to slow down their performance by oral recitation of the stimuli; this exercise is known as pacing. A final method of improving performance involves reducing the number of stimuli on the page so that there is more space between the stimuli that are to be cancelled. The task is made easier or harder by making the stimuli less or more dense.

There is little doubt that the retraining programs developed and tested so far have improved the performance of individuals with VIP disorders. Figures 5.1–5.3 give examples of pre- and posttest patient performances on cancellation, arithmetic, and copying tasks. In addition to this important practical outcome, several other findings of theoretical importance have emerged from studies of the effects of retraining that have been conducted in our laboratory (see Diller, 1976; Diller & Gordon, 1981a, 1981b; Diller & Weinberg, 1977; Weinberg et al., 1977, 1979). These findings are

1. A deficit in visual scanning is the basis of the visual information processing (VIP) disorders of RBD patients. VIP impairments are observed not only on neuropsychological test performances but also in day-to-day ("real life") behavior as well (e.g., reading, writing, copying, etc.).

2. The scanning deficit is not simply either present or absent; its severity varies widely among patients. A reliable classification of the severity of VIP impairments may be derived from measuring patient performance on visual cancellation tasks. Individuals with all degrees of impairment benefit from treatment, although those most severely impaired improve the most. This seeming differential impact of training on mildly and severely impaired patients may actually be artificial as it could be a function of a low ceiling on

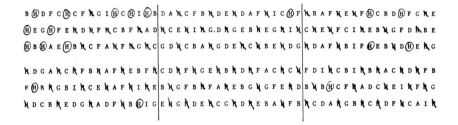

(a)

(b)

FIGURE 5.1   (a) At the time of pretesting, the patient makes 18 errors of omission; 12 of these errors are on the left side of the page. (b) Approximately 5 weeks later, after receiving about 20 hours of training, the patient successfully cancels all targets. Note that competence is achieved without sacrificing time.

some tasks. Mildly impaired patients by definition cannot improve as much as severely impaired patients. The tests are, in effect, too easy for the mildly impaired (Weinberg *et al.*, 1977, 1979).

3. Certain principles form the basis of the training programs that we have developed. These principles include: anchoring (acknowledgment of left-side stimuli before commencing a task); density (wider spacing of stimuli to reduce errors); pacing (slowing of the response to prevent impulsive behavior); feedback (provision of information about the correctness of the response); information load (instructions to cancel two stimuli or to make

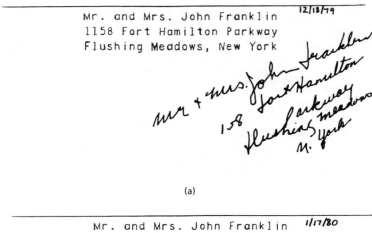

Mr. and Mrs. John Franklin   12/18/79
1158 Fort Hamilton Parkway
Flushing Meadows, New York

(a)

Mr. and Mrs. John Franklin   1/17/80
1158 Fort Hamilton Parkway
Flushing Meadows, New York

(b)

FIGURE 5.2   (a) At pretraining the patient miscopies the address (leaves out the first *1* on the left and the period after *Mr.*). Note also the shift to the right side of the page and the collision of words. (b) Posttraining, 4 weeks later, the patient still displays mild spatial organization problems but accurately copies the text and no longer shifts to the right side of the page.

cancellation contingent on other stimuli, complications that increase error). These principles have been incorporated into all VIP training programs that have been developed in our laboratory. These principles and the training programs themselves are described in greater detail elsewhere (Diller, 1976; Diller *et al.*, 1974; Diller & Gordon, 1981a, 1981b; Weinberg *et al.*, 1977, 1979).

4. Competence in the processing of visual information is layered. Individuals must acquire the skills needed for gross scanning of the environment before learning to locate words at the beginning of a line. Thus, patients are provided with exercises on the scanning machine before being given printed material. The mastery of scanning printed material, in turn, must precede learning to appreciate location in space (another manifestation of the VIP deficit is RBD patients' difficulty in estimating distances in external space).

$$\begin{array}{r} 5 \\ +1 \\ \hline 6 \end{array}$$

$$\left(\begin{array}{r} 5 \\ -4 \\ \hline 9 \end{array}\right)$$

$$\begin{array}{r} 75 \\ +8 \\ \hline 83 \end{array}$$

$$\left(\begin{array}{r} 84 \\ -36 \\ \hline 120 \end{array}\right)$$

$$\begin{array}{r} 452 \\ 137 \\ +245 \\ \hline 834 \end{array}$$

$$\begin{array}{r} 48 \\ 2853 \\ 724 \\ 82 \\ +6215 \\ \hline 9922 \end{array}$$

$$\begin{array}{r} 420 \\ \times 4 \\ \hline 1680 \end{array}$$

$$\begin{array}{r} 420.3 \\ \times 29 \\ \hline 3782.7 \\ 8406 \\ \hline 12188.7 \end{array}$$

(a)

$$\begin{array}{r} 5 \\ +1 \\ \hline 6 \end{array}$$

$$\begin{array}{r} 5 \\ -4 \\ \hline 1 \end{array}$$

$$\begin{array}{r} 75 \\ +8 \\ \hline 83 \end{array}$$

$$\begin{array}{r} 84 \\ -36 \\ \hline 48 \end{array}$$

$$\begin{array}{r} 452 \\ 137 \\ +245 \\ \hline 834 \end{array}$$

$$\begin{array}{r} 48 \\ 2853 \\ 724 \\ 82 \\ +6215 \\ \hline 9922 \end{array}$$

$$\begin{array}{r} 420 \\ \times 4 \\ \hline 1680 \end{array}$$

$$\begin{array}{r} 420.3 \\ \times 29 \\ \hline 3782 7 \\ 8406 \\ \hline 12188.7 \end{array}$$

(b)

FIGURE 5.3 (a) At pretesting two simple arithmetic errors were made. These mistakes were the result of neglecting to see the plus or minus sign on the left side of the example. (b) At posttesting, approximately 4 weeks later, no errors are made.

This secondary difficulty cannot be treated until the patient has been taught to compensate for his or her primary scanning problem. The hierarchical arrangement (in this case, relearning) of skills was empirically demonstrated in one of our studies (Weinberg *et al.*, 1979), which showed that training RBD patients to orient themselves in external space when combined with training in academic skills was more effective than training in academic skills alone. The neuropsychological test performances of RBD patients receiving the combined treatment program exceeded those of patients receiving a single treatment (Weinberg *et al.*, 1979).

5. Analysis of data derived from computerized axial tomography (CAT) scans shows clearly that gains made by RBD patients receiving VIP training programs were not only independent of the degree of the initial VIP impairment but of the locus and extent of brain damage as well. Furthermore, these gains were maintained for at least 4 months following termination of treatment. In contrast, during this same period, not only did the performance of the RBDs in the control group remain stable but the VIP impairments of some became worse.

6. RBD patients have elevated negative affect scores as measured by the Multiple Affect Adjective Checklist (Zuckerman & Lubin, 1965) that are not related to the locus and extent of the brain damage and are not affected by perceptual intervention.

INDIFFERENCE AND AROUSAL DIFFICULTIES

Indifference or Aprosodia

Since the 1950s there has been increasing interest in the proposition that the cerebral hemispheres are asymmetric with regard to emotion and arousal as well as cognition. It has been alleged that RBD patients are characterized by indifference and denial of affect whereas LBD patients regard their strokes as catastrophic and suffer from anxiety (Gainotti, 1972). Cicone, Wapner, and Gardner (1980) defined the indifference reaction as "a set of behaviors, including an indifference to or denial of physical problems, a forced joviality coupled with a tendency to indulge in 'gallows' and sexual humor, and a general tendency toward social and emotional inappropriateness [p. 145]." The indifference of RBD patients was noted first by Babinski (1914) and then was reaffirmed in clinical studies by Denny-Brown, Meyer, and Horenstein (1952), Gainotti (1972), and Hécaen (1962).

Two reviews (Sackeim, Greenberg, Weiman, Gur, Hungerbuhler, & Geschwind, 1982; Tucker, 1981) have provided evidence to support earlier findings of hemispheric asymmetries in affective responsiveness. Tucker (1981) has stated that an intact right hemisphere is *required* for the interpretation of emotional stimuli. Ross (Ross, 1981, 1982; Ross & Mesulam, 1979; Ross & Rush, 1981) has clinical data suggesting that RBD patients are not indifferent, but have difficulty in both expressing and comprehending affect. Ross has called this disorder *aprosodia*. Researchers, unaware of the aprosodic disorder, have often observed this difficulty as indifference.

Other investigators have supplied additional evidence supporting Ross's interpretation of this behavioral disturbance. For example, Wechsler (1973) found that RBD patients had poor memory for stories with emotional content. In addition, two studies by Heilman and his co-workers (Heilman, Scholes, & Watson, 1975; Tucker, Watson & Heilman, 1977) showed that RBD patients with VIP disorders had difficulty comprehending the affective components of speech. Patients with RBD did poorly on tasks that required them to name emotions and to discriminate affective tones. Thus, the affective comprehension deficit disrupts the patient's ability to understand the manner in which affect is expressed (Heilman, Schwartz, & Watson, 1978). The affective expression deficit associated with aprosodia causes the patient "difficulty in expressing emotion through normal tone of voice inflections in everyday interactions [Ross & Mesulam, 1979, p. 147]." It should be noted that Gardner, Ling, Flamm, and Silverman (1975) found that, on a task involving the comprehension of humor, the use of captions aided RBD patients to understand cartoons. The verbal cue provided by the caption was needed to facilitate the processing of the affect. They noted further that RBD patients either laughed at every item or emitted little response even when laughter was appropriate. Faglioni, Spinnler, and Vignolo (1969) found that RBD patients out-performed LBD patients in auditory discrimination of meaningful sounds. This finding, another example of meaningful content facilitating the performance of RBD patients, supported that of Gardner *et al.* (1975).

Another study of the emotional reactions of RBD patients was reported by Cicone *et al.* (1980). They found that RBD patients had difficulty recognizing faces, discriminating facial expressions, and choosing the appropriate emotion needed to describe a scene presented either visually or orally. The difficulty in choosing the correct emotion was due only in part to a VIP disorder; the VIP part of the deficit was caused by an inability to recognize pictures of faces, a visual task. The difficulty also was related to a misinterpretation of the meanings of situations. These findings tend to support Werner's (1957) belief that affective processes are inseparable from cognitive processes. Discovery of the inability of RBD patients to make appropriate inferences about the meanings of situations sheds new light on the extent of their information processing deficits (Birch, Belmont, & Karp, 1964, 1965, 1967).

Arousal Disorders

There is reason to believe that in addition to their VIP disorders and affective expression and comprehension difficulties, some RBD patients are also plagued by an arousal disorder. The evidence for this deficit is derived from several sources. For example, slow visual reaction times have been noted by De Renzi and Faglioni (1965). Heilman *et al.* (1978) noted that their sample of RBD patients, in addition to appearing hypokinetic, also had reduced galvanic skin responses (GSR). This observation of hypokinesis is in accord with the finding of Ben-Yishay, Diller, Mandelberg, Gordon, and Gerstman (1971) that RBD patients make fewer maneuvers on the WAIS Block Design Subtest than either LBD patients or normal controls.

A small number of RBD patients studied by Heilman and his colleagues (Heilman, 1979; Heilman *et al.*, 1978; Valenstein & Heilman, 1979) manifested an information processing deficit characterized as an arousal–attentional disorder. The primary evidence for this disorder stems from the observation of flattened affect, VIP deficits, hypokinesis, and hypo-arousal coexisting in these patients (Heilman *et al.*, 1978). The existence of this syndrome, however, is contradicted by (*a*) Gainotti's (1972) finding that although emotional "indifference" is strongly associated with VIP deficits, it does not necessarily stem from visual–perceptual problems and (*b*) Cicone *et al.*'s (1980) report that only a part of the difficulty experienced by their RBD patients in choosing appropriate emotions to describe a scene was attributable to a VIP disorder. Our experience suggests that although those RBD patients with VIP disorders also have affective comprehension–expression disorders, the two deficits are orthogonal to each other. Thus, those with severe VIP deficits will have an affective comprehension–expression deficit *but* the affective disorder may or may not be severe. Only about 25% of the RBD patients seen in our laboratory without a VIP problem have difficulty in affective comprehension or expression. As Valenstein and Heilman (1979) noted, emotions are associated with both arousal and cognition. Affective memory can be impaired by either arousal or cognitive (abstraction) problems, and therefore emotional disorders are possible even in the absence of arousal or perceptual difficulties. It is possible to speculate that several specific deficits exist in RBD patients (e.g., arousal, inability to label affect, etc.). Whether they have one deficit or many, however, it is easy to understand that RBDs are poorly equipped to handle the complex demands of social discourse.

DEPRESSION

The relationship between depression and the location of brain damage is a controversial issue. That is, is depression associated with RBD or LBD? Are LBDs more depressed than RBDs? Additionally, it is not known whether the depression of RBD patients is part of the already described affective communication disorder, aprosodia, or a separate deficit related to an individual's reaction to the stroke. For example, frequent unprovoked crying is often observed among patients with RBD. Yet these patients frequently answer "I don't know" when asked the reason for their crying. Unaware that such crying is a consequence of their stroke that will dissipate with time, patients automatically associate crying with sadness (i.e., depression).

There are conflicting reports regarding the relationship between RBD and depression. Gainotti (1972) observed that the incidence of depression was equivalent in RBD and LBD patients. This parity was also reported by Dikmen and Reitan (1974, 1977), who measured depression using the MMPI. In contrast, both Black (1975) and Gasparrini, Satz, Heilman, and Coolidge (1978), also using the MMPI, found elevated levels of depression in their samples of LBD patients but not in their samples of RBD patients. Studies of psychiatric patients diagnosed as depressed have shown evidence of right hemisphere dysfunction in these patients (Goldstein, Filskov, Weaver, & Ives, 1977) and recovery of right hemisphere functioning with elevation in mood level following electroconvulsive therapy (Kronfol, Hamsher, Digre, & Waziri, 1978).

Thus, the evidence as to whether depression is primarily associated with RBD or LBD is not clear. Despite these conflicting data, our research group has found that levels of depression, measured by the Multiple Affect Adjective Checklist, MAACL, (Zuckerman & Lubin, 1965) exhibited by our RBD patients 4 months following their hospital discharge are significantly higher than those of a matched group of nondisabled adults as well as those of individuals with breast, lung, or skin cancer or spinal cord injury (Table 5.2). The levels of MAACL depression in the RBD patients were 1.5 to 2 times

TABLE 5.2
MAACL Depression Scores of Four Groups of Individuals

Group	N	Mean
I. Nondisabled adults (age 60–80)		
A. Males	24	10.1
B. Females	58	12.0
II. Cancer patients (6 mo postsurgery)		
A. Breast cancer	36	13.4
B. Melanoma	56	12.0
C. Lung cancer	21	14.5
III. Spinal cord injured patients		
A. 1 yr postinjury	66	14.6
B. 2 yr postinjury	29	11.8
IV. RBD patients		
A. 4 mo postdischarge	30	19.8

greater than those of the other groups. Additionally, the presence of depression was found to be independent of the presence of a VIP disorder. In order to validate the elevated depression scores against behavioral manifestations of depression, the typical daily activities of 29 RBD patients (4 months postdischarge) were compared to those of a matched (age, sex, marital status, vocational status) sample of 85 nondisabled adults. The measures of activity were the Activity Pattern Indicators (APIs), developed by the Rehabilitation Indicators Project (Brown, Diller, Fordyce, Jacobs, & Gordon, 1980). The APIs time usage measures describe activity participation during 2 typical days (Brown, 1982; Szalai, 1972). Figures 5.4–5.6 show that the activity patterns of RBD (i.e., left hemiplegic) patients were significantly different ($p < .01$) from those of the nondisabled. Relative to the normal controls, the RBDs did fewer different things (diversity), slept 10% more (inactivity), spent 8% less time participating in household tasks, and spent half as much time in social activities or in activities that involved social participation. As would be expected, RBD patients spent more time at home (93% vs. 75%) and five times less time traveling than did those in the nondisabled sample. Conversely, there is more than a three-fold difference (7% versus 25%) in activities performed away from home. These differences in time usage are independent of age. The patterns of inactivity (e.g., sleep, resting, social isolation), are associated with depression; they have been noted by others (Feibel & Springer, 1982); Gresham, Fitzpatrick, Wolf, McNamara, Kannel, & Dawber, 1975; Gresham, Phillips, Wolf, McNamara, Kannel, & Dawber, 1979; Labi, Phillips, & Gresham, 1980). Gresham and his colleagues view the residual disability among stroke survivors as a social one that has been

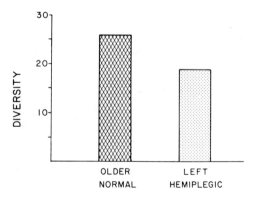

FIGURE 5.4   Diversity of activity in a matched group of older normal ($N = 85$) and left hemiplegic ($N = 29$) individuals.

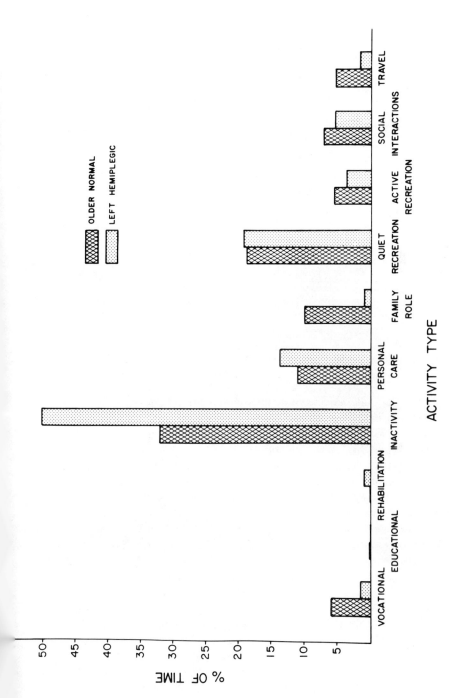

FIGURE 5.5 Percentage of time spent, by activity type, in a matched group of older normal ($N = 85$) and left hemiplegic ($N = 29$) individuals.

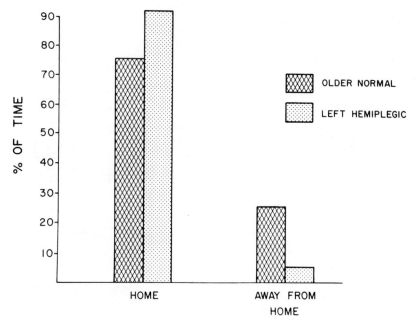

FIGURE 5.6   Percentage of time spent, by location of activity, in a matched group of older normal (N = 85) and left hemiplegic (N = 29) individuals.

found to be independent of degree of motor impairment and the number of associated medical problems.

Beck (1963) and Kovacs (1980) have noted that depression results in part from a misapplication of the abstraction process. That is, events are seen as either black or white; conclusions are either too narrow or too broad. It is indeed surprising that many RBD patients fit Beck's clinical description of depressed people. However, for RBD patients, depression may result from a cognitive disorder associated with brain damage as opposed to the inappropriate perception of day-to-day events. The extent to which the depression found in RBD patients is related to the other deficits (i.e., VIP, arousal, and affect communication) is not known. Indeed, the affect communication disorder may mask an RBD patient's depression, as the examiner may have difficulty interpreting the patient's behavior as that of depression because the patient is perceived as indifferent or because there is an absence of affect in the patient's verbal statements (Ross & Rush, 1981). Ross and Rush have suggested that clinicians heed the RBD patient's words and ignore the manner in which the affect is communicated.

When we try to design treatment that will remediate these elevated levels of depression, several thoughts come to mind. Wright (1960), discussing the

impact of physical disability, developed ideas that are also useful in understanding the depression of RBD patients. One way of confronting such depression is to contain the loss. For example, a motor impairment that limits
the patient's ability to walk may lead the RBD patient to feel that he or she is
no longer a person. Clinical experience suggests that talk alone cannot
achieve catharsis and thereby alleviate the depression. However, acknowl-
edging the loss, identifying the actual role and function lost, and focusing on
remaining skills and assets can generate awareness on the part of the patient
of being larger than the loss. The patient says, in effect, "If I can't walk, I'm
nobody." The psychologist responds, "Aren't you more than someone who
walks?" (Diller & Gordon, 1981b). The goal of this approach then, is to help
the patient to realize that impairment does not destroy assets that allow him
or her to live life to its fullest. These tactics may be viewed as applications of
cognitive therapy to alter disturbed or overmagnified cognitions toward impairment. Indeed, Kovacs and Beck (1978) include self-denigration as part of
the depressive thought disorder. If the problems of RBD patients are in part
cognitive, the approaches to treatment offered by Beck and his colleagues
(Beck, Rush, Shaw, & Emery, 1979) may prove effective.

Labi *et al.* (1980) offer another view; they have argued that feelings of
stigma experienced by stroke victims may be one cause of their avoidance of
social interaction with their former peers. This speculation is supported by
the work of Hyman (1971, 1972), who found that feelings of stigma among
stroke patients were negatively associated with motivation, functional improvement in medical rehabilitation, and the resumption of social roles
(household and leisure activities) upon their return home. This phenomenon
also has been observed in paraplegics (Cogswell, 1968). Thus, it appears that
patients who feel stigmatized devalue their social status.

Conclusion

The deficits that confront the stroke victim are complex and pervasive,
affecting almost all areas of life. The breadth of the associated disturbances
makes the period of adjustment both long and difficult. Helping patients to
cope successfully with the effect of a stroke requires recognition not only of
the patients' obvious physical limitations but also of their cognitive and
affective disorders, which are not as obvious or as readily understood. Research has documented that the stroke victims are helped by medical rehabilitation. Work reviewed in this chapter has shown that the VIP disturbances of RBD are amenable to treatment. We must now turn our attention
to developing effective treatments for the affective disorders associated with
RBD that have heretofore not only resisted diagnosis but also remediation.

References

Anderson, E., Anderson, T. P., & Kottke, F. J. Stroke rehabilitation: Maintenance of achieved gains. *Archives of Physical Medicine and Rehabilitation*, 1977, *58*, 345–352.

Babinski, J. Contribution a l'etude des troubles mentaux dans l'hemiplegie organique cerebrale (anosognosie). *Review Neurologic* (Paris), 1914, *27*, 845–848.

Barth, J. T., & Boll, T. J. Rehabilitation and treatment of central nervous system dysfunction: A behavioral medicine perspective. In C. K. Prokop & L. A. Bradley (Eds.), *Medical psychology: Contributions to behavioral medicine.* New York: Academic Press, 1981.

Bay, E. Principles of classification and their influence on our concepts of aphasia. In A. V. S. deReuck & M. O'Connor (Eds.), *Disorders of language.* London: Churchill, 1964.

Beck, A. T. Thinking and depression: I. Idiosyncratic content and cognitive disorders. *Archives of General Psychiatry*, 1963, *9*, 324–333.

Beck, A. T., Rush, A. J., Shaw, B. F., & Emery, G. *Cognitive therapy of depression.* New York: Guilford Press, 1979.

Benson, D. F. Psychiatric problems in aphasia. In M. T. Sarno & O. Hook (Eds.), *Aphasia assessment and treatment.* New York: Masson, 1980.

Ben-Yishay, Y., Diller, L., Mandelberg, I., Gordon, W., & Gerstman, L. J. Similarities and differences in block design performance between older normal and brain injured persons: A task analysis. *Journal of Abnormal Psychology*, 1971, *78*, 17–25.

Birch, H. G., Belmont, I., & Karp, E. The relation of single stimulus threshold to extinction to double simultaneous stimulation. *Cortex*, 1964, *1*, 19–39.

Birch, H. G., Belmont, I., & Karp, E. The prolongation of inhibition in brain-damaged patients. *Cortex*, 1965, *1*, 397–409.

Birch, H. G., Belmont, I., & Karp, E. Delayed information processing and extinction following cerebral damage. *Brain*, 1967, *93*, 113–130.

Black, F. W. Unilateral brain lesions and MMPI performance: A preliminary study. *Perceptual and Motor Skills*, 1975, *40*, 87–93.

Brown, M. *Actual and perceived differences in activity patterns of able-bodied and disabled men.* Unpublished doctoral dissertation, New York University, 1982.

Brown, M., Diller, L., Fordyce, W., Jacobs, D., & Gordon, W. Rehabilitation indicators: Their nature and uses for assessment. In B. Botton & D. W. Cook (Eds.), *Rehabilitation client assessment.* Baltimore: University Park Press, 1980.

Cicone, M., Wapner, W., & Gardner, H. Sensitivity to emotional expressions and situations in organic patients. *Cortex*, 1980, *16*, 145–158.

Cogswell, B. E. Self-socialization: Readjustment of paraplegics in the community. *Journal of Rehabilitation*, 1968, *34*, 11–13.

Darley, F. The efficacy of language rehabilitation in aphasia. *Journal of Speech and Hearing Disorders*, 1972, *3*, 37.

Denny-Brown, D., Meyer, J. S., & Horenstein, S. The significance of perceptual rivalry resulting from parietal lesions. *Brain*, 1952, *75*, 433–471.

De Renzi, E., & Faglioni, P. The comparative efficiency of intelligence and vigilance tests in detecting hemispheric cerebral damage. *Cortex*, 1965, *1*, 410–433.

Dikmen, S., & Reitan, R. M. MMPI correlates of localized cerebral lesions. *Perceptual and Motor Skills*, 1974, *39*, 831–840.

Dikmen, S., & Reitan, R. M. MMPI correlates of adaptive ability deficits in patients with brain lesion. *Journal of Nervous and Mental Disease*, 1977, *165*, 247–254.

Diller, L. A model of cognitive retraining in rehabilitation. *Journal of Clinical Psychology*, 1976, *29*, 74–79.

Diller, L., Ben-Yishay, Y., Gerstman, L., Goodkin, R., Gordon, W., & Weinberg, J. Studies in cognition and rehabilitation in hemiplegia. Institute of Rehabilitation Medicine, New York-University Medical Center, 50, 1974. (Monograph)

Diller, L., & Gordon, W. A. Interventions for cognitive deficits in brain injured adults. *Journal of Consulting and Clinical Psychology*, 1981, 49, 822–834. (a)

Diller, L., & Gordon, W. A. Rehabilitation and clinical neuropsychology. In S. B. Filskov & T. J. Boll (Eds.), *Handbook of clinical neuropsychology*. New York: Wiley, 1981. (b)

Diller, L., & Weinberg, J. *Learning in hemiplegia*. Paper presented at the meeting of the American Psychological Association, St. Louis, September 1962.

Diller, L., & Weinberg, J. Evidence for accident-prone behavior in hemiplegic patients. *Archives of Physical Medicine and Rehabilitation*, 1970, 51, 358–362.

Diller, L., & Weinberg, J. Hemi-inattention in rehabilitation: The evolution of a rational treatment program. In E. A. Weinstein & R. P. Freidland (Eds.), *Advances in Neurology* (Vol. 18). New York: Raven Press, 1977.

Executive Summary of the National Research Strategy for Neurological and Communication Disorders (DHEW Publication No. 791911). Washington, D.C.: National Institutes of Health, 1979.

Faglioni, P., Spinnler, H., & Vignolo, L. A. Contrasting behavior of right and left hemisphere damaged patients on a discriminative and a semantic task of auditory recognition. *Cortex*, 1969, 5, 366–389.

Feibel, J. H., & Springer, C. J. Depression and failure to resume social activities. *Archives of Physical Medicine and Rehabilitation*, 1982, 63, 276–278.

Feigenson, J. S. Stroke rehabilitation: Effectiveness, benefits, and cost. Some practical considerations. *Stroke*, 1979, 10, 1–4.

Feigenson, J., McCarthy, M., Meese, P., Feigenson, W., Greenberg, S., Rubin, E., & McDowell, F. Stroke rehabilitation I: Factors predicting outcome and length of stay—an overview. *New York State Journal of Medicine*, 1977, 77, 1426–1430.

Folstein, M. F., Maiberger, R., & McHugh, P. R. Mood disorder as a specific complication of stroke. *Journal of Neurology, Neurosurgery and Psychiatry*, 1977, 40, 1018–1020.

Gainotti, G. Emotional behavior and hemispheric side of the lesion. *Cortex*, 1972, 8, 41–55.

Gardner, H., Ling, P. K., Flamm, L., & Silverman, J. Comprehension and appreciation of humorous material following brain damage. *Brain*, 1975, 98, 399–412.

Gardner, H., & Winner, E. Artistry and aphasia. In M. T. Sarno (Ed.), *Acquired aphasia*. New York: Academic Press, 1981.

Gasparrini, B., & Satz, P. A treatment for memory problems in left hemisphere CVA patients. *Journal of Clinical Neuropsychology*, 1979, 2, 137–151.

Gasparrini, W. G., Satz, P., Heilman, K. M., & Coolidge, F. L. Hemispheric asymmetries of affective processing as determined by the MMPI. *Journal of Neurology, Neurosurgery and Psychiatry*, 1978, 41, 470–473.

Geschwind, N. Disconnection syndromes in animals and man. *Brain*, 1965, 88, 237–294; 586–644.

Goldstein, K. *Language and language disturbances*. New York: Grune & Stratton, 1948.

Goldstein, S. G., Filskov, S. B., Weaver, L. A., & Ives, J. Neuropsychological effects of electroconvulsive therapy. *Journal of Clinical Psychology*, 1977, 33, 798–806.

Goodglass, H., & Kaplan, E. *The assessment of aphasia and related disorders*. Philadelphia: Lea & Febiger, 1972.

Gresham, G. E., Fitzpatrick, T. E., Wolf, P. A., McNamara, P. M., Kannel, W. B., & Dawber, T. R. Residual disability in survivors of stroke: The Framingham study. *The New England Journal of Medicine*, 1975, 293, 954–956.

Gresham, G. E., Phillips, T. F., Wolf, P. A., McNamara, P. M., Kannel, W. B. & Dawber, T.

R. Epidemiologic profile of long-term stroke disability: The Framingham study. *Archives of Physical Medicine and Rehabilitation*, 1979, *60*, 487–491.

Hécaen, H. Clinical symptomatology in right and left hemisphere lesions. In V. B. Mountcastle (Ed.), *Interhemispheric relations and cerebral dominance*. Baltimore: Johns Hopkins University Press, 1962.

Heilman, K. M. Neglect and related disorders. In K. M. Heilman & E. Valenstein (Eds.), *Clinical neuropsychology*. New York: Oxford University Press, 1979.

Heilman, K. M., Scholes, R., & Watson, R. T. Auditory affective agnosia. *Journal of Neurology, Neurosurgery and Psychiatry*, 1975, *38*, 69–72.

Heilman, K. M., Schwartz, H. D., & Watson, R. T. Hypoarousal in patients with the neglect syndrome and emotional indifference. *Neurology*, 1978, *28*, 229–232.

Holland, A., & Sonderman, J. Effects of a program based on the token test for teaching comprehension skills to aphasics. *Journal of Speech and Hearing Research*, 1974, *17*, 589–598.

Hyman, M. D. The stigma of stroke. *Geriatrics*, 1971, *26*, 132–141.

Hyman, M. D. Social psychological determinants of patients' performance in stroke rehabilitation. *Archives of Physical Medicine and Rehabilitation*, 1972, *53*, 217–226.

Kertesz, A. *Aphasia and associated disorders*. New York: Grune & Stratton, 1979.

Kertesz, A. *Western Aphasia Battery*. London, Ontario: University of Western Ontario, 1980.

Kertesz, A., & McCube, P. Recovery patterns and prognosis in aphasia. *Brain*, 1977, *100*, 1–18.

Kovacs, M. Cognitive therapy in depression. *Journal of the American Academy of Psychoanalysis*, 1980, *8*, 127–144.

Kovacs, M., & Beck, A. T. Maladaptive cognitive structures in depression. *American Journal of Psychiatry*, 1978, *135*, 525–533.

Kronfol, Z., Hamsher, K. de S., Digre, K., & Waziri, R. Depression and hemispheric functions: Changes associated with unilateral ECT. *British Journal of Psychiatry*, 1978, *132*, 560–567.

Labi, M. L. C., Phillips, T. F., & Gresham, G. E. Psychosocial disability in physically restored long-term stroke survivors. *Archives of Physical Medicine and Rehabilitation*, 1980, *61*, 561–565.

Leftoff, S. Learning functions for unilaterally brain damaged patients for serially and randomly ordered stimulus material: Analysis of retrieval strategies and their relationship to rehabilitation. *Journal of Clinical Neuropsychology*, 1981, *4*, 301–315.

Luria, A. R. *Higher cortical functions in man*. New York: Basic Books, 1966.

Robinson, R. G. Differential behavior and biochemical effects of right and left hemispheric cerebral infarction in the rat. *Science*, 1979, *205*, 707–710.

Robinson, R. G., & Benson, D. F. Depression in aphasic patients: Frequency, severity, and clinical-pathological correlations. *Brain and Language*, 1981, *14*, 282–291.

Robinson, R. G., Shoemaker, W. J., Schlumpf, M., Valk, T., & Bloom, F. Effect of experimental cerebral infarction in rat brain on catecholamines and behavior. *Nature*, 1975, *255*, 332–334.

Ross, E. D. The aprosodias. *Archives of Neurology*, 1981, *38*, 561–569.

Ross, E. D. The divided self. *The Sciences*, 1982, *22*, 8–12.

Ross, E. D., & Mesulam, M. M. Dominant language functions of the right hemisphere? Prosody and emotional gesturing. *Archives of Neurology*, 1979, *36*, 144–148.

Ross, E. D., & Rush, J. Diagnosis and neuroanatomical correlates of depression in brain-damaged patients. *Archives of General Psychiatry*, 1981, *38*, 1344–1354.

Sackeim H. A., Greenberg, A. A., Weiman, A. L., Gur, R. C., Hungerbuhler, J. P., & Geschwind, N. Hemispheric asymmetry in the expression of positive and negative emotions: Neurological evidence. *Archives of Neurology*, 1982, *39*, 210–218.

Sarno, J. Emotional aspects of aphasia. In M. T. Sarno (Ed.), *Acquired Aphasia*. New York: Academic Press, 1981.

Sarno, J., & Sarno, M. T. *Stroke: A guide for patients and their families* (Rev. ed.). New York: McGraw-Hill, 1979.

Sarno, M. T. Review of research in aphasia: Recovery and rehabilitation. In M. T. Sarno & O. Hook (Eds.), *Aphasia: Assessment and treatment*. New York: Masson, 1980.

Sarno, M. T. Recovery and rehabilitation in aphasia. In M. T. Sarno (Ed.), *Acquired aphasia*. New York: Academic Press, 1981. (a)

Sarno, M. T. (Ed.). *Acquired aphasia*. New York: Academic Press, 1981. (b)

Sarno, M. T., & Levita, E. Recovery from treated aphasia during the first year post-stroke. *Stroke*, 1979, *10*, 663–670.

Seron, X., Deloche, G., Bastard, V., Chassin, G., & Hermand, N. Word finding difficulties and learning transfer in aphasic patients. *Cortex*, 1979, *15*, 149–155.

Spreen, O., & Risser, A. Assessment of aphasia. In M. T. Sarno (Ed.), *Acquired aphasia*. New York: Academic Press, 1981.

Szalai, A. *The use of time*. The Hague: Mouton, 1972.

Truscott, L., Kretschmann, C. M., Toole, J. F., & Pajak, T. F. Early rehabilitative care in community hospitals: Effect on quality of survivorship following a stroke. *Stroke*, 1974, *5*, 623–629.

Tucker, D. M. Hemispheric specialization and emotion. *Psychological Bulletin*, 1981, *89*, 19–46.

Tucker, D. M., Watson, R. T., & Heilman, K. M. Discrimination and evocation of affectively untoned speech in patients with right parietal disease. *Neurology*, 1977, *27*, 947–950.

Valenstein, E., & Heilman, K. M. Emotional disorders resulting from lesions of the central nervous system. In K. M. Heilman & E. Valenstein (Eds.), *Clinical neuropsychology*. New York: Oxford University Press, 1979.

Wechsler, A. F. The effect of organic brain disease on recall of emotionally charged versus neutral narrative test. *Neurology*, 1973, *23*, 130–135.

Weinberg, J., Diller, L., Gordon, W. A., Gerstman, L. J., Lieberman, A., Lakin, P., Hodges, G., & Ezrachi, O. Visual scanning training effect in reading related tasks in acquired right brain damage. *Archives of Physical Medicine and Rehabilitation*, 1977, *58*, 479–486.

Weinberg, J., Diller, L., Gordon, W. A., Gerstman, L. J., Lieberman, A., Lakin, P., Hodges, G., & Ezrachi, O. Sensory awareness and spatial organization in people with right brain damage. *Archives of Physical Medicine and Rehabilitation*, 1979, *60*, 491–496.

Weinstein, S., & Teuber, H. L. Effects of penetrating brain injury on intelligence scores. *Science*, 1957, *125*, 1036–1037.

Weisenburg, T., & McBride, K. *Aphasia: A clinical psychological study*. New York: Commonwealth Fund, 1935.

Werner, H. The concept of development from a comparative and organismic point of view. In D. B. Harris (Ed.), *The concept of development*. Minneapolis: University of Minnesota Press, 1957.

Wright, B. A. *Physical disability: A psychological approach*. New York: Harper & Row, 1960.

Zuckerman, M., & Lubin, B. *Manual for the Multiple Affect Adjective Checklist*. San Diego: Education and Industrial Testing Services, 1965.

6

A Competency-Based Approach to Coping with Cancer

BETH E. MEYEROWITZ
RICHARD L. HEINRICH
CYNDIE COSCARELLI SCHAG

Introduction

The diagnosis and treatment of cancer create serious psychosocial as well as medical problems. The extent and duration of these problems may be strongly influenced by the methods patients use to cope with the disease. Research that identifies and assesses effective and ineffective coping strategies used by cancer patients is critically important in understanding and modifying the impact of cancer. Despite the importance of studying effective and adaptive coping responses, however, relatively little research has addressed this issue directly. Additionally, much of the literature that does focus on coping with cancer has methodological and theoretical drawbacks. This chapter begins with an overview of the literature. Special emphasis is placed on the research regarding denial, because that coping mechanism has been the one most frequently identified in patients. Later in the chapter we discuss a model for research on coping that overcomes some of the problems in the current literature and that has important implications for furthering knowledge and developing treatment programs. Findings relevant to this approach are reviewed.

Impact of Cancer

Estimates show that each year 700,000 Americans are diagnosed as having cancer (American Cancer Society, 1978) and that 25% of the people in this country will contract the disease during their lifetimes (Sobel, 1979). Such statistics indicate that cancer is and will continue to be a major health problem, affecting most households in the nation. In addition to its impact on the physical health of patients, the disease also creates considerable psychosocial problems. A number of studies have indicated that virtually all patients can expect cancer to have a major psychological impact on their lives. In fact, some authors have suggested that the psychological trauma that results from the diagnosis and treatment of cancer can be as potentially damaging to the patient as the cancer itself (Harrell, 1972).

Until recently there has been a relative dearth of information regarding this psychosocial impact, in part because of the poor prognoses of most cancer patients. For the most part investigators restricted their research to patients in hospitals and studied reactions to cancer and to dying. As a result of recent advances in diagnosis and treatment, more and more individuals are being cured, are having extended remissions, and are living outside of hospitals. These advances have allowed clinicians and researchers to study the ways patients live with cancer and the day-to-day impact it has on their lives.

Although research describing the impact of the diagnosis and treatment of cancer has been reviewed elsewhere (Meyerowitz, 1980), a brief overview is provided to orient the reader to the problems with which cancer patients must cope. The consensus in the literature, based largely on either perceptions of medical personnel or self-report by cancer patients, is that cancer and its treatment normally have a major impact on the lives of the patients. Typically, the effect of the disease is multifaceted, with behavioral, cognitive, and affective consequences. Specifically, research has indicated that most cancer patients experience (a) emotional distress, including some degree of depression, anxiety, and/or anger; (b) physical symptomatology, including both psychosomatic disturbances and direct effects of the disease and its treatments; (c) some disruption in everyday life patterns, including marital and/or sexual relationships and general level of activity; and/or (d) considerable fears regarding disease progression and death (see Meyerowitz, 1980). The presence of some of these reactions is considered to be a normal response to the stress of facing cancer and its medical treatments. In fact, several authors believe that the complete absence of these reactions should be viewed with concern (e.g., Peck, 1972).

Although a number of generalizations about the effects of cancer have been made, there has been considerable variation in the degree and type of psychosocial impact reported (Wortman & Dunkel-Schetter, 1979). Some patients report overwhelming life-style disruption and emotional distress from which they never fully recover, whereas others appear to experience a relatively smooth adjustment. A number of person-related and disease-related variables have been postulated to explain these differences in quality of life after cancer diagnosis. For example, significant relationships have been found between aspects of quality of life and patient's age (e.g., Katz, Kellerman, & Siegel, 1980), premorbid personality (e.g., Hinton, 1975), social environment (e.g., Northouse, 1981), site of disease (e.g., Louhivouri & Hakama, 1979), progression of disease (e.g., Silberfarb, Maurer, & Crouthamel, 1980), time since diagnosis (e.g., Maguire, 1978), and administration of treatment (e.g., Forester, Kornfeld, & Fleiss, 1978).

These patient and disease characteristics account for some of the variability in the quality of patients' lives. However, one of the most frequently cited and potentially important determinants of individual differences is coping. Not only has the method of coping with cancer been suggested as critical in patient adjustment, but also coping is one area (unlike demographic variables, for example) in which intervention and modification may be possible.

Coping Mechanisms

DEFENSE MECHANISMS

Much of the literature on coping with cancer was stimulated by a frequent observation made by early researchers (e.g., Shands, Finesinger, Cobb, & Abrams, 1951; Sutherland, 1952). In describing the reactions of cancer patients, these writers noted that many patients appeared to use defense mechanisms in adjusting to their disease. These authors suggested that cancer patients were under such severe stress that previously successful means of coping were likely to be disrupted, and that defenses that in other life situations might be maladaptive could be required to cope with the overwhelming anxiety caused by the disease and its treatment. In fact, psychologically healthy patients were often observed to use coping mechanisms that were usually observed in neurotic patients. Furthermore, these responses appeared to enhance adjustment. Based on these observations, researchers asked two questions: what are the frequently occurring coping mechanisms, and are they, in fact, successful and adaptive?

Authors have listed and described a number of defensive styles, basing their findings on observation (e.g., Mastrovito, 1974; Milton, 1973) and on patient interviews (e.g., Katz, Weiner, Gallagher, & Hellman, 1970; Peck,

1972). The defenses that have been identified vary somewhat from study to study—including, for example, displacement, projection, suppression, regression, and identification, among others. The variation from study to study may be partially the result of the failure of most authors to define or operationalize their terms adequately; thus the behaviors labeled as a given defense in one study may receive a different label in another study. Also, these studies have observed patients with different cancers, prognoses, and treatments. Such important differences may lead patients to use different coping mechanisms. Despite the difficulties with these studies, one defense mechanism, denial, has emerged in virtually every study. In fact, denial was so frequently observed that much of the research on coping has focused on that one defense. For that reason, the remainder of this review section does the same.

DENIAL

Not only was denial repeatedly identified by researchers and clinicians, nearly every author found it to be quite common in patients facing the diagnosis and treatment of cancer. For example, Katz et al. (1970) interviewed 30 women hospitalized for breast lump biopsies. They found that over one-third of the women tested were using denial, more than twice as many as were reported to be using any of the other defenses that these authors identified. In interviews with 50 patients beginning radiation therapy, Peck (1972) also found denial to be an extremely common means of coping. Even patients in remission have been found to use denial. Sanders and Kardinal (1977) interviewed 6 adult leukemia patients who were in clinical remission. They found denial to be common to all subjects. O'Malley, Koocher, Foster, and Slavin (1979) interviewed 115 childhood cancer patients (i.e., patients who had received their diagnosis before the age of 18) who were at least 60 months postdiagnosis and had been disease-free for over 1 year. Denial was identified as a universally used coping mechanism among these patients as well.

These studies, then, support the clinical observations that defense mechanisms, particularly denial, are common in cancer patients with a wide range of personal and disease characteristics. Clinical claims that this coping mechanism can be effective in the case of cancer patients (e.g., Mastrovito, 1974) have also received some empirical support. In the Katz et al. study (1970) indices of adrenocortical activity and interview ratings of levels of unpleasant affect and disruption in life functioning were obtained from the 30 women hospitalized for breast lump biopsies. The authors used these measures of disruption to assess the adequacy of the defense mechanisms identified in patients. Denial along with stoicism–fatalism and prayer–faith were reported as the means of coping associated with the lowest levels of physiological and psychological disruption. Although these data are consistent with observations of cancer patients, it must be noted that these subjects were not diagnosed as having cancer at the time of data collection. In fact, Polivy (1977) found that breast lump biopsy patients coped differently from cancer patients. She obtained a series of measures of body image and self-image from mastectomy patients, benign breast lump biopsy patients, and surgical control patients. Only the mastectomy patients were reported to have used denial, a coping mechanism that lasted for several months following the operation. The apparent discrepancy between the Katz *et al.* and Polivy findings may result from differences in operational definitions for denial, differences in the aspects of psychological well-being that were assessed, and/or differences in the time at which measures were taken.

Two studies tested the relationship between denial and the psychological well-being of cancer patients directly. In the O'Malley *et al.* (1979) study described previously, psychiatric symptom formation was assessed in the 115 surviving childhood cancer patients. All patients used denial to some extent, but the levels of denial of some patients were not high enough to deal with the pervasive anxiety associated with having had cancer. These patients were the ones most likely to show evidence of psychiatric symptomatology. The authors concluded that "the effective use of denial facilitates long-term adjustment [p. 615]." A similar result was obtained by Moses and Cividali (1966). They analyzed the effects of differential levels of awareness on 30 cancer patients whom they interviewed several times concerning their thoughts and feelings about cancer. The authors found a significant relationship between intermediate awareness, defined as a "suspicion of [cancer] to clear-cut intellectual awareness of cancer [p. 987]" and free-floating anxiety and fear. Patients using intermediate awareness were believed to be using defense mechanisms that were only partially successful, and they were thus more likely to experience anxiety and discomfort than patients who were either successful in denial or who were not even attempting to deny.

These final studies make explicit what many other authors have implied: that there are effective and ineffective ways to use denial. Authors generally regard denial as a relatively temporary and selective process used to defend against certain highly stressful aspects of cancer at different times in the adaptation process (Mastrovito, 1974). However, questions about which aspects of cancer may be safely denied, when, and by whom have not been addressed adequately. Furthermore, those data that do exist are contradictory in many instances. For example, some authors have found that denial serves as only a short-term means of coping during an immediate crisis period (e.g., Mastrovito, 1974; Polivy, 1977) whereas others have identified denial as adaptive for years following diagnosis and treatment (e.g., O' Malley *et al.*, 1979).

Difficulties in ascertaining the optimal levels of and uses for denial may be indicative of methodological and conceptual shortcomings in this area of research. Perhaps the most basic unanswered question is "What is denial?" Denial, an intrapsychic and frequently pathologic mechanism, is extremely difficult to define operationally and to quantify accurately. Different definitions have been used in virtually every study, making comparisons and generalizations of questionable value. A wide range of specific responses have been labeled *denial*, so authors draw conclusions about denial based on very different patient behaviors. Important distinctions among coping responses may be lost. For example, Dansak and Cordes (1979) suggest that authors have failed to distinguish between denial and suppression, categorizing voluntary lack of communication with medical staff as denial.

However, even if a reliable and valid operational definition for denial could be agreed upon, further questions would remain. Implicit in the description of denial as a selective process is the assumption that only some things can or should be denied. Yet researchers have provided little empirical information about what patients deny and for what purposes. Moreover, their focus on defensive processes such as denial assumes that a cancer patient differs from a physically healthy patient only in the frequency with which she or he uses typical defense mechanisms.

CANCER-RELATED STRESSORS

In order to provide data regarding the selective use of coping strategies, cancer cannot be viewed as one, unitary stressor with which patients cope. People do not cope psychologically with the disease of cancer, but with the *impact* of cancer. Cancer, then, does not represent a single stressor that patients deny either successfully or unsuccessfully. The impact of cancer is made up of numerous potentially distressing and disruptive situations, feelings, and thoughts that, taken together, form the overall impact of the disease. When one person faces the disease, he or she will be facing diverse problematic situations (e.g., specific problems involving job discrimination, fears of death, interpersonal difficulties) and the strategies required to cope most effectively may differ with the specific problem situation and the individual dealing with it.

Although researchers have failed to view cancer as a multifaceted group of stressors, they have identified cancer as a stressor that may demand specific coping responses.[1] Additionally, they have suggested that certain behaviors, such as minimizing and avoiding some of the problems created by cancer, might help patients cope with the disease.

Future research should extend the situation-specific approach to coping to include identification of both the actual daily problems of patients and the specific responses to each of those problems. Not only might this approach serve to minimize some of the definitional and conceptual difficulties noted in past research, it could also have greater clinical applicability. Data regarding defense mechanisms offer very little information relevant to the development of psychosocial treatment programs. It is unclear how to teach denial or whether such instruction would be in the long-term best interest of the patient. The aspects of denial that are effective in coping with specific cancer-related problems must be operationally defined. For example, suggestions that involve making an active response (e.g., stay busy with your family) might be more helpful to distressed patients, but such suggestions are premature prior to research indicating the potential efficacy of such a response. As Hamburg (1974) has said, "Behavioral scientists could help many people cope with their predicaments if investigators could build a substantial inventory of (1) common problem situations [and] (2) feasible strategies [p. 23]." Rather than viewing coping in terms of intrapsychic defensive processes, then, coping can be seen as a set of overt and covert behavioral responses to changes in the body and the environment.

A Competency-Based Model of Coping

A model for future research in this area has been provided by Goldfried and D'Zurilla (1969). Although their work involved assessing competence in college freshmen, their sequential criterion analysis recently has been suggested as a model for assessing coping with chronic illness (Turk, 1979; Turk, Sobel, Follick, & Youkilis, 1980). Goldfried and D'Zurilla (1969) described their conception of coping as one that

> rather than being based on personality characteristics, or underlying dynamics, is defined operationally by the individual's interactions with his environment. The basic unit in our

[1]Denial also has been observed frequently in patients with other life-threatening illnesses (e.g., Hackett & Cassem, 1974; Hamburg, 1974). It is not clear whether that denial is the same as the defense observed in cancer patients or the specific coping responses vary among stressors (i.e., diseases). The differences in definitions and the variations in disease-related problems make comparisons of questionable value. Identification of the specific situations with which the patient is coping may allow for cross-disease comparisons on similar problems.

conceptualization of competence is the *effective response* of the individual to specific life situations. . . . it is defined as a response or pattern of responses to a problematic situation [p. 158].

They go on to state that:

> For any given situation, it is clear that there may be more than one effective (or ineffective) way of handling the situation. Indeed, in our own work on assessing effectiveness among college freshmen, we have been struck with the uniqueness with which individuals are capable of handling situations effectively (or ineffectively) [p. 161].

Clearly, then, these authors recommend surveying both problematic situations and variations in responses to each of these situations. This approach is also justified by the findings of other research. Sidle, Moos, Adams, and Cady (1969) asked college students to describe all the coping strategies they might use in dealing with three situations presented by the researchers. They also gave students the same three situations, each with a list of 10 response options. These options were to be rated according to the likelihood of performing each one. Their findings suggested that both person and situation variables were important in explaining coping in that some problems tended to elicit certain strategies and some people were more likely to use a given strategy. Therefore, a complete analysis requires data regarding the situation and the individual responding to it. In another study, Folkman and Lazarus (1980) followed 100 adults in the community over the course of a year to see how they coped with the stressful events of daily living. Coping was described as either problem- or emotion-focused, and in 98% of the stressful events reported subjects used both approaches. The authors concluded that "on the whole, coping patterns are not greatly determined by person factors, nor are they determined entirely by situation factors [p. 229]." To understand these relationships more fully the authors recommend in the future assessing specific coping strategies rather than grouping all responses into only problem- or emotion-focused categories.

The Goldfried and D'Zurilla (1969) competency-based model involves three stages that can be applied to the evaluation of coping and living with cancer. First, specific, day-to-day stressors must be identified. By and large, prior coping research in the cancer area has failed to differentiate among possible stressors, grouping together as equivalent the impacts of widely diverse components of cancer among patients with very different diseases. Second, a wide variety of patients must be questioned to determine the range of responses that are typically made to each problematic situation. Responses may vary according to the situation and the patient's physical and psychological characteristics. Finally, the relative efficacy of each possible response must be measured. A response or group of responses that is effective in one situation may be ineffective in another situation. Through this procedure, intervention programs could be developed to teach new patients those responses that proved effective for patients facing similar problems. In addition to its applied value, this procedure could, perhaps more important-ly, contribute to the development of theoretical perspectives on cancer and coping that are well grounded in relevant data (see Glaser & Strauss, 1967). The literature relevant to each stage of the model is presented in the follow-ing sections.

PROBLEM SPECIFICATION

The initial step in understanding coping is to identify those situations, thoughts, and feelings with which the individual must cope. Cancer is not a single disease. Variations in diagnosis, site, stage, prognosis, time, and treat-ment can lead to quite different problems. The patient does not cope with the disease of cancer, but with the specific day-to-day problems it causes.

There is a large body of literature describing the impact of cancer on the lives of patients. This literature has made significant contributions to the specification of problems by suggesting the general areas in which problems may occur. The problem areas that have been identified include physical disability (Craig, Comstock, & Geiser, 1974), family and marital disruption (Jamison, Wellisch, & Pasnau, 1978), sexual difficulties (Derogatis & Kour-lesis, 1981; Maguire, 1978), self-esteem reduction (Quint, 1963), cognitive impairment (Weizman, Eldar, Shoenfeld, Hirschorn, Wijsenbeck, & Pinkhas, 1979), social–recreational disruption (McAleer & Kluge, 1978), employment problems (McAleer & Kluge, 1978), and psychological distress (Craig & Abeloff, 1974; Maguire, 1978).

This literature describing problem areas is a combination of clinical re-ports, personal impressions, and systematic research. These studies, and a number of others reporting comparable data, vary greatly in the soundness of their methodology. Frequently, differences in cancer site, prognosis, and time since operation are disregarded. Also, there are many instances in which the problem catagories lack operational definitions. Despite these difficulties, this group of studies provides useful guidelines to direct future research on problem specification.

Although most studies have explored the general areas of difficulty experi-enced by patients, some researchers have gained greater specificity by nar-rowing their focus to the physical problems resulting from particular treat-ment interventions. For example, the reduction in arm mobility related to mastectomy (Eisenberg & Goldenberg, 1966), the loss of bowel control asso-ciated with colostomy (Sutherland, Orbach, Dyk, & Bard, 1952), the in-crease in gastric distress caused by chemotherapy (Nerenz, Leventhal,

Love, & Ringler, 1980), and the anticipatory nausea and vomiting linked to chemotherapy (Burish & Lyles, 1979) have been explored.

Recently researchers have begun to combine the two approaches to problem identification previously described by extending the specification of problems beyond physical distress to include many of the general areas identified as troublesome in previous research. Habeck, Blandford, Sacks, and Malec (1981) asked an interdisciplinary team to generate a list of key problem areas based on their clinical experience and on the cancer literature. Seventeen areas were identified, including a wide range of physical, financial, legal, interpersonal, emotional, and spiritual needs. Inpatients, outpatients, and family members were interviewed and asked to describe the severity of patient problems in each area of need. Within some categories problems were listed quite specifically (for example, needs for physical rehabilitation), and in other areas only very general difficulties were assessed (such as problems with interpersonal relationships). Based on the interviews the authors were able to rank order the 20 most pressing needs for both inpatients and outpatients. Although the sample was not large enough to allow for stratification of the results by performance status, cancer site, treatment regimen, or other potentially important patient and disease characteristics, the authors identified a core group of needs for their patient sample. These problems included specific difficulties in the general areas of physical, psychological, social, and vocational functioning.

Another group of researchers used a problem specification approach as the basis of a treatment intervention for breast, lung, and melanoma patients (Gordon, Freidenbergs, Diller, Hibbard, Wolf, Levine, Lipkins, Ezrachi, & Lucido, 1980). In problem-oriented, structured interviews, these authors assessed 122 psychosocial problems covering 13 areas of life functioning. Specially trained oncology counselors then treated 157 patients. The problem specification for each patient guided the choice of the individual's treatment. Although the authors have not published the specified information from their structured interviews, they reported that the impact of cancer and the adjustment to it were different for patients in the three cancer site groups, suggesting that cancer cannot be viewed as one disease.

Follick (1978) used a similar approach to studying a subpopulation of cancer patients with ostomies (a surgical procedure through which an artificial opening is created in the abdominal wall for the excretion of bodily wastes). Initially, he administered an open-ended questionnaire to ostomy patients in which they were asked to identify the problems they experienced in each of seven areas. Structured interviews were also conducted with patients and their spouses. Based on these findings, a questionnaire was mailed to ostomy patients. Results from 131 patients (a return rate of 33%) demonstrated the potential usefulness of problem specification. For example, in the area of social activities 70% of the patients reported changes following surgery. Of these people, however, only 31% stated they had experienced *decreases* in social activities, a fact that could not have been determined if more detailed information had not been sought. Further specification indicated that of the 31% of patients who reported decreases in social activities, 62% experienced increased anxiety in social settings. This increase in anxiety occurred despite the fact that only 12% of these people reported that the reactions of other people had actually been problematic. These data could prove extremely useful in understanding the problems of patients and in developing treatment interventions.

The potential importance of problem specification is further demonstrated by an inventory of problems which two of the present authors are developing (Heinrich, Schag, and Ganz, manuscript in preparation). A self-report measure, the Cancer-Inventory of Problem Situations (C-IPS), was developed based on interviews with patients, nurses, and oncologists and on a review of the literature. The C-IPS is a list of 131 problem statements for which patients indicate the degree of application to themselves. Items fall into the following areas: sleeping, eating, finances, physical ability, activity, transportation, self-care, communication with medical staff, control in medical stiuations, anxiety in medical situations, side effects of treatment, cognitive ability, prosthetic devices, pain, physical appearance, family and friends, worry, employment, marriage, sexuality, and social relationships. Data have been collected from 57 cancer patients who vary according to cancer site, stage, and severity.

Table 6.1 shows the patient responses for two problem areas: communication with medical staff and communication with family and friends. At this stage of development of the problem survey instrument, questions are asked at both a general level (e.g., asking doctors questions) and at a specific level (e.g., asking the doctors if I am improving). Learning that patients have difficulty communicating is a first step, but characterizing the exact nature of the communication problem and the specific situation in which that problem occurs is also important. Do the patients have difficulty asking questions or understanding answers? Is the problem specific to physicians or does it extend to all medical personnel or to family members? Do the communication problems center on cancer-related topics or is all communication problematic for many patients?

As the data in Table 6.1 illustrate, problem specification may begin to answer these questions. For example, 86% of patients report some difficulty communicating with family or friends. Although the anecdotal literature is consistent with this general finding, the assumption is often made that these problems are related to people decreasing their social contacts with the patient. In the present study, however, only 11% of patients responded that

TABLE 6.1

Percentages of Patients Reporting Difficulties on Two Subsections of the Cancer-Inventory of Problem Situations[a]

Problem statement	Percentage of patients reporting applicability
Communication with physicians and nurses	72
I have:	
Difficulty asking doctors questions	39
Difficulty asking nurses questions	35
Difficulty expressing my feelings to the doctors	42
Difficulty expressing my feelings to the nurses	37
Difficulty asking my doctor if I am improving	37
Difficulty asking my doctor about my treatments	39
Difficulty telling my doctor that I want another doctor's opinion	21
Difficulty getting information from my doctor about my disease	33
Difficulty understanding what the doctors tell me about my treatment or disease	44
Difficulty understanding what the nurses tell me about my treatment or disease	33
Difficulty telling my doctor about my symptoms	32
I have found that:	
The medical team withholds information from me about my disease	26
Doctors don't explain what they are doing to me	30
Nurses don't explain what they are doing to me	25
Communication with family and friends	86
I have:	
Difficulty telling my friends or relatives to come over less often	18
Difficulty telling my friends or relatives to leave when I do not feel well	30
Difficulty asking my friends or relatives to do something fun with me	26
Difficulty meeting new friends	26
I have found that:	
I do not know what to say to my family or friends	37
Friends or relatives tell me I'm looking good when I'm not	55
Friends or relatives withhold information from me	12
Friends or relatives avoid talking about my disease	51
Friends or relatives talk too much about my disease	25
Family and friends avoid seeing me	11
Relatives and/or friends visit too often	7
Relatives and/or friends do not visit often enough	40

[a] $N = 57$ patients, Karnofsky status = 4–9 (Karnofsky & Burchenal, 1949).

family and friends avoided them. A far more common complaint was that friends or relatives tell patients that they are looking good when the patients believe that they look sick. This concern, endorsed by over half of the patients, is rarely mentioned in the literature. As this example illustrates, failure to specify problems can result in misleading conclusions regarding the coping needs of patients.

In assessing problem situations, care must be taken to avoid making either under- or overestimates. Both the occurrence and the severity of problems should be tapped. If patients are asked to identify situations that are problematic for them, the occurrence of potentially difficult situations may be underestimated. For example, a patient who has had a problem and coped with it effectively is unlikely to report future occurrences of the same situation as problematic. On the other hand, problems may be overestimated if patients are asked to indicate whether a particular situation (defined a priori as problematic) has occurred without rating its severity. Some patients may have the problem but not be bothered by it. A thorough assessment could include data regarding both the frequency of potentially problematic situations and the extent to which these situations are seen as problematic.

Implicit in the need to rate both frequency and severity is the more general difficulty involved in deciding when a situation becomes problematic. Individual differences must be considered in that what is problematic for one patient may create no difficulties for another. Data should be collected to allow for an investigation of the association between problems and relevant person and disease characteristics. Also, patients may not always be the best judges of when a problem occurs. Physicians, patients, and family members are not always in agreement in their judgments of the problematic nature of a situation. In that the goal of this stage of the competency-based model is to identify a wide range of potentially problematic situations, all of these possible sources of information should be tapped. Finally, problem specification may not reveal the many factors influencing and maintaining problems. For example, patients who do not ask their physicians questions may be silent for several reasons. One patient may ask no questions because he or she has no questions to ask, another patient may have questions but be too fearful of hearing certain answers to ask the questions, and a third patient may be discouraged from asking questions by an unsupportive physician. These distinctions can be extremely important in developing treatment interventions, but are not required in developing an extensive list of cancer-related problems. For the purpose of problem specification, then, any situation judged to be troublesome by any informed rater for any reason is worth exploring.

The research cited up to this point has focused entirely on specifying patient problems. Cancer affects people in addition to the patient. Research has demonstrated that the spouses (Wellisch, Jamison, & Pasnau, 1978), widows (Vachon, Freedman, Formo, Rogers, Lyall, & Freeman, 1977), parents (Chodoff, Friedman, & Hamburg, 1964), children (Grandstaff, 1976), and nurses (Koocher, 1979) of cancer patients must also cope with the disease. In fact, the problems associated with cancer extend beyond the lives of the people dealing directly with the disease. People who avoid breast self-exams for fear of finding lumps, who postpone medical consultation for cancer-related symptoms, or who avoid contact with cancer patients based on unfounded beliefs about the disease all have cancer problems. The competency-based model of problem specification could be applied to these difficulties as well.

RESPONSE ENUMERATION

Following the identification of cancer-related problems, the competency-based approach to studying coping requires the enumeration of possible responses. The goal of this phase is to gather a comprehensive list of the coping strategies to be used for each problem that was previously specified. To obtain maximal information, potential responses should be elicited longitudinally from a diverse patient population. A critical component of such an investigation involves collecting data from patients who report no difficulty with a particular problem. In fact, a major advantage of this approach is the opportunity it provides for researchers to learn about a wide range of *successful* responses from cancer patients.

Obviously, obtaining a comprehensive enumeration of responses for every problem facing cancer patients would be an overwhelming task. Nonetheless, clinically useful data could be obtained by beginning with those problematic situations that have been identified as especially frequent and/or disruptive (for example, the lists of 20 in- and outpatient problems obtained by Habeck *et al.*, 1981). Aside from its clinical significance, such data could also be theoretically useful; problem areas identified by this procedure could be selected for future research based on their relevance to various theoretical perspectives on cancer and coping, such as attribution and social comparison theories. (For a discussion of these and other perspectives, see Taylor, 1982.)

Most of the research relevant to this phase of the model has been reviewed in "Coping Mechanisms." In some studies, researchers approached the task of response enumeration by identifying the variety of coping mechanisms observed in patients, without reference to the specific problems to which patients were responding. Despite the drawbacks of this approach, as discussed earlier, these studies often resulted in useful lists of typical patient responses. Patients and the people working with them might learn that coping responses that are unusual and maladaptive in many situations (e.g., denial) are common among cancer patients.

A second approach to studying coping has been to choose one category of coping responses that has been frequently observed in patients and to study it in greater depth. A primary example of this approach was provided previously in discussion of the denial research. Another example of a coping response that has been studied in some depth is information seeking. For example, Bean, Cooper, Alpert, and Kipnis (1980) interviewed 33 patients receiving chemotherapy to determine the extent to which they asked questions or sought information. Of the patients, 78% said that they asked questions of medical personnel and the vast majority of these people (89%) felt that they had received sufficient information. The authors concluded that, in general, the patients showed a notable lack of interest in obtaining further information. However, another study examining information seeking obtained somewhat different findings. Messerli, Garamendi, and Romano (1980) mailed questionnaires to mastectomy patients who had received their operations within the preceding 5 years. Over 86% of these patients reported having unanswered questions regarding their treatments. Very few reported that they had asked questions of their doctors, either because they did not know what to ask (47%) or because they were too upset to ask (28%). The findings in these studies illustrate the important postulates of the competency-based approach. A specific coping response may or may not be expressed depending upon the demands of the situation, the cancer variables, and the person. It cannot be assumed that all patients will use information-seeking coping responses. These two studies suggest the need for further research to determine the range and frequency of information-seeking responses in a variety of cancer patients and situations.

RESPONSE EVALUATION

The final step in the systematic assessment of coping is the evaluation of each response in terms of its relative efficacy. Determining specific criteria for response evaluation is a complex task, requiring measurement of both the success and the adaptiveness of the response. A successful response is one that serves to achieve a specific goal or to decrease the problematic nature of the situation to which the patient is responding, particularly the emotional distress associated with the problem. An adaptive response is one that is judged to be in the best interest of the patient. Obviously, the most effective response will be both successful and adaptive. With cancer patients, however, these criteria often operate separately. For example, a chemotherapy patient can *successfully* reduce nausea and vomiting by refusing chemotherapy treatments, but that response is most likely a *maladaptive* one from the perspective of the long-term good of the patient. In fact, problems with treatment adherence are often the result of patients choosing successful, but maladaptive, resolutions to therapy-related problems. On the other hand, the postmastectomy patient who finds a lump in her contralateral breast and contacts her physician may have chosen an adaptive response, but be completely unsuccessful in reducing her fears. In this latter situation another response may be required by the patient to minimize fear (e.g., temporary denial or relaxation exercises).

The evaluation of the success of a response is an empirical one: has the problem been resolved or not? Determining adaptiveness, however, requires making a value judgment regarding the patient's best interest. These decisions will often be complex and assessors (e.g., patient, family, physician) may disagree. Not only are different value judgments involved, but the various interests of the patient may be in conflict (e.g., psychological versus physical well-being; long-term versus short-term results).

Most research has tended to focus on the success of responses such as denial in minimizing emotional distress. Because these studies, as reviewed earlier, have failed to identify the specific problems that are being responded to and the specific response that is being tested, success was typically measured by correlating reports of denial with reports of distress. Despite the problems with much of the denial research (see "Coping Mechanisms"), studies suggesting the potential efficacy of selective denial should not be disregarded. It is striking that so many authors, using independent observations, agree that some degree of denial is a common and healthy response in adapting to cancer. In fact, Mastrovito (1974) has suggested that the complete absence of selective denial may result in chronic anxiety, depression, and tension. Further research is required to identify those specific responses that are indicative of denial and the specific problems for which it is successful.

Whereas most research has focused on the success of denial, the evaluation of adaptiveness often is dealt with by a disclaimer to the effect that denial is useful as long as it does not interfere with patients' acceptance of treatment. Most authors consider any response that might threaten survival to be maladaptive, yet few studies have systematically assessed the relationship between coping and longevity. Two studies that examine the association between psychological adjustment and life-span begin to question this relationship. Derogatis, Abeloff, and Melisaratos (1979) found that, of 35 women being treated for metastatic breast cancer, those patients who lived longer tended to have higher psychological distress levels. In another study (Rogentine, van Kammen, Fox, Docherty, Rosenblatt, Boyd, & Bunney, 1979) 64 malignant melanoma patients were asked to rate the amount of adjustment required in coping with the illness. Patients who relapsed within 1 year reported requiring significantly less adjustment than was required by patients who remained in remission. Despite a number of methological problems with these studies (e.g., Krant, 1981), the results suggest that successful coping responses may not always be adaptive. Much further research specifically directed toward this possibility is needed before any implications for clinical interventions can be drawn.

Weisman and his colleagues, the Project Omega Group, have succeeded in overcoming some of the problems in previous research on response evaluation (Weisman, 1976; Weisman & Worden, 1977; Weisman, Worden, & Sobel, 1980). The researchers investigated the psychological distress experienced by newly diagnosed patients, developed a screening instrument predicting patients at high risk for distress, and evaluated two different treatment interventions aimed at reducing the psychological vulnerability of high-risk patients. In each of these phases of the research, coping strategies were assessed in relation to the daily problems of patients. Patients' coping responses were evaluated by a trained clinician during a clinical interview in which patients reported their experiences, problems, and resources. Specifically, the clinician attempted to elicit situations that had been or were problematic for the individual and the strategies that were used to resolve the difficulties. The clinician then classified the patient's coping strategies into one or more of 15 categories of problem-solving behaviors that had been identified in previous research with noncancer patients. Finally, the clinician evaluated how effective the patient's coping responses had been on a four-point scale of problem resolution. A problem was considered resolved if it no longer distressed the patient and the patient's behavior did not reflect distress. Using this method the Omega group found that good copers (i.e., patients who resolved problems and had little distress) used a wider range of coping responses and tended to use more confrontation, redefinition of problems, and compliance with authority. The poor copers, on the other hand, tended to use behaviors categorized as suppression–passivity and stoic submission.

Despite the fact that these researchers were not attempting a competency-based analysis of coping responses, they did demonstrate the usefulness of some components of the model. For example, coping responses were rated in relation to specific problems to which patients were adjusting in their day-to-day lives. Additionally, it appears that an attempt was made to consider both success and adaptiveness in rating problem resolutions, although the criteria were not clearly delineated. No a priori assumptions were made regarding the efficacy of responses. These determinations were made empirically.

The method of assessment used in this research is consistent with some aspects of a competency-based approach to coping, but there are several major differences. First, the overall goal of the Omega Project was to identify and treat patients at high risk for psychosocial vulnerability, whereas the competency-based model seeks to enumerate effective responses to specific problems. By discovering competent responses from patients who use them, the researcher gains some idea of new strategies that can be taught to patients who have problems in the specific area in question. Patients need not be identified as good or poor copers. Virtually all patients have difficulty in reducing some problems and cope well with others. The specific problems facing any patient can be assessed and responses that have been effective for similar problems can be taught. Second, the Omega Project's study on coping was more general than a problem-specific approach would suggest. These researchers categorized coping responses into 15 general categories and assumed that all responses could be classified within this finite group. They also implicitly assumed that the same coping responses could be used for a very wide range of problems. Response enumeration, on the other hand, assumes that although some responses may be applied across some situations, some problems may need specific coping responses. Questionnaires developed to encompass all possible responses to any problem must be quite general, requiring diverse behaviors to be grouped together.

Future Directions

Cancer causes a wide variety of problems and virtually every patient faced with the disease experiences distress or disruption in some area. The ways in which patients cope with these problems will influence their postdiagnostic quality of life. A competency-based model (Goldfried & D'Zurilla, 1969; Turk *et al.*, 1980) has been proposed to investigate the specific daily problems facing cancer patients and effective strategies for coping with those problems. These data may have immediate applicability to cancer patients. Patients, their families, and the medical personnel working with them could anticipate and prepare for the problematic situations likely to arise for specific individuals. Data also could be provided relating coping responses to person and situation variables. Merely increasing the response options available to patients is likely to be valuable.

The proposed model would also provide data relevant to the development of psychosocial treatment programs for cancer patients. Although a competency-based assessment has not been completed, two research groups have provided excellent demonstrations of the applicability of some components of the model to developing general approaches to intervention (Gordon *et al.*, 1980; Weisman *et al.*, 1980). Other therapy outcome research has focused on identifying a specific problem facing a number of patients and on teaching one or two strategies for coping with that problem. For example, very carefully planned and highly effective interventions have been developed for the anticipatory nausea and vomiting associated with chemotherapy (e.g., Burish & Lyles, 1979). These studies are reviewed by Burish and Lyles, Chapter 7.

Specific information regarding the relative efficacy of coping response options can lead to data-based therapy programs that could be fitted to both the problematic situations and the individual facing them. Problem-specific therapies could be developed from these findings because treatments could be matched to the needs of the patient. Help could be given not only to generally highly distressed patients, but also to patients with specific and circumscribed problems. Since virtually all patients do experience some problems, these findings might have wide-ranging applicability. However, treatment efficacy cannot be assumed and therapy outcome research is required. Multiple base-line studies testing the relative impact of several coping strategies in dealing with specific problems may prove useful.

Data regarding problematic situations might suggest changes to be made in the environments of patients as well as therapy programs to be developed. Some of the problems facing cancer patients are not direct results of the disease itself. The interpersonal stigma associated with cancer, the climate of some hospitals and clinics, the possibility of job discrimination, and many other factors add to the psychosocial impact of cancer. In some instances it may be possible to deal directly with finding solutions to these problems rather than helping patients learn to adjust to them.

Finally, the competency-based approach can provide data for the development and refinement of theory regarding coping with cancer. One cannot assume that psychological theory developed with other populations (e.g., psychiatric patients or college students) will necessarily provide a comprehensive account of the experiences of cancer patients. Existing theoretical perspectives have provided useful insights in the cancer area. Nevertheless, such theory-guided research restricts a priori the kinds of hypotheses that are investigated. In contrast, the competency-based model provides a systematic and comprehensive means of generating data that permits the specification of critical research questions and relevant theoretical perspectives. Such an approach should prove useful in helping to refine and modify existing theory, making it more applicable to cancer-related phenomena (e.g., Taylor, 1982), and could ultimately lead to the development of new theoretical approaches that are solidly grounded in relevant data.

References

American Cancer Society. *Cancer facts and figures.* New York: Author, 1978.

Bean, G., Cooper, S., Alpert, R., & Kipnis, D. Coping mechanisms of cancer patients: A study of 33 patients receiving chemotherapy. *CA—A Cancer Journal for Clinicians,* 1980, *30,* 256–259.

Burish, T. G., & Lyles, J. N. Effectiveness of relaxation training in reducing the aversiveness of chemotherapy in the treatment of cancer. *Journal of Behavior Therapy and Experimental Psychiatry,* 1979, *10,* 357–361.

Chodoff, P., Friedman, S. B., & Hamburg, D. A. Stress, defenses and coping behavior: Observations in parents of children with malignant disease. *American Journal of Psychiatry,* 1964, *120,* 743–749.

Craig, T. J., & Abeloff, M. D. Psychiatric symptomatology among hospitalized cancer patients. *American Journal of Psychiatry,* 1974, *131,* 1323–1327.

Craig, T. J., Comstock, G. W., & Geiser, P. B. The quality of survival in breast cancer: A case-control comparison. *Cancer,* 1974, *33,* 1451–1457.

Dansak, D. A., & Cordes, R. S. Cancer: Denial or suppression? *International Journal of Psychiatry in Medicine,* 1979, *9,* 257–262.

Derogatis, L., Abeloff, M. D., & Melisaratos, N. Psychological coping mechanisms and survival time in metastatic breast cancer. *Journal of the American Medical Association,* 1979, *242,* 1504–1508.

Derogatis, L. R., & Kourlesis, S. M. An approach to evaluation of sexual problems in the cancer patient. *CA—A Cancer Journal for Clinicians,* 1981, *31,* 46–50.

Eisenberg, H. S., & Goldenberg, I. S. A measurement of quality of survival of breast cancer patients. In J. L. Hayward & R. D. Bulbrook (Eds.), *Clinical evaluation of breast cancer.* London: Academic Press, 1966.

Folkman, S., & Lazarus, R. S. An analysis of coping in a middle-aged community sample. *Journal of Health and Social Behavior,* 1980, *21,* 219–239.

Follick, M. J. *Problem specification by ostomy patients.* Paper presented at the annual meeting of the Association for the Advancement of Behavior Therapy, Chicago, November 1978.

Forester, B. M., Kornfeld, D. S., & Fleiss, J. Psychiatric aspects of radiotherapy. *American Journal of Psychiatry,* 1978, *135,* 960–963.

Glaser, B. G., & Strauss, A. L. *The discovery of grounded theory: Strategies for qualitative research.* Chicago: Aldine, 1967.

Goldfried, M. R., & D'Zurilla, T. J. A behavioral-analytic model for assessing competence. In C. D. Spielberger (Ed.), *Current topics in clinical and community psychology* (Vol. 1). New York: Academic Press, 1969.

Gordon, W. A., Freidenbergs, I., Diller, L., Hibbard, M., Wolf, C., Levine, L., Lipkins, R., Ezrachi, O., & Lucido, D. Efficacy of psychosocial intervention with cancer patients. *Journal of Consulting and Clinical Psychology,* 1980, *48,* 743–759.

Grandstaff, N. W. The impact of breast cancer on the family. *Frontiers of Radiation Therapy and Oncology,* 1976, *11,* 145–156.

Habeck, R. V., Blandford, K. K., Sacks, R., & Malec, J. *The WCCC cancer rehabilitation and continuing care needs assessment study report.* Unpublished report, University of Wisconsin, Madison, 1981.

Hackett, T. P., & Cassem, N. H. Development of a quantitative rating scale to assess denial. *Journal of Psychosomatic Research,* 1974, *18,* 93–100.

Hamburg, D. A. Coping behavior in life-threatening circumstances. *Psychotherapy and Psychosomatics,* 1974, *23,* 13–25.

Harrell, H. C. To lose a breast. *American Journal of Nursing*, 1972, *72*, 676–677.

Heinrich, R. L., Schag, C. C., & Ganz, P. A. Living with cancer: The cancer inventory of problem situations. Manuscript in preparation.

Hinton, J. The influence of previous personality on reactions to having terminal cancer. *Omega*, 1975, *6*, 95–111.

Jamison, K., Wellisch, D. K., & Pasnau, R. O. Psychosocial aspects of mastectomy: I. The woman's perspective. *American Journal of Psychiatry*, 1978, *135*, 432–436.

Karnofsky, D. A., & Burchenal, J. H. The clinical evaluation of chemotherapy agents in cancer. In C. M. MacCleod (Ed.) *Evaluation of chemotherapeutic agents*. New York: Columbia University Press, 1949.

Katz, E. R., Kellerman, J., & Siegel, S. E. Behavioral distress in children with cancer undergoing medical procedures: Developmental considerations. *Journal of Consulting and Clinical Psychology*, 1980, *48*, 356–365.

Katz, J. L., Weiner, H., Gallagher, T. F., & Hellman, L. Stress, distress and ego defenses: Psychoendocrine response to impending breast tumor biopsy. *Archives of General Psychiatry*, 1970, *23*, 131–142.

Koocher, G. P. Adjustment and coping strategies among the caretakers of cancer patients. *Social Work and Health Care*, 1979, *5*, 145–150.

Krant, M. J. Coping psychologically with breast cancer. *Journal of the American Medical Association*, 1981, *245*, 31–32.

Louhivuori, K. A., & Hakama, M. Risk of suicide among cancer patients. *American Journal of Epidemiology*, 1979, *109*, 59–65.

Maguire, P. Psychiatric problems after mastectomy. In P. C. Brand & P. A. van Keep (Eds.), *Breast cancer: Psycho-social aspects of early detection and treatment*. Baltimore: University Park Press, 1978.

Mastrovito, R. C. Cancer: Awareness and denial. *Clinical Bulletin*, 1974, *4*, 142–146.

McAleer, C. A., & Kluge, C. A. Counseling needs and approaches for working with a cancer patient. *Rehabilitation Counseling Bulletin*, 1978, *21*, 238–245.

Messerli, M. L., Garamendi, C., & Romano, J. Breast cancer: Information as a technique of crisis intervention. *American Journal of Orthopsychiatry*, 1980, *50*, 728–731.

Meyerowitz, B. E. Psychosocial correlates of breast cancer and its treatments. *Psychological Bulletin*, 1980, *87*, 108–131.

Milton, G. W. Thoughts in mind of a person with cancer. *British Medical Journal*, 1973, *4*, 221–223.

Moses, R., & Cividali, N. Differential levels of awareness of illness: Their relation to some salient features of cancer patients. *Annals of the New York Academy of Sciences*, 1966, *125*, 984–994.

Nerenz, D. R., Leventhal, H., Love, R. R., & Ringler, K. *Factors contributing to emotional distress during cancer chemotherapy*. Paper presented at the meeting of the American Psychological Association, Montreal, September 1980.

Northouse, L. L. Mastectomy patients and the fear of cancer recurrence. *Cancer Nursing*, 1981, *4*, 213–225.

O'Malley, J. E., Koocher, G., Foster, D., & Slavin, L. Psychiatric sequelae of surviving childhood cancer. *American Journal of Orthopsychiatry*, 1979, *49*, 608–616.

Peck, A. Emotional reactions to having cancer. *American Journal of Roentgenology*, 1972, *114*, 591–599.

Polivy, J. Psychological effects of mastectomy on a woman's feminine self-concept. *Journal of Nervous and Mental Disease*, 1977, *164*, 77–87.

Quint, J. C. The impact of mastectomy. *American Journal of Nursing*, 1963, *63*, 88–92.

Rogentine, G. N., van Kammen, D. P., Fox, B. H., Docherty, J. P., Rosenblatt, J. E., Boyd, S.

C., & Bunney, W. E. Psychological factors in the prognoses of malignant melanoma: A prospective study. *Psychosomatic Medicine*, 1979, *41*, 647–655.

Sanders, J. B., & Kardinal, C. G. Adaptive coping mechanisms in adult acute leukemia patients in remission. *Journal of the American Medical Association*, 1977, *238*, 952–954.

Shands, H. C., Finesinger, J. E., Cobb, S., & Abrams, R. D. Psychological mechanisms in patients with cancer. *Cancer*, 1951, *4*, 1159–1170.

Sidle, A., Moos, R., Adams, J., & Cady, P. Development of a coping scale: A preliminary study. *Archives of General Psychiatry*, 1969, *20*, 226–232.

Silberfarb, P. M., Maurer, L. H., & Crouthamel, C. S. Psychosocial aspects of neoplastic disease: I. Functional status of breast cancer patients during different treatment regimes. *American Journal of Psychiatry*, 1980, *137*, 450–455.

Sobel, H. J. Review of the current literature: Coping with cancer. *Behavioral Medicine Newsletter*, 1979, *1*, 6–9.

Sutherland, A. M. Psychological impact of cancer surgery. *Public Health Reports*, 1952, *67*, 1139–1143.

Sutherland, A. M., Orbach, C. E., Dyk, R. B., & Bard, M. The psychological impact of cancer and cancer surgery: I. Adaptation to the dry colostomy; Report and summary of findings. *Cancer*, 1952, *5*, 857–872.

Taylor, S. E. Social cognition and health. *Personality and Social Psychology Bulletin*, 1982, *8*, 549–562.

Turk, D. C. Factors influencing the adaptive process with chronic illness: Implications for intervention. In I. G. Sarason & C. D. Spielberger (Eds.), *Stress and Anxiety* (Vol. 6). Washington, D.C.: Hemisphere, 1979.

Turk, D. C., Sobel, H. J., Follick, M. J., & Youkilis, H. D. A sequential criterion analysis for assessing coping with chronic illness. *Journal of Human Stress*, 1980, *6*(2), 35–40.

Vachon, M. L. S., Freedman, K., Formo, A., Rogers, J., Lyall, W. A. L., & Freeman, S. J. J. The final illness in cancer: The widow's perspective. *Canadian Medical Association Journal*, 1977, *117*, 1151–1154.

Weisman, A. D. Early diagnosis of vulnerability in cancer patients. *The American Journal of the Medical Sciences*, 1976, *271*, 187–196.

Weisman, A. D., & Worden, J. W. *Coping and vulnerability in cancer patients: A research report*. Cambridge, Mass.: Authors, 1977.

Weisman, A. D., Worden, J. W., & Sobel, H. J. *Psychosocial screening and intervention with cancer patients*. Cambridge, Mass.: Authors, 1980.

Weizman, A., Eldar, M., Shoenfeld, Y., Hirschorn, M., Wijsenbeck, H., & Pinkhas, J. Hypercalcaemia-induced psychopathology in malignant disease. *British Journal of Psychiatry*, 1979, *135*, 363–366.

Wellisch, D. K., Jamison, K. R., & Pasnau, R. O. Psychological aspects of mastectomy: II. The man's perspective. *American Journal of Psychiatry*, 1978, *135*, 543–546.

Wortman, C. B., & Dunkel-Schetter, C. Interpersonal relationships and cancer: A theoretical analysis. *Journal of Social Issues*, 1979, *35*, 120–155.

7

Coping with the Adverse Effects of Cancer Treatments*

THOMAS G. BURISH
JEANNE NARAMORE LYLES

Introduction

Few diseases—perhaps none—are feared as much as cancer. It is estimated (American Cancer Society, 1980) that approximately one in five people living in the United States currently has or will develop cancer, and that the great majority of these individuals will die from their cancer. Recent data also suggest that two out of three families in the United States have or will have at least one member with cancer. Taken together, these statistics suggest that most Americans, including most people reading this chapter, either will develop and die from cancer themselves or will watch someone in their families develop and die from cancer.

Because of the ubiquitous and devastating nature of cancer, the federal government and private agencies have spent billions of dollars trying to find ways of curing the disease or at least of prolonging the lives of people who have cancer. These treatment-oriented endeavors have been very success- ful; as a result, the life expectancy of most cancer patients today is consider- ably longer than it was 5 or 10 years ago and several forms of cancer are considered curable. But these gains have not come without a cost. Many forms of cancer treatment are painful, have repulsive and aversive side

*The authors thank Stephen A. Maisto and Michael P. Carey for their helpful comments on an earlier draft of the manuscript. The writing of this chapter was supported in part by Grant No. CA 25516 from the National Cancer Institute.

effects, and place great financial and personal demands on patients and their families. The costs of treatment are sometimes so overwhelming that patients choose a hastened and inevitable death rather than continue to undergo the hell they have come to know as cancer treatment (e.g., Gorzynski & Holland, 1979; McArdle, Calman, Cooper, Hughson, Russell, & Smith, 1981). Whitehead (1975), for example, described the cost of chemotherapy, a commonly used cancer treatment:

> After one or more courses [of chemotherapy], patients may begin to vomit on the morning of their treatment, or upon arrival at the physician's office, in anticipation of the injection, attesting to the abhorrence with which they regard the treatment. They confess to feeling ill for three weeks or more out of every four and may become deeply depressed and suicidal [p. 200].[1]

As discussed later in this chapter, reactions to other forms of cancer treatments can be equally devastating. Cancer differs from most other chronic diseases, therefore, in that its treatment can be as aversive as or more aversive than the symptoms of the disease. It is for this reason that a chapter on coping with the treatments for cancer is included in this volume.

The chapter is divided into four major sections. Each of the first three sections covers the literature on psychosocial issues and behavioral intervention strategies relevant to one of the major forms of adult cancer treatment: surgery, chemotherapy, and radiation therapy.[2] However, it should be emphasized that many cancer patients receive more than one type of treatment and thus experience the side effects described in several sections in this chapter. In the final section, general issues relevant to coping with any form of cancer treatment are discussed.

Surgery

Surgery is the preferred treatment for many types of cancer (e.g., breast cancer, colorectal cancer; American Cancer Society, 1980). Patients undergoing surgery may encounter a variety of problems related to disfigurement and loss of body tissue or organs, changes in body images, and postoperative rehabilitation. Some of these problems, such as those associated with inadequate preparation for surgery, are similar to those encountered with other forms of surgery and have been reviewed in detail elsewhere (e.g., Kendall

---

[1]Reprinted, by permission of the *New England Journal of Medicine* (293; 199–200, 1975).

[2]Little research has been conducted on the adverse consequences of more recently developed treatment procedures such as immunotherapy and thermotherapy; in general they appear to produce fewer and less potent side effects. Therefore, no separate sections of the chapter are devoted to these treatment modalities.

& Watson, 1981). Although all types of cancer surgery can cause problems in coping, this chapter focuses on those types of surgery that are most commonly performed and that result in especially difficult challenges to normal sexual, social, and bodily functioning: surgical procedures for breast, genital, urinary, colorectal, and head and neck cancers.

BREAST CANCER

Breast cancer and its surgical treatment by removing part or all of the breast tissue (a procedure referred to as *mastectomy*) have received more attention in the psychosocial cancer literature than any other topic. Approximately one in every four women with cancer has breast cancer, making it by far the most common type of cancer in women (American Cancer Society, 1980). The majority of women with breast cancer will receive one of three general types of mastectomies: (a) a *simple or total mastectomy* in which the entire breast is removed; (b) a *modified radical mastectomy* in which the breast and axillary lymph nodes are removed; or (c) a *radical mastectomy* in which the breast, axillary nodes, and pectoral muscles are removed. Following a mastectomy, most patients experience depression, anxiety, and reduced self-esteem. Many patients can take up to a year to regain normal functioning in these areas, and a small percentage of patients take considerably longer or never adequately adjust (Meyerowitz, 1980; Morris, Greer, & White, 1977).

In addition to the anxiety and depression mentioned above, the surgical treatment of breast cancer usually produces a variety of other problems, sometimes of serious proportions. One of the most common problems is impaired self-image. Following a mastectomy, many women, especially those for whom appearance and shapeliness have been of great importance (Bard & Sutherland, 1955; Holland, 1976), "feel worthless, ugly, defeminized, socially and sexually unacceptable [Bronner-Huszar, 1971, p. 134]." Single women in particular may fear that because of their mastectomy they will never be seen as attractive to men (Holland, 1973). As might be expected, some data suggest that the more radical the mastectomy, the greater the resultant decrease in self-image and self-esteem (Blum, 1980).

A second major problem involves impaired sexual functioning. For some patients, such as those receiving adrenalectomy, there may be a physiological basis for the loss of interest in sexual activity (Holland, 1976), but for most patients the problems are largely psychological in nature. Fears of being rejected or found undesirable may cause patients to withdraw from sexual activity. For example, Clifford, Clifford, and Georgiade (1980) found that 30% of the mastectomy patients in their sample reported a decrease in the frequency of sexual intercourse, 27% reported reduced sexual satisfaction, and 62% reported a general negative change in overall sexual functioning. Many mastectomy patients also refuse or find it difficult to reveal the scar to their partners; this can exacerbate a partner's concerns about the repulsiveness of the scar or the possibility of hurting the patient by touching or pressing against the scarred area (Holland & Mastrovito, 1980; Witkin, 1975).

Impaired sexual functioning is sometimes indicative of one of the most frequently reported consequences of mastectomy: disturbed marital relationships (e.g., Lee & Maguire, 1975; Meyerowitz, 1980; Silberfarb, Maurer, & Crouthamel, 1980). Patients frequently complain of a lack of understanding or support from their spouses and of a decreased ability to communicate with them (e.g., Clifford *et al.*, 1980). Although a mastectomy patient may feel unhappy in her marriage, she may nevertheless avoid ending the relationship because of her fear of being found unacceptable to other men. As a result, she can find herself in a very stressful and fragile situation.

A fourth major category of problems includes those that are more directly related to the physical effects of surgery. For example, many postmastectomy patients experience reduced arm mobility and lymphedema (swelling of the arm) on the side where the surgery was performed (e.g., Eisenberg & Goldenberg, 1966; Silberfarb *et al.*, 1980). Healey (1971) found that 34% of a sample of 271 mastectomy patients still experienced reduced range of shoulder motion after 1 to 4 years and that 34% also experienced lymphedema. Of those with lymphedema, 95% were self-conscious about it and more than 50% had difficulty fitting clothes. For 28 women the combination of reduced range of motion and lymphedema was so disabling that they had trouble completing activities of daily living such as combing hair and hooking bras.

Because of the plethora of problems that can result from mastectomies, there has been an increasing amount of controversy over whether such a radical treatment is necessary and/or worth the decreased quality of life it often causes, especially for women in whom the cancer has not yet spread to the lymph nodes or other tissue (Sanger & Reznikoff, 1981). For example, Harris, Levene, and Hellman (1980) have suggested that radiation therapy without surgery may be an acceptable alternative to mastectomy for cases of early breast cancer. Although there is little question that mastectomies can cause a variety of problems, it should be kept in mind that many other types of cancer treatments cause equally or more serious problems. It has even been reported that some women feel that the distress of a mastectomy is minor compared to the side effects they later experience from chemotherapy (Holland & Mastrovito, 1980). As Holland (1976) and others have pointed out, until data regarding the cost of alternative treatment strategies, including long-term survival rates, become available, it is premature to denounce mastectomy as an unacceptable or inhumane procedure.

Because it appears that mastectomies will continue to be performed on many women, attention should be devoted to identifying ways of preventing and ameliorating problems resulting from the surgery. In a few areas considerable research has already been conducted and successful treatments identified. For example, several investigators have suggested that disability resulting from reduced arm and shoulder range of motion and lymphedema can be avoided or at least minimized by proper rehabilitation procedures such as physical therapy, shoulder and arm movement exercises, and wearing elastic sleeves designed to minimize swelling (e.g., Goldsmith & Alday, 1971; Healey, 1971). Breast prostheses or reconstructive surgery may reduce the sense of loss and disfigurement so often experienced (e.g., Clifford & Clifford, 1981; Holland & Mastrovito, 1980). In the psychosocial area, however, relatively little treatment-oriented research has been carried out, and most of the literature consists of clinical observations, anecdotes, autobiographical accounts, and speculation. Of the relatively small number of research investigations that do exist, most are flawed by methodological problems such as failure to include control procedures, poorly defined measurement techniques, and retrospective data collection. However, at least one relatively well-designed study has been reported (Maguire, Tait, Brooke, Thomas, & Sellwood, 1980). Maguire and his colleagues assigned 152 patients to either a treatment group or a no-treatment control group. The treatment group received individual counseling by a specialist nurse both before and after surgery. Patients' functioning levels were determined by an interview and a shortened version of the Brown–Birley Life Events Schedule shortly after surgery, 3 months postsurgery, and 12–18 months postsurgery. The 3-month evaluation revealed that the counseling procedure had little effect: 39% of the treatment group and 43% of the control group were experiencing significant anxiety, depression, and/or sexual problems. However, although unable to ameliorate these problems, the nurse usually could recognize them and as a result refer these patients for psychiatric help. Overall, 75% of the patients in the treatment group whose data indicated that they were having serious problems were referred by the medical staff for help. These referrals were apparently quite important. By the 12–18 month followup only 12% of the counseling group were still experiencing psychological problems, whereas 39% of the control patients still had significant difficulties. Unfortunately, the authors provided little detail about the nature of either the counseling intervention or the psychiatric help provided as a result of the referrals.

Although this and other intervention strategies (e.g., Gordon, Freidenbergs, Diller, Hibbard, Wolf, Levine, Lipkins, Ezrachi, & Lucido, 1980; Schwartz, 1977; Winick & Robbins, 1976, 1977) provide little solid data on how to treat or prevent the adverse psychological effects of breast cancer, they are relatively consistent in suggesting that interventions of some type can have a positive effect; however, considerably more and better research is needed to determine the active ingredients of these interventions, how they can best be provided, and what their limitations are likely to be.

GENITAL CANCERS

Approximately 76,000 new cases of gynecological cancers are diagnosed each year, making them the second most common type of cancer in women (American Cancer Society, 1980). As with breast cancer, surgical procedures are often the treatment of choice. The most common operation is a hysterectomy, which is usually performed for cancer of the uterus. A radical vulvectomy is often performed for vulvar cancer, although for extensive disease a pelvic exenteration (involving surgical removal of the vagina, uterus, fallopian tubes, ovaries, part of the vulva, bladder, and rectum) may be performed. Women receiving this procedure must also cope with the difficulties resulting from two required ostomies.

The most common concerns of women following gynecological surgery involve sexuality. In some cases the capacity for sex is *physically* impaired or lost as a result of the surgery. For example, vaginal shortening may follow radical hysterectomy, impairing comfort during sexual intercourse (Andersen & Hacker, in press). Premenopausal patients may also mourn the loss of childbearing activity and dread the onset of the symptoms of menopause (e.g., Drellich, Bieber, & Sutherland, 1956; Holland, 1973). Perhaps the greatest difficulties, however, are *psychological* in nature. Following gynecological surgery, patients often feel sexually unattractive, fearing rejection by their partners and refusing to allow them to see the surgical site (e.g., Holland, 1973; Sewell & Edwards, 1980). These feelings of embarrassment and decreased self-esteem can contribute to reduced sexual interest and capacity for orgasm. Some women, aware of recent evidence linking some types of genital cancers with factors such as early sexual activity, multiple partners, and herpes infections, feel guilt and shame over the possibility of being personally responsible for their cancer (e.g., Andersen & Hacker, in press). In response to the patient's behavior, sexual partners may also withdraw from continued sexual activity with them, wary of hurting the patient or fearful of catching cancer venereally (Krant, 1981). Unfortunately, some partners also show repulsion to the impairment, contributing further to the patient's despair.

Although research on adjustment to gynecological surgery is sparse and methodologically weak, the available data support the expected conclusion that many patients have adjustment problems. For example, Sewell and Edwards (1980) collected data on 46 women 6 months postoperatively; they found that most of these patients reported negative changes in body image, sexual relationships, and frequency of intercourse, with patients who underwent more radical procedures (i.e., exenteration) reporting more severe difficulties. Other authors have reported similar findings (e.g., Abitbol & Davenport, 1974; Decker & Schwartzman, 1962; Seibel, Freeman, & Graves, 1980; Vincent, Vincent, Greiss, & Linton, 1975).

Impairment in social and marital functioning may also follow gynecological surgery. For example, Drellich et al. (1956) found that anxiety and irritability are common after surgery and that many women experience feelings of being useless and unattractive and of prematurely aging. Sewell and Edwards (1980) reported that 6 months after surgery many women had family and marital problems, with younger patients tending to have more disruptions than older patients in relationships with significant others.

Regrettably, as is the case with other cancer sites, gynecological cancer patients often receive little help adjusting to their difficulties. For example, Vincent et al. (1975) found that the majority of patients they sampled did not receive any information regarding sexual adjustment to their surgery. A recent study by Capone, Westie, and Good (1980), however, suggests that intervention programs may help to overcome such adjustment problems to gynecological surgery. The authors met with patients both before and after surgery in order to provide support, correct misinformation (e.g., that intercourse will cause a recurrence of disease) and give accurate information, and encourage a return to preoperative levels of functioning. None of the patients involved was medically or anatomically prevented from resuming sexual relations. The authors reported that at 3, 6, and 12 months postsurgery, fewer than 50%, 33%, and 20%, respectively, of the intervention patients reported a reduction or cessation in intercourse compared with more than 75%, 75%, and 50%, respectively, of the untreated control patients. Several authors have also suggested that sex therapy and reconstructive surgery may be beneficial to gynecological cancer patients (e.g., Andersen & Hacker, in press; Krant, 1981); however, the effectiveness of these procedures remains to be investigated.

Men may also face significant physical and psychological distress after genital cancer surgery. Cancer of the prostate accounts for 17% of cancers in males, making it the second most common site of cancer in men after the lungs (American Cancer Society, 1980). Men may experience significant sexual difficulties following surgery, including temporary or permanent loss of capacity for erection and ejaculation (Holland, 1973; von Eschenbach,

1980). Nerve and tissue damage secondary to surgery varies depending upon the site and extent of surgery. As with gynecological cancer patients, male patients may experience distress regarding the loss of function and fears regarding their continued attractiveness to their sexual partners (Furlow, 1980; Gorzynski & Holland, 1979). Self-doubt, depression, and anxiety may reduce sex drive and further inhibit a successful adjustment.

Little research has been carried out to help find ways of improving postsurgery coping in male patients with genital cancer. Furlow (1980) has suggested that with organic impotence penile prostheses may be considered, and reported that patients and partners are usually satisfied with this intervention. Furlow (1980) and others (e.g., Gorzynski & Holland, 1979) have also suggested that for both organic and psychogenic impotence, sex therapy and preoperative sperm banking may be helpful; however, no data regarding the psychological benefits of these procedures have been reported. As with most areas of cancer coping, considerable research on the development of effective intervention strategies is needed.

URINARY AND COLORECTAL CANCERS

Several types of urinary and colorectal or bowel cancers result in blockage of the bladder or portions of the intestine or in their removal by some type of surgical procedure. As a result, another type of surgical procedure is carried out to create an opening in the abdominal wall, called an *ostomy* or *stoma*, for the elimination of feces or urine (Donovan & Pierce, 1976; Kirkpatrick, 1980). There are various types of ostomies. For example, in an ileostomy the stoma is made from the small intestine, whereas in a colostomy it is made from the large intestine. With a urostomy a loop of the ileum is used for the elimination of urine. In some cases the ostomies are temporary and in others they are permanent. In either case they can create considerable physical and psychological problems for the patient.

Significant levels of depression, including feelings of despair and worthlessness, are common following any type of ostomy (e.g., Sutherland, Orbach, Dyk, & Bard, 1952). Patients may experience feelings of shame and dirtiness as they are forced to deal openly with bodily wastes. Patients are also often shocked initially by the swollen, sore, red appearance of the ostomy before it heals (Dericks, 1974; Dietz, 1980), and they may be reluctant to look at it, let others see it, or accept responsibility for its care (e.g., Holland, 1973; Rodriguez, 1981). Not surprisingly, therefore, one of the greatest adjustments necessary to ostomies may be learning to care for them properly. For example, most ostomy patients must learn to wear and care for the appliance or bag into which urine and/or other matter empties, and some patients must learn to irrigate or flush out their intestine in order to promote movement of the stool. In each of these areas, initial attempts at self-care can be very stressful. For example, initial attempts at irrigation can result in painful bloating and cramping (Sutherland *et al.*, 1952). Embarrassment may also result from flatus, as colostomates and ileostomates cannot control the escape of gas. Some patients become very reclusive following ostomy surgery, and others become overly compulsive about cleanliness and self-care. For example, Sutherland *et al.* (1952) described patients who spent more than 6 hours in the bathroom daily irrigating their stomas.

Even if a patient adjusts adequately to the physical restrictions and maintenance required by the ostomy, other problems can result, perhaps the most common of which are sexual in nature. In males, sexual functioning is impaired in about 50% of colostomy patients and in almost all patients after bladder removal (Kirkpatrick, 1980). Dyk and Sutherland (1956) found that of a sample of 22 males, only 3 did not report some degree of impotence and a decrease in frequency of intercourse. Similarly, most of the women they interviewed reported a decrease in sexual activity. Unlike males, however, women generally do not sustain physical damage that would prevent the return to sexual activity or cause sterility (Dericks, 1974).

The physical complications that interfere with sexual functioning may be compounded by other factors. Patients commonly report negative body image, lowered self-esteem, and fear of injury (e.g., Dericks, 1974; Holland, 1973). Concerns regarding the loss of sexual attractiveness are also often exacerbated by actual rejection by sexual partners or by the partners' commonly experienced fears of hurting the patients that result in treating them gingerly. In fact, stomas are not fragile and patients are unlikely to be hurt during sexual activity (Donovan & Pierce, 1976). For many patients, adequate psychoeducational support may be sufficient to promote recovery of sexual functioning; for others, sex therapy may be an appropriate intervention (Rodriguez, 1981). Reconstructive surgery should also be considered where appropriate (Dericks, 1974).

Functioning following ostomy may also be impaired in a variety of other ways. For example, patients frequently report postoperative weakness resulting in slow return to normal daily activities including employment, and as a result financial pressures may arise (e.g., Rodriguez, 1981). Dyk and Sutherland (1956) reported that ostomy patients frequently complain of family difficulties, with other family members finding factors such as the patient's extensive use of the bathroom facilities annoying. Patients also reported receiving insufficient support and care from spouses who blame the patient for the negative changes in the family. Unfortunately, there are no reports of well-controlled empirical research on helping ostomy patients cope with the myriad of problems that often confront them.

HEAD AND NECK CANCERS

Surgery for cancer of the head and neck can be emotionally devastating because of its effects on social attractiveness and communication (Dietz, 1980; Holland, 1973). With removal of bone and muscle through surgery, basic functions such as speaking, eating, and swallowing may be impaired (Curtis & Zlotolow, 1980). As a result, patients may experience significant difficulties in social and vocational functioning. Reconstructive surgery and rehabilitation techniques such as speech therapy may aid many patients in regaining function and self-esteem, although complete recovery is often an unrealistic goal (Curtis & Zlotolow, 1980; Dietz, 1980).

There is little written of either an empirical or clinical nature on coping with the psychological difficulties resulting from head and neck surgery. However, a report by Nigl (1979) suggests that EMG biofeedback and deep muscle relaxation training may be useful in some situations. Nigl gave seven relaxation training sessions to a 62-year-old patient who had not eaten solid food for more than 3 years following radical oral surgery and postsurgery radiation therapy. The patient sustained nerve and muscle damage during surgery, and could not perform basic functions such as eating and swallowing effectively. Nigl reported that following biofeedback and relaxation training, the patient once again began eating solid food, and that this improvement was maintained at 1- and 4-month follow-up testing. Secondary benefits included increased self-esteem and self-confidence and reduced hopelessness. These results suggest that in some cases behavioral interventions may help to improve physical and psychological functioning in head and neck surgery patients. Clearly, however, additional research employing larger groups of patients and adequate control procedures is needed.

SUMMARY

The treatment of cancer by surgery can produce significant psychological and physical distress for patients, including major disruptions in emotional health, life-style, social and vocational functioning, sexual functioning, appearance, self-image, and physical capabilities. Although these difficulties can result to a greater or lesser degree from all types of cancer surgery, they appear to be especially prevalent in patients who have had surgery for breast, gynecological, genital, urinary, colorectal, or head and neck cancers.

Although there is little research evidence on effective ways of reducing the distress of cancer surgery, clinical observations suggest that many of the factors contributing to psychological distress and poor postoperative adjustment are susceptible to intervention. For example, training and communication skills to promote improved social and sexual functioning and relaxation techniques to reduce anxiety may be beneficial. Stress may also be reduced through follow-up care including group therapy, adequate rehabilitation, and appropriate referrals for professional help (e.g., for sex therapy). It should be kept in mind, however, that although such interventions seem warranted on clinical grounds, there is little empirical evidence to support their use. Indeed, perhaps the major conclusion of a review of the surgery literature must be that the distress caused by various forms of cancer surgery urgently warrants behavioral research in the areas of prevention and rehabilitation.

Chemotherapy

DESCRIPTION OF TREATMENT AND SIDE EFFECTS

Chemotherapy has become a common treatment for many types of cancers. In contrast to the 1960s, when chemotherapy was frequently considered a last resort for cancers that did not respond to other forms of treatment, chemotherapy is now often considered a preferred treatment approach (Krakoff, 1981). Moreover, some forms of cancer, if discovered early enough, are considered to be curable with chemotherapy (e.g., acute lymphoblastic leukemia and testicular cancer). Unfortunately, however, chemotherapy can produce some of the most adverse side effects of any form of cancer treatment.

Chemotherapy is a systemic treatment involving the administration of chemicals that are toxic to rapidly dividing cells, such as those that compose cancerous tissue, and therefore helps to arrest or retard the malignant disease process. Regrettably, however, these toxic chemicals do not limit their action to cancerous cells. As Dempster, Balson, and Whalen (1976) have explained, "in essence, malignant cells are more susceptible to toxic agents . . . than normal tissue. The result can be described as an attempt to poison the malignant cells before the normal tissues are seriously affected by toxic substances. This can become a close race [p. 2]."

As a result of its effects on normal tissues, even a "successful" course of chemotherapy can produce a variety of adverse side effects, including decreased immunity to other diseases, changes in liver enzymes, hair loss, fatigue, loss of appetite, stomatitis, nausea, vomiting, diarrhea, temporary or permanent frigidity or impotence, change in skin color, and negative affects such as anxiety and depression (e.g., Golden, 1975; Greer, 1979; Peterson & Popkin, 1980). Each of these side effects, including emotional states such as anxiety and depression, are produced by the direct pharmacological properties of the anticancer drugs. Unfortunately, no medications have yet been identified that can adequately control these side effects in most cancer patients. Thus, there are several relatively severe and largely unavoidable *pharmacological* side effects that are reliably produced by various cancer chemotherapies.

In addition to these pharmacological side effects, many patients develop *conditioned* negative responses to their chemotherapy; that is, the sights, smells, and even thoughts associated with chemotherapy can begin to elicit responses such as anxiety, nausea, and vomiting (e.g., Morrow, 1982; Nesse, Carli, Curtis, & Kleinman, 1980). For example, Redd, Andresen, & Minagawa (1982) reported that one of their patients became nauseated in a restaurant when she happened to see her chemotherapy nurse, and several of our patients have reported becoming nauseated and vomiting at home the evening before their chemotherapy as they began to think about the ordeal they would go through the next day. Unfortunately, these conditioned side effects can be as debilitating as or more debilitating than the pharmacological side effects of the drugs.

The pharmacological and conditioned side effects of cancer chemotherapy can be exceptionally aversive. In fact, some patients become suicidal because of them, and others refuse to undergo continued treatments, fully aware that a hastened death is the probable consequence of their decision (e.g., Seigel & Longo, 1981; Whitehead, 1975). Thus, in a clinical sense, the successful chemotherapeutic treatment of cancer depends not only upon developing drugs that are effective against specific cancers, but also upon finding methods of reducing the adverse consequences of these drugs. This would make the increased quantity of life gained through chemotherapy more worthwhile to the patient than the decreased quality of life that results during treatment.

Most pharmacological and behavioral research aimed at reducing the side effects of cancer chemotherapy has focused on the common and sometimes disabling side effects of nausea, vomiting, and the negative affects (e.g., anxiety and depression) that are commonly observed in chemotherapy patients. The results of this research are discussed next.

PHARMACOLOGICAL RESEARCH

A large number of laboratory and clinical studies have been conducted to identify drugs that might be effective in reducing the nausea and vomiting caused by many chemotherapy protocols. Because of the scope, technical nature, and large number of these studies, a critical review of this literature is not included in the present chapter. However, two general points should be made regarding this research. First, despite the considerable efforts made in this area, no antiemetic drug has emerged that is regarded as adequate in controlling the side effects of chemotherapy (Chang, 1981; Frytak & Moertel, 1981; Seigel & Longo, 1981). Second, past failures in identifying successful drug treatments for chemotherapy side effects should not be taken as a comment on the future likelihood of developing effective antiemetic agents. Several researchers have identified potentially effective antiemetic drugs (e.g., delta-9-tetrahydrocannabinol: Poster, Penta, Bruno, & Macdonald, 1981; high dose metoclopramide: Gralla, Itri, Pisko, Squillante, Kelsen, Braun, Bordin, Braun, & Young, 1981; and multidrug therapies: Peroutka & Snyder, 1982); further research on these and other drugs is urgently needed. It should be noted, however, that even if these drugs are proven to be effective in reducing such side effects as nausea and vomiting, most of them appear to have several side effects, including fatigue, loss of muscle coordination, hallucinations, psychological highs and lows, and specific organ toxicities. For some patients these side effects can outweigh potential benefits. Thus, although the search for effective pharmacological treatment should continue, it should not dampen the enthusiasm or acceptance of the pursuit of alternative approaches to controlling side effects of chemotherapy, such as the behavioral approaches described in the next section.

BEHAVIORAL RESEARCH

The failure of antiemetic medications to control chemotherapy-induced nausea and vomiting combined with the observation that many cancer patients display what appears to be *conditioned* nausea and vomiting prior to the actual chemotherapy infusion have led a growing number of researchers to use behavioral techniques to relax the patient and, it is hoped, reduce adverse reactions to chemotherapy. Five types of behavioral interventions have been reported in the literature: hypnosis, progressive muscle relaxation training with relaxation imagery, systematic desensitization, electromyographic (EMG) biofeedback, and stress management training.

Hypnosis was one of the first behavioral procedures used to decrease the side effects of chemotherapy. The early hypnosis studies (e.g., Dempster *et al.*, 1976; LaBaw, Holton, Tewell, & Eccles, 1975) were uniformly positive in suggesting that the procedure was effective in reducing nausea and vomiting. However, these studies did not employ adequate experimental designs, and their conclusions were based primarily on subjective observations by the authors and patients rather than on objective scales or quantifiable assessment techniques. Fortunately, a more methodologically rigorous study by

Redd *et al.* (1982) has confirmed and extended the implications of these earlier reports. Using a multiple base-line design, Redd *et al.* individually hypnotized six female cancer patients both before and during their chemotherapy treatments. Results indicated that hypnosis reduced each patient's ratings of nausea before and during chemotherapy and completely suppressed anticipatory vomiting. When three patients missed hypnosis training before a chemotherapy session, anticipatory nausea and vomiting returned.

Several studies conducted in our clinic have employed progressive muscle relaxation training and guided relaxation imagery with cancer chemotherapy patients. Although the designs of these studies have varied from a single subject case report (Burish & Lyles, 1979) to experimental designs containing an attention control and/or a no-treatment control group (Burish & Lyles, 1981; Lyles, Burish, Krozely, & Oldham, 1982), similar dependent variables and treatment procedures have been used. Patients were studied during 5 to 11 consecutive chemotherapy sessions, which were divided into base-line, treatment, and follow-up. Dependent measures included physiological responses (pulse rate and blood pressure), affect checklists (anxiety, hostility, and depression), patient ratings of nausea and anxiety, nurse rating of nausea and anxiety, and nurse reports of emesis. These measures were collected before, during, and/or after each chemotherapy session. Results consistently indicated that the relaxation training procedure was significantly more effective than the control procedures in reducing patients' physiological arousal, anxiety, depression, and nausea during and after chemotherapy. The observer ratings were consistent with the patients' self-reports.

Morrow and Morrel (1982) compared systematic desensitization to a Rogerian-oriented counseling condition and a no-treatment control condition in a well-designed study involving 60 cancer patients who reported anticipatory (prechemotherapy) nausea and vomiting. Patients in the two treatment conditions were given two experimental sessions in the therapist's office between their fourth and fifth chemotherapy treatments. Ratings of the intensity, frequency, and duration of anticipatory nausea and vomiting were taken during patients' third and fourth (base-line) and fifth and sixth (follow-up) sessions. Results indicated that systematic desensitization was significantly more effective than either of the other conditions in reducing the severity and duration of anticipatory nausea and vomiting. No significant differences were found between the counseling and no-treatment control conditions.

Multiple-site EMG biofeedback has been combined with progressive muscle relaxation training in one case study investigation (Burish, Shartner, & Lyles, 1981). The study included three base-line, four treatment, and three follow-up sessions conducted during 10 consecutive chemotherapy treatments. Results indicated that, compared to base-line, during training and follow-up the patient showed reductions in physiological arousal (EMG, pulse rate, and systolic blood pressure) and reported feeling less anxious and nauseated.

One other behavioral technique used to control the side effects of chemotherapy was Meichenbaum's (1977) stress inoculation training procedure. Moore and Altmaier (1981) taught this procedure to nine chemotherapy patients during six training sessions. The authors reported no objective data but suggested that patients showed fewer anxiety-related behaviors following the training sessions.

Overall, studies assessing effectiveness of behavioral approaches to reducing the adverse side effects of cancer chemotherapy, especially conditioned nausea and vomiting, are remarkably consistent and promising in outcome. As Redd and Andrykowski (1982) have pointed out, these results are especially noteworthy because they have been generated by several different procedures employed by numerous therapists working in different clinics with patients having different types of cancer receiving different chemotherapy protocols. Nonetheless, although promising, this research is in its early stages, and considerable additional investigation is needed. In particular, four important issues can be identified that have been inadequately studied but that are important to the large-scale clinical application of behavioral techniques.

First, although the behavioral procedures employed were generally effective during the treatment sessions, there are few data on the generalization of treatment effects beyond the treatment sessions. That is, do patients actually learn a *self-control* technique? Unfortunately, several of the better controlled studies suggest that the treatment intervention does not generalize at all (e.g., Redd & Andrykowski, 1982) or only moderately well (Lyles *et al.*, 1982), although there is at least one study (Morrow & Morrell, 1982) in which relatively strong generalization effects were observed on a short-term basis (i.e., during the two chemotherapy sessions following the final behavioral treatment session). Generalization might be improved by several techniques. For example, it may be helpful to decrease gradually the role of the therapist and to increase the responsibility for and autonomy of the patient in self-relaxation. Second, periodic booster sessions could be provided by the therapist following the completion of the formal training program. Third, the nurse who administers the chemotherapy or someone who is with the patient during chemotherapy (e.g., a spouse) might be taught to help the patient in relaxing and carrying out the behavioral technique in question. Finally, a cue-controlled procedure might be taught in which feelings of anxiety or nausea serve as constant cues automatically eliciting the behavioral self-control procedure. Cue-controlled learning would help assure that the behavioral technique is applied in the appropriate situation.

Second, the treatment procedures employed to date have generally been costly in professional time and training. Spending several hours of professional time over the course of several individual training sessions is an expensive and impractical approach considering the number of therapists available, the number of chemotherapy patients that are having problems, and the potential monetary costs involved. More efficient techniques such as group training, the use of audiotapes, and the training of spouses, friends, or volunteers as therapists are needed. Also, research is needed to help identify variables that would enable a clinician to predict which types of patients are and are not likely to respond to different behavioral intervention strategies. Such research would allow a better matching of patient and treatment variables, and thus would be an initial step toward more individualized and efficient patient care.

Third (and relevant to issues of efficacy), additional research is needed to identify patients at risk for developing adverse conditioned responses to chemotherapy and then to develop procedures that might *prevent* the development of such responses. Recent multivariate analyses, for example, suggest that patients who develop conditioned nausea and vomiting tend to have more severe posttreatment vomiting, to be younger, and to be receiving specific types of chemotherapy protocols (Cohen, Sheehan, Ruckdeschel, & Blanchard, 1982; Morrow, 1982). Others have suggested that increased levels of anxiety and depression and the use of inhibitory coping styles are associated with the development of anticipatory nausea and vomiting (Altmaier, Ross, & Moore, 1982). Clearly, both psychological and physiological factors contribute to individual responses to chemotherapy treatment. Hopefully, several of these factors are open to modification such that the development of unnecessarily adverse responses to chemotherapy can be prevented.

Finally, it should be noted that some chemotherapy patients receiving behavioral interventions actually become conditioned to the relaxation procedure, and as a result the behavioral intervention exacerbates rather than ameliorates the problem. Similar observations have been made regarding antiemetic medications (e.g., Kutz, Borysenko, Come, & Benson, 1980). It is unclear why such conditioning occurs in some patients, but obviously this is a question that deserves further study.

CONFINEMENT TO GERM-FREE ENVIRONMENTS

Another source of stress to some patients receiving chemotherapy derives from their complete and prolonged physical isolation in a gnotobiotic or germ-free environment. Because chemotherapy can greatly reduce the body's ability to resist disease, chemotherapy patients frequently acquire various infections; in fact, infections are a leading cause of death in cancer chemotherapy patients (Kellerman, Siegel, & Rigler, 1980). In order to reduce the risk of infection in patients with severely reduced immunocompetence, isolation in germ-free environments is sometimes employed. Two basic types of protected environments are used: (a) a plastic tent erected around a normal hospital bed; and (b) a small room kept sterile by blowing air through cleansing filters arranged in parallel layers, commonly referred to as a laminar airflow unit. In either case, the protected environment eliminates skin-to-skin contact with other people, confines movement to a very small area, and raises the possibilities of both sensory isolation and social deprivation.

There has been much speculation about the stressfulness of prolonged stays in germ-free environments (sometimes greater than 200 days; Kohle, Simons, Weidlich, Dietrich, & Durner, 1971), and there are reports of patients refusing to begin or continue to stay in these environments (e.g., Holland, Plumb, Yates, Harris, Tuttolomondo, Holmes, & Holland, 1977; Kohle et al., 1971). However, there are few objective data on the degree of psychological stressfulness that isolation produces. Moreover, the research that has been done does not support many of the speculations.

Although several articles have been published on patients' responses to isolation in germ-free environments (e.g., Gordon, 1975; Kohle et al., 1971), only a few contain objective data. In one of these investigations, Holland et al. (1977) studied 52 adults who received chemotherapy for relapse of acute leukemia and were confined to laminar airflow rooms. Psychological functioning was measured by means of a diary and forced-choice questionnaires completed by the patient, a clinical interview, clinical records, and rating scales completed by the attending nurses. The results were encouraging: no symptoms of sensory deprivation (e.g., heightened anxiety or hallucinations) were observed, and no consistent isolation-related changes were found in scales measuring negative affects, delirium, or psychoses. Although some patients appeared to have some difficulty adapting to the new environment during the first 48 to 72 hours, their discomfort was relatively minor and decreased after this initial period passed. The most frequent complaint was not being able to touch other people.

In another investigation reporting objective data, Kellerman et al. (1980) studied 14 children with a median age of approximately 7 years who were confined to a laminar airflow unit for a median of 87.5 days. The children had a variety of advanced-staged malignant solid tumors for which they were receiving treatment. Dependent measures included standard IQ tests, a behavior rating scale completed by the attending nurses, and clinical observations. In agreement with the findings of Holland et al. (1977), results indicated no consistent pattern of intellectual decrement and no long-term or debilitating psychological effects. Most of the children did show some depression upon entry to the unit and again between the seventh and ninth weeks, but these effects were not severe and were relatively short-lived.

Overall, the data suggest that protective isolation is not a significant source of additional stress for cancer chemotherapy patients who are willing to undergo it. However, this conclusion must be regarded as tentative until additional research employing adequate control groups (e.g., matched inpatients not in protective isolation) is completed. It should also be noted that the patients in both the Holland *et al.* and Kellerman *et al.* studies seemed to receive considerable support from the medical staff and had liberal visitation with parents and family (although, of course, no skin contact). It is likely that protective isolation *can* cause considerable distress if such supportive care is not provided.

SUMMARY

Although commonly used and often effective in prolonging the cancer patient's life, chemotherapy frequently produces a host of adverse side effects of which negative affect, nausea, and vomiting have been given the most attention. Unfortunately, antiemetic medication has so far proven unsatisfactory in controlling these side effects, although several promising drug therapies have been identified. Behavioral techniques such as hypnosis, progressive muscle relaxation training, systematic desensitization, EMG biofeedback, and stress management training have also been employed, especially with conditioned responses, and have generally been found to be effective. However, there is a need for additional research in order to increase the generalization of the treatment effect, create a practical means of providing behavioral techniques on a large scale, and develop early intervention preventive measures. Finally, there is considerable concern that the protective isolation techniques sometimes used with chemotherapy patients may cause problems associated with sensory and social deprivation. However, the few existing data on this topic suggest that this need not be the case if adequate support is provided by the medical staff.

Radiation Therapy

DESCRIPTION OF TREATMENT AND SIDE EFFECTS

Like chemotherapy, radiation therapy is a widely used treatment for a variety of cancers. According to Krisch and Goodman (1981), for example, over 50% of all cancer patients receive some form of radiation therapy.

Although radiation is often effective in destroying cancerous tissue, it can also cause a number of adverse side effects, including some so severe that patients voluntarily decide to terminate the treatment (Frytak & Moertel, 1981).

There are two basic types of radiation therapy: external beam therapy and internal therapy. External beam therapy is the most commonly used type of radiation treatment and involves directing a beam of ionizing radiation (e.g., X rays or radium) at an area of malignant tissue in order to destroy the tissue. The beam of radiation can usually be directed with considerable accuracy to the proper area and depth to destroy the tumor and minimize, but rarely eliminate, the destruction of normal tissue (Krisch & Goodman, 1981; Prosnitz, 1971). Thus, unlike chemotherapy, external beam radiation is generally considered a specific rather than a systemic treatment.

Internal radiation therapy is used less frequently than external beam therapy and involves the placement of a radioactive isotope into the body. This form of radiation may be used for a small, localized tumor as, for example, in bladder and cervical cancer (Donovan & Pierce, 1976; National Cancer Institute, 1980). Because the literature relevant to psychosocial issues and behavioral interventions with radiation patients focuses almost exclusively on external beam treatment, internal radiation treatment is not discussed further in this chapter. However, it should be noted that many of the problems cited for external beam radiation are also descriptive of internal radiation treatment.

The medical basis for the use of radiation with cancer patients is that radiation interferes with cell division in rapidly multiplying cells such as those composing cancerous tissue (Creech, 1975). However, in addition to destroying malignant tissue, radiation also affects normal tissue, which can cause a variety of side effects. Common physical side effects of radiation therapy include fatigue, skin irritation and peeling, burns, and hair loss in the irradiated area. Radiation therapy for head and neck cancer may damage the mucous membranes in the mouth and throat area, resulting in problems such as congestion, change or loss of taste, dysphagia, considerably increased dental caries, periodontal infections, and bone necrosis (e.g., Donaldson, 1982). With abdominal radiation or radiation over a large area, nausea, vomiting, anorexia, and bone marrow depression may result. For example, approximately 79% of patients receiving radiation to the trunk area report some degree of nausea and vomiting, with resulting loss of appetite and weight (Welch, 1980). Unfortunately, as with chemotherapy, this nausea and vomiting cannot usually be adequately controlled by antiemetic medication (Frytak & Moertel, 1981; Harris, 1978). Finally, abdominal and pelvic radiation may cause diarrhea, sexual dysfunction, and sterility (e.g., Andersen & Hacker, in press; Donaldson, 1977).

In general, the specific side effects experienced by radiation patients are a function of two variables: (a) the particular area of the body, or field, that is radiated; and (b) the dose of radiation administered (Donaldson, 1982). The side effects usually begin after the first treatment and increase in severity with additional treatments as the tolerance of normal tissue to withstand the radiation is approached and surpassed. Radiation treatments are not given if it is determined that a medically unacceptable level of damage to normal tissue, especially to major organs, would result. Thus, although patients do sometimes voluntarily elect to terminate their treatment because of the side effects, radiation therapy is rarely life-threatening.

LITERATURE REVIEW

From a behavioral perspective, radiation therapy has received considerably less empirical attention than chemotherapy. In fact, the great majority of material published in the area is largely descriptive in nature, and covers the various problems that radiation patients encounter during the course of their treatment and stresses the need for the development of methods to prevent or ameliorate these problems. In view of the extant literature, the radiation section of the chapter is organized by problem areas that have been identified rather than by treatments that have been developed.

Problems in Patient Education

Most of the reported problems associated with radiation treatment in cancer patients appear to involve inadequate preparation or education. In some cases, patients apparently receive little or no relevant information, while in other cases the information is presented in such a complex fashion or at such a stressful time that patients fail to understand and remember it. Prior research suggests that several repetitions of various types of information may often be required before a cancer patient is able to understand and recall the information (e.g., Isler, 1971; Rotman, Rogow, DeLeon, & Heskel, 1977). Unfortunately, in most of the literature in the radiation area, it is unclear whether patients' reports of inadequate information were due to a lack of presentation or to an inadequate presentation and repetition of the material. Regardless, the result is the same: an unprepared and confused patient whose treatment becomes much more frightening and aversive than necessary.

Perhaps the most frequent information problems cited in the radiation literature involve patient complaints about inadequate preparation prior to the onset of their treatment. Patients reporting for radiation often deny that they were informed of their diagnosis (Peck, 1972; Peck & Boland, 1977; Rotman *et al.*, 1977). For example, Peck found that only 14 of 50 patients reporting for radiation stated that they had been told directly by their referring physician that they had cancer. Even if cancer patients do know their diagnoses, however, they frequently do not understand the intent of the radiation about to be administered (e.g., Isler, 1971; Mitchell & Glicksman, 1977). Radiation is often seen by patients as a last-ditch effort (e.g., Creech, 1975; Holland, Rowland, Lebovits, & Rusalem, 1979). For example, in one sample of radiation patients, 94% associated radiation therapy with inoperability of their tumors and hence with poor prognoses (Peck & Boland, 1977). In reality, however, radiation therapy is frequently used with curative intent (e.g., Krisch & Goodman, 1981; Prosnitz, 1971). When the prognosis is good, it thus appears that unnecessary anxiety and depression can be avoided if this information, appropriately couched in terms that avoid guarantees, is conveyed to the patient until the patient understands it. If radiation is being used with palliative intent only, it appears that conveying this information would at least help to avoid confusion and to help the patient begin to cope with and prepare for the course of the treatment and disease.

In addition to concerns regarding the intent of radiation therapy, patients hold many misconceptions about the specific nature of radiation and the equipment used to deliver treatment. One of the publications of the National Cancer Institute (1980) graphically describes this problem: "The prospect of receiving an invisible treatment from a large machine in a room with no other human being present is understandably frightening [p. 29]." For example, Peck and Boland (1977) found that, especially at first, many patients fear that the machine will fall on them. Other patients, well aware of advertisements cautioning against the use of X rays and other forms of radiation, fear that the treatment itself will cause another type of cancer to develop (Peck & Boland, 1977). Actually, the dangers of radiation causing cancer in other parts of the body are minimal because of the high level of accuracy of the beam and careful shielding with lead of surrounding areas. Finally, confusion between external beam radiation therapy and other types of radiation may cause family and friends to fear that the patient is radioactive and hence to avoid him or her (Rotman et al., 1977; Vachon & Lyall, 1976). This behavior is in turn likely to increase the patient's feelings of isolation and abandonment. In fact, patients are not radioactive except with the less frequently used internal radiation therapy, and even in this situation the therapy is generally short-term, the patient is hospitalized and contacts with others are minimized, and following removal of the isotope no radioactivity remains (Prosnitz, 1971). Clearly, much of the anxiety and confusion characteristic of many radiation patients and their families could be eliminated if adequate psychoeducational preparation for radiation therapy were routinely provided.

A final educational problem concerns the specific side effects of radiation therapy. Many patients commonly have exaggerated fears regarding possible pain, disfigurement, loss of bodily and sexual functioning, and harm to major organs that might result from the treatment (National Cancer Institute, 1980; Peck & Boland, 1977; Rotman *et al.*, 1977). The harboring of these unrealistic fears can have at least three possible consequences. First, unnecessary stress may result simply because the anticipated side effects are much worse than the actual side effects. Second, additional stress may accrue because the patient cannot appropriately predict and plan for the actual side effects of the treatment (Holland, 1977). Research has repeatedly suggested that if the patient is informed about and can predict the likelihood of the possible side effects of the medical treatment, the side effects will be more tolerable than if such understanding and prediction is not present (e.g., Egbert, Battit, Welch, & Bartlett, 1964). Finally, patients may misinterpret the presence of side effects to mean that they are not responding to treatment and that their disease is progressing or getting worse, again increasing the levels of anxiety or hopelessness (e.g., Peck & Boland, 1977). In fairness, it should be noted that many physicians have expressed concerns that forewarning patients of the possible side effects of radiation will increase the likelihood of these side effects occurring. However, the data do not appear to support this view. Instead, it appears that patients are usually unlikely to complain of problems that did not occur, even if these problems were mentioned as possible results of the treatment (Holland, 1977; Peck & Boland, 1977; Welch, 1980). Moreover, data collected by Mitchell and Glicksman (1977) confirm that if given a choice, most patients prefer more complete explanations and realistic expectations prior to beginning treatment.

Problems Associated with Physical Side Effects

Regardless of whether the physical side effects of radiation are accurately anticipated, they can be very stressful to the patient. For example, gastrointestinal problems such as nausea and vomiting occur with several types of radiation therapy, and in some cases can lead to conditioned gastrointestinal symptoms similar to those experienced by chemotherapy patients. Unlike the chemotherapy area, however, little research has been conducted on this problem with radiation patients. Fortunately, however, on the basis of one case study that has been conducted with a radiation patient (Hamberger, 1982), it appears that the relaxation techniques used with chemotherapy patients may be equally effective with radiation patients. The study involved a patient who had received over 30 cobalt radiation therapy sessions following bladder removal and ostomy construction for the treatment of bladder cancer. The patient experienced stomach pain, nausea, and vomiting during the radiation treatments, and several months after the treatments terminated began to reexperience these symptoms for no apparent organic reason. The patient was given one progressive muscle relaxation training session in the therapist's office and was asked to practice relaxing regularly at home, which he reported doing. The reports of the patient and his spouse indicated that relaxation training produced an immediate cessation of the gastric attacks and that this effect was maintained at a 1-year follow-up. As in the chemotherapy area, these results suggest that relaxation training techniques may be effective in reducing treatment-related nausea and vomiting. Clearly, however, additional work employing larger patient samples and adequate control procedures is needed in the radiation area.

A common side effect of radiation to the head and neck area involves dental problems. For example, radiation can decrease salivary flow and affect tissues in the bones, leading to rampant dental caries and to infections that can result in osteoradionecrosis and consequent masticatory disability and facial disfigurement (e.g., Driezen, Daley, & Drane, 1977; Frank, Herdly, & Philippe, 1965). Fortunately, selected removal of diseased teeth or those with poor prognoses prior to radiation, combined with postradiation preventive dental care programs (e.g., good oral hygiene, use of topical fluoride solutions, regular dental appointments), appear to be effective in reducing the incidence of dental disease. However, many patients do not comply with preventive dental care programs set up for them, and as a result, serious side effects emerge. Thus, there is a strong need for research aimed at increasing compliance with dental hygiene programs that are necessary to minimize the adverse consequences of radiation treatment to the head and neck areas.

SUMMARY

In reviewing the radiation area, Rotman *et al.* (1977) concluded that "few therapeutic modalities in medicine induce more misunderstanding, confusion, and apprehension than the use of irradiation in cancer treatment [p. 744]." Our review supports this conclusion. It appears that radiation patients are often not informed or inadequately informed about the reason they are receiving radiation therapy and its nature, side effects, or likely outcome, and as a result the radiation experience is more intimidating, confusing, and stressful than necessary. Since data (e.g., Mitchell & Glicksman, 1977; Welch, 1980) suggest that patients are hesitant to approach physicians and other medical personnel with their complaints or needs for additional information, it appears that members of the treatment team should take considerable responsibility for educating and preparing patients for radiation treatment.

In addition to improving patient preparation for radiation therapy, research is needed either to develop ways of helping patients cope with the side effects of radiation (e.g., nausea and vomiting) or to comply with the successful treatment techniques that have already been developed (e.g., dental care programs). In some cases treatment approaches already developed to deal with similar side effects associated with other medical treatments (e.g., the use of relaxation training for chemotherapy-induced nausea and vomiting) may be effective in the radiation area, whereas in other cases new treatment techniques may need to be developed. In either case, the severity and frequency of radiation-induced side effects warrant considerably increased research efforts.

General Issues

Although there are specific problems and issues relevant to each type of cancer treatment, there are also several general issues that are common to all cancer treatments. Several of these general issues are discussed in this final section.

First, the literature reviewed in this chapter clearly illustrates that despite the ubiquitousness of cancer and the devastating nature of many cancer treatments, there is a *dearth of well-controlled empirical research or well-developed theoretical positions* relevant to the topic of coping with cancer treatments. The majority of published articles contain anecdotes, clinical observations, personal accounts, case studies, or subjective impressions based on limited observation. Few of these articles even meet the criteria of a good descriptive study; for example, most do not contain detailed observations objectively documented over the course of a treatment experience. The few experimental studies that are reported often contain serious problems with population sampling (size and representativeness), demand characteristics, adequate control groups, and reliable and valid dependent measures. Clearly, progress in helping people cope with the stresses of cancer treatments depends not only on additional research, but more importantly on better quality research.

Second, although there is a literature on preparing people for psychotherapy (e.g., Holmes & Urie, 1975) and noxious medical or surgical procedures (e.g., Langer, Janis, & Wolfer, 1975), there is a surprising dearth of empirical or clinical work on *how to best prepare people, especially adults, for various cancer treatments*. How do you prepare a woman for the loss of a breast as a result of radical mastectomy? What should a radiation or chemotherapy patient be told about the likely side effects of treatment? How much information should be given or at least offered? Is it better to begin treatment immediately after the diagnosis is made or wait until a patient is able to understand and appreciate to some extent what will occur? McCue

(1980) has recently reviewed the literature on preparing children for noxious medical procedures, and has suggested several possible applications to the pediatric cancer area in particular. A similar review and analysis is necessary for the adult cancer literature. As is true in other areas, adequate preparation should help to reduce the negative impact of many forms of cancer treatment.

Third, in each of the literatures associated with various cancer treatments, the issue of *personal control* repeatedly arises. Cancer treatments rarely give control and responsibility to the patient, and commonly take them away. Except perhaps for minor adjustments in diet, cancer patients generally are not told to do anything except just take their treatment, and wait. They are also rarely given any choices: they are generally told they *need* a *specific* treatment, and that they are *scheduled* to receive it on a *certain* day. Is this the best approach? Would patients benefit psychologically and do no worse physically if they participated actively in making decisions regarding their treatment? Is the attraction of many unconventional cancer treatments (e.g., megavitamins, various diets, "natural" medicines, ritualistic prayers and incantations) due in large part to their giving some feeling of control and responsibility back to the patient?

Certainly, there is evidence that people in general (e.g., Averill, 1973) and cancer patients in particular (e.g., Achterberg, Simonton, & Matthews-Simonton, 1976) desire considerable control over their lives. Moreover, several researchers have suggested that the success of various behavioral interventions in helping cancer patients cope with their treatment may be due in large part to the confidence and positive emotional state produced by increased feelings of control (e.g., Lyles *et al.*, 1982; Morrow & Morrel, 1982). However, it is also clear that some people in some situations prefer not to have control and the responsibility that comes with it. There are some cancer patients who prefer that the medical staff make the decisions concerning what treatments should be given, when, and for how long. Thus, although in general it seems wise to give control to patients where possible, it should not be forced upon patients who do not desire it or are not prepared for it. Additional research identifying areas where control can be given and people who would benefit from having it seems warranted.

Fourth, although the focus of this chapter has been on the aversiveness of cancer treatments, it should also be recognized that *terminating treatment may also cause problems*. We and others (e.g., Gorzynski & Holland, 1979; Krant, 1981) have noticed that some patients show increased anxiety and depression when their radiation or chemotherapy ends because they fear that without the treatment their tumor may grow again or new tumors may arise. Thus, bad as it was, the treatment was nevertheless desired because it was viewed as an active agent likely to prolong life. Some of our chemotherapy patients have even welcomed nausea and vomiting because they believed that the sicker they became, the more effective the chemotherapy was in arresting their disease. Several patients also seem to dread the termination of treatment because it may lead to a cessation of the supportive relationships they have established with the medical staff administering the treatments. Thus, it should be recognized that the administration of cancer treatments may lead to one set of coping problems but their cessation may lead to another set. Unfortunately, no published empirical work is available identifying methods of helping cancer patients cope with the increased fears that often arise at the termination of treatment.

Fifth, it should be recognized that *cancer treatments also cause coping problems for patients' families and the medical staff involved in administering the treatments.* For example, Binger, Ablin, Feuerstein, Kushner, Zoger, & Mikkelsen (1969) found that in 50% of the families of a leukemic child, at least one family member needed psychiatric help to cope with the situation; and Stewart, Yarkin, Meyerowitz, Harvey, and Jackson (1982) found that the stresses experienced by nurses working in an outpatient cancer chemotherapy clinic were significantly greater than those experienced by nurses in cardiac, intensive care, or operating room units. A review of this literature is beyond the scope of this chapter; several issues relevant to this topic are discussed by Masters, Cerreto, and Mendlowitz in Chapter 14.

Sixth, the degree to which peer group support can enhance successful coping should be evaluated in a controlled manner. Patient support groups have developed throughout the country, based upon the premise that fellow cancer patients can provide unique empathy, information, and hope and often can present a model of successful coping. Perhaps the best-known group is Reach to Recovery for breast cancer patients, but many other groups are also active (e.g., the Lost Cord Society for laryngectomees). Given the widespread presence of these groups, investigations of their efficacy are warranted. In addition, it may be possible to use these networks to implement other methods of coping.

Finally, it should be recognized that although it is sometimes possible to identify specific stressors associated with cancer treatments, in actuality *the stresses of coping with cancer treatments and of having the disease of cancer are intertwined.* As pointed out by Meyerowitz, Heinrich, and Schag in chapter 6, it is the composite of many separate stresses that make cancer such a dreaded and difficult disease to cope with. Nonetheless, it can be safely predicted that with continued advances in the extent to which cancer treatments can "cure" the patient and extend life expectancy, the greatest challenge to cancer patients will increasingly become learning to live with— and cope with—their treatment.

References

Abitbol, M. M., & Davenport, J. H. Sexual dysfunction after therapy for cervical carcinoma. *American Journal of Obstetrics and Gynecology*, 1974, *119*, 181–189.

Achterberg, J., Simonton, O. C., & Matthews-Simonton, S. *Stress, psychological factors, and cancer*. Fort Worth, Texas: New Medicine Press, 1976.

Altmaier, E. M., Ross, W., & Moore, K. A pilot investigation of the psychologic functioning of patients with anticipatory vomiting. *Cancer*, 1982, *49*, 201–204.

American Cancer Society. *Cancer 1981: Facts and figures*. New York: Author, 1980.

Andersen, B. L., & Hacker, N. F. Treatment for gynecologic cancer: A review of the effects on female sexuality. *Health Psychology*, in press.

Averill, J. R. Personal control over aversive stimuli and its relationship to stress. *Psychological Bulletin*, 1973, *80*, 286–303.

Bard, M., & Sutherland, A. M. Psychological impact of cancer and its treatment. 4. Adaptation to radical mastectomy. *Cancer*, 1955, *8*, 656–672.

Binger, C. M., Ablin, A. R., Feuerstein, R. C., Kushner, J. H., Zoger, S., & Mikkelsen, C. Childhood leukemia: Emotional impact on patient and family. *New England Journal of Medicine*, 1969, *280*, 414–418.

Blum, L. S. *The psychology of mastectomy: Time to move on*. Paper presented at the meeting of the American Psychological Association, Montreal, September 1980.

Bronner-Huszar, J. The psychological aspects of cancer in man. *Psychosomatics*, 1971, *12*, 133–138.

Burish, T. G., & Lyles, J. N. Effectiveness of relaxation training in reducing the aversiveness of chemotherapy in the treatment of cancer. *Journal of Behavior Therapy and Experimental Psychiatry*, 1979, *10*, 357–361.

Burish, T. G., & Lyles, J. N. Effectiveness of relaxation training in reducing adverse reactions to cancer chemotherapy. *Journal of Behavioral Medicine*, 1981, *4*, 65–78.

Burish, T. G., Shartner, C. D., & Lyles, J. N. Effectiveness of multiple-site EMG biofeedback and relaxation training in reducing the aversiveness of cancer chemotherapy. *Biofeedback and Self-Regulation*, 1981, *6*, 523–535.

Capone, M. A., Westie, K. S., & Good, R. S. Sexual rehabilitation of the gynecologic cancer patient: An effective counseling model. *Frontiers of Radiation Therapy and Oncology*, 1980, *14*, 123–129.

Chang, J. C. Nausea and vomiting in cancer patients: An expression of psychological mechanisms? *Psychosomatics*, 1981, *22*, 707–709.

Cohen, R. E., Sheehan, A., Ruckdeschel, J. C., & Blanchard, E. B. *The prediction of post-treatment and anticipatory nausea and vomiting associated with antineoplastic chemotherapy*. Paper presented at the meeting of the Society of Behavioral Medicine, Chicago, March 1982.

Clifford, E., & Clifford, M. Psychological perspectives of mastectomy and breast reconstruction. *Resident and Staff Physician*, 1981, *27*, 49–55.

Clifford, E., Clifford, M., & Georgiade, N. G. Breast reconstruction following mastectomy: 2. Marital characteristics of patients seeking the procedure. *Annals of Plastic Surgery*, 1980, *5*, 344–346.

Creech, R. H. The psychologic support of the cancer patient: A medical oncologist's viewpoint. *Seminars in Oncology*, 1975, *2*, 285–292.

Curtis, T. A., & Zlotolow, I. M. Sexuality and head and neck cancer. *Frontiers of Radiation Therapy and Oncology*, 1980, *14*, 26–34.

Decker, W. H., & Schwartzman, E. Sexual function following treatment for carcinoma of the cervix. *American Journal of Obstetrics and Gynecology*, 1962, *83*, 401–405.

Dempster, C. R., Balson, P., & Whalen, B. T. Supportive hypnotherapy during the radical treatment of malignancies. *International Journal of Clinical and Experimental Hypnosis*, 1976, *24*, 1–9.

Dericks, V. C. The psychological hurdles of new osteomates: Helping them up . . . and over. *Nursing '74*, 1974, *4*, 52–55.

Dietz, J. H. Adaptive rehabilitation in cancer: A program to improve quality of survival. *Postgraduate Medicine—Cancer Rehabilitation*, 1980, *68*, 145–153.

Donaldson, S. S. Nutritional consequences of radiotherapy. *Cancer Research*, 1977, *37*, 2407–2413.

Donaldson, S. S. Effects of therapy on nutritional status of the pediatric cancer patient. *Cancer Research* (Supplement), 1982, *42*, 729s–736s.

Donovan, M. I., & Pierce, S. G. *Cancer care nursing*. New York: Appleton-Century-Crofts, 1976.

Drellich, M. G., Bieber, I., & Sutherland, A. M. The psychological impact of cancer and cancer surgery. 6. Adaptation to hysterectomy. *Cancer*, 1956, *9*, 1120–1126.

Driezen, S., Daley, T., & Drane, J. Prevention of xerostomia-related dental caries in irradiated cancer patients. *Journal of Dental Research*, 1977, *56*, 99–104.

Dyk, R. B., & Sutherland, A. M. Adaptation of spouse and other family members to the colostomy patient. *Cancer*, 1956, *9*, 123–138.

Egbert, L. D., Battit, G. E., Welch, C. E., & Bartlett, M. K. Reduction of postoperative pain by encouragement and instruction of patients: A study of doctor–patient rapport. *New England Journal of Medicine*, 1964, *270*, 820–827.

Eisenberg, H. S., & Goldenberg, I. S. A measurement of quality of survival of breast cancer patients. In J. L. Hayward & R. D. Bulbrook (Eds.), *Clinical evaluation of breast cancer*. London: Academic Press, 1966.

Frank, R. M., Herdly, J., & Philippe, E. Acquired dental defects and salivary gland lesions after irradiation for carcinoma. *Journal of the American Dental Association*, 1965, *70*, 868–883.

Frytak, S., & Moertel, C. G. Management of nausea and vomiting in the cancer patient. *Journal of the American Medical Association*, 1981, *245*, 393–396.

Furlow, W. L. Sexual consequences of male genitourinary cancer: The role of sex prosthetics. *Frontiers of Radiation Therapy and Oncology*, 1980, *14*, 104–107.

Golden, S. Cancer chemotherapy and management of patient problems. *Nursing Forum*, 1975, *12*, 279–303.

Goldsmith, H. S., & Alday, E. S. Role of the surgeon in the rehabilitation of the breast cancer patient. *Cancer*, 1971, *28*, 1672–1675.

Gordon, A. Psychological aspects of isolator therapy in acute leukaemia. *British Journal of Psychiatry*, 1975, *127*, 588–590.

Gordon, W. A., Freidenbergs, I., Diller, L., Hibbard, M., Wolf, C., Levine, L., Lipkins, R., Ezrachi, O., & Lucido, D. Efficacy of psychosocial intervention with cancer patients. *Journal of Consulting and Clinical Psychology*, 1980, *48*, 743–759.

Gorzynski, J. G., & Holland, J. C. Psychological aspects of testicular cancer. *Seminars in Oncology*, 1979, *6*, 125–129.

Gralla, R. J., Itri, L., Pisko, S., Squillante, A., Kelsen, D., Braun, D., Bordin, L., Braun, T., & Young, C. Antiemetic efficacy of high-dose metoclopramide: Randomized trials with placebo and prochlorperazine in patients with chemotherapy-induced nausea and vomiting. *New England Journal of Medicine*, 1981, *305*, 905–909.

Greer, S. Psychological inquiry: A contribution to cancer research. *Psychological Medicine*, 1979, *9*, 81–89.

Hamberger, L. K. Reduction of generalized aversive responding in a posttreatment cancer patient: Relaxation as an active coping skill. *Journal of Behavior Therapy and Experimental Psychiatry*, 1982, *13*, 229–233.

Harris, J. G. Nausea, vomiting, and cancer treatment. *CA—A Cancer Journal for Clinicians*, 1978, *28*, 194–201.

Harris, J. R., Levene, M. B., & Hellman, S. Primary radiation therapy for early breast cancer. *Frontiers of Radiation Therapy and Oncology*, 1980, *14*, 83–89.

Healey, J. E. Role of rehabilitation medicine in the care of the patient with breast cancer. *Cancer*, 1971, *28*, 1666–1671.

Holland, J. Psychologic aspects of cancer. In J. F. Holland & E. Frei (Eds.), *Cancer medicine*. Philadelphia: Lea & Febiger, 1973.

Holland, J. The clinical course of breast cancer: A psychological perspective. *Frontiers of Radiation Therapy and Oncology*, 1976, *11*, 133–145.

Holland, J. Psychological aspects of oncology. *Medical Clinics of North America*, 1977, *61*, 737–748.

Holland, J. C., & Mastrovito, R. Psychologic adaptation to breast cancer. *Cancer*, 1980, *46*, 1045–1052.

Holland, J., Plumb, M., Yates, J., Harris, S., Tuttolomondo, A., Holmes, J., & Holland, J. F. Psychological response of patients with acute leukemia to germ-free environments. *Cancer*, 1977, *40*, 871–879.

Holland, J. C., Rowland, J., Lebovits, A., & Rusalem, R. Reactions to cancer treatment: Assessment of emotional response to adjuvant radiotherapy as a guide to planned intervention. *The Psychiatric Clinics of North America*, 1979, *2*, 347–358.

Holmes, D. S., & Urie, R. G. Effects of preparing children for psychotherapy. *Journal of Consulting and Clinical Psychology*, 1975, *43*, 311–318.

Isler, C. Radiation therapy: 2. The nurse and the patient. *RN Magazine*, 1971, *34*, 48–51.

Kellerman, J., Siegel, S., & Rigler, D. Special treatment modalities: Laminar airflow rooms. In J. Kellerman (Ed.), *Psychological aspects of childhood cancer*. Springfield, Ill.: Thomas, 1980.

Kendall, P. C., & Watson, D. Psychological preparation for stressful medical procedures. In C. K. Prokop & L. A. Bradley (Eds.), *Medical psychology: Contributions to behavioral medicine*. New York: Academic Press, 1981.

Kirkpatrick, J. R. The stoma patient and his return to society. *Frontiers of Radiation Therapy and Oncology*, 1980, *14*, 20–25.

Kohle, K., Simons, C., Weidlich, S., Dietrich, M., & Durner, A. Psychological aspects in the treatment of leukemia patients in the isolated-bed system "life island." *Psychotherapy and Psychosomatics*, 1971, *19*, 85–91.

Krakoff, I. H. Cancer chemotherapeutic agents. *CA—A Cancer Journal for Clinicians*, 1981, *31*, 4–14.

Krant, M. J. Psychosocial impact of gynecologic cancer. *Cancer*, 1981, *48*, 608–612.

Krisch, R. E., & Goodman, R. L. Introduction: Recent developments and future prospects in radiation therapy. *Seminars in Oncology*, 1981, *8*, 1–2.

Kutz, I., Borysenko, J., Come, S., & Benson, H. Paradoxical emetic response to antiemetic treatment in cancer patients. *New England Journal of Medicine*, 1980, *303*, 1480.

LaBaw, W., Holton, C., Tewell, K., & Eccles, D. The use of self-hypnosis by children with cancer. *The American Journal of Clinical Hypnosis*, 1975, *17*, 233–238.

Langer, E. J., Janis, I. L., & Wolfer, J. Reduction of psychological stress in surgical patients. *Journal of Experimental Social Psychology*, 1975, *11*, 155–165.

Lee, E. C., & Maguire, G. Emotional distress in patients attending a breast clinic. *British Journal of Surgery*, 1975, *62*, 162.

Lyles, J. N., Burish, T. G., Krozely, M. G., & Oldham, R. K. Efficacy of relaxation training and guided imagery in reducing the aversiveness of cancer chemotherapy. *Journal of Consulting and Clinical Psychology*, 1982, *50*, 509–521.

Maguire, P., Tait, A., Brooke, M., Thomas, C., & Sellwood, R. Effect of counselling on the psychiatric morbidity associated with mastectomy. *British Medical Journal*, 1980, *281*, 1454–1456.

McArdle, C. S., Calman, K. C., Cooper, A. F., Hughson, A., Russell, A., & Smith, D. The social, emotional and financial implications of adjuvant chemotherapy in breast cancer. *British Journal of Surgery*, 1981, *68*, 261–264.

McCue, K. Preparing children for medical procedures. In J. Kellerman (Ed.), *Psychological aspects of childhood cancer.* Springfield, Ill.: Thomas, 1980.

Meichenbaum, D. *Cognitive behavior modification: An integrative approach.* New York: Plenum, 1977.

Meyerowitz, B. E. Psychosocial correlates of breast cancer and its treatments. *Psychological Bulletin*, 1980, *87*, 108–131.

Mitchell, G. W., & Glicksman, A. S. Cancer patients: Knowledge and attitudes. *Cancer*, 1977, *40*, 61–66.

Moore, K., & Altmaier, E. M. Stress inoculation training with cancer patients. *Cancer Nursing*, 1981, *4*, 389–393.

Morris, T., Greer, H. S., & White, P. Psychological and social adjustment to mastectomy: A two-year follow-up study. *Cancer*, 1977, *40*, 2381–2387.

Morrow, G. R. Prevalence and correlates of anticipatory nausea and vomiting in chemotherapy patients. *Journal of the National Cancer Institute*, 1982, *68*, 585–588.

Morrow, G. R., & Morrell, C. Behavioral treatment for the anticipatory nausea and vomiting induced by cancer chemotherapy. *New England Journal of Medicine*, 1982, *307*, 1476–1480.

National Cancer Institute, National Institutes of Health, U.S. Department of Health and Human Services. *Coping with cancer: A resource for the health professional* (NIH Publication No. 80-2080). Washington, D.C.: U.S. Government Printing Office, 1980.

Nesse, R. M., Carli, T., Curtis, G. C., & Kleinman, P. D. Pretreatment nausea in cancer chemotherapy: A conditioned response? *Psychosomatic Medicine*, 1980, *42*, 33–36.

Nigl, A. J. Electromyograph training to increase oral cavity functioning in a postoperative cancer patient. *Behavior Therapy*, 1979, *10*, 423–427.

Peck, A. Emotional reactions to having cancer. *American Journal of Roentgenology, Radium Therapy, and Nuclear Medicine*, 1972, *114*, 591–599.

Peck, A., & Boland, J. Emotional reactions to radiation treatment. *Cancer*, 1977, *40*, 180–184.

Peroutka, S. J., & Snyder, S. H. Antiemetics: Neurotransmitter receptor binding predicts therapeutic actions. *Lancet*, 1982, *I*, 658–659.

Peterson, L., & Popkin, M. Neuropsychiatric effects of chemotherapeutic agents for cancer. *Psychosomatics*, 1980, *21*, 141–153.

Poster, D. S., Penta, J. S., Bruno, S., & Macdonald, J. S. Delta-9-tetrahydrocannabinol in clinical oncology. *Journal of the American Medical Association*, 1981, *245*, 2047–2051.

Prosnitz, L. R. Radiation therapy: 1. Treatment for malignant disease. *RN Magazine*, 1971, *34*, 42–47.

Redd, W. H., Andresen, G. V., & Minagawa, R. Y. Hypnotic control of anticipatory emesis in patients receiving cancer chemotherapy. *Journal of Consulting and Clinical Psychology*, 1982, *50*, 14–19.

Redd, W. H., & Andrykowski, M. A. Behavioral intervention in cancer treatment: Controlling aversion reactions to chemotherapy. *Journal of Consulting and Clinical Psychology*, 1982, *50*, 1018–1029.

Rodriguez, D. B. Rehabilitation of the ostomy patient. *Cancer Bulletin*, 1981, *33*, 22–24.

Rotman, M., Rogow, L., DeLeon, G., & Heskel, N. Supportive therapy in radiation oncology. *Cancer*, 1977, *39*, 744–750.

Sanger, C. K., & Reznikoff, M. A comparison of the psychological effects of breast-saving procedures with the modified radical mastectomy. *Cancer*, 1981, *48*, 2341–2346.

Schwartz, M. D. An information and discussion program for women after a mastectomy. *Archives of Surgery*, 1977, *112*, 276–281.

Seibel, M. M., Freeman, M. G., & Graves, W. L. Carcinoma of the cervix and sexual function. *Obstetrics and Gynecology*, 1980, *55*, 484–487.

Seigel, L. J., & Longo, D. L. The control of chemotherapy-induced emesis. *Annals of Internal Medicine*, 1981, *95*, 352–359.

Sewell, H. H., & Edwards, D. W. Pelvic genital cancer: Body image and sexuality. *Frontiers of Radiation Therapy and Oncology*, 1980, *14*, 35–41.

Silberfarb, P. M., Maurer, L. H., & Crouthamel, C. S. Psychosocial aspects of neoplastic disease: 1. Functional status of breast cancer patients during different treatment regimens. *American Journal of Psychiatry*, 1980, *137*, 450–455.

Stewart, B., Yarkin, K., Meyerowitz, B. E., Harvey, J., & Jackson, L. Psychological stress associated with outpatient oncology nursing. *Cancer Nursing*, 1982, *5*, 383–387.

Sutherland, A. M., Orbach, C. E., Dyk, R. B., & Bard, M. Psychological impact of cancer and cancer surgery. 1. Adaptation to dry colostomy; preliminary report and summary of findings. *Cancer*, 1952, *5*, 857–872.

Vachon, M. L. S., & Lyall, W. A. L. Applying psychiatric techniques to patients with cancer. *Hospital and Community Psychiatry*, 1976, *27*, 582–584.

Vincent, C. E., Vincent, B., Greiss, F. C., & Linton, E. B. Some marital-sexual concomitants of carcinoma of the cervix. *Southern Medical Journal*, 1975, *68*, 552–558.

von Eschenbach, A. C. Sexual dysfunction following therapy for cancer of the prostate, testis, and penis. *Frontiers of Radiation Therapy and Oncology*, 1980, *14*, 42–50.

Welch, D. A. Assessment of nausea and vomiting in cancer patients undergoing external beam radiotherapy. *Cancer Nursing*, 1980, *3*, 365–371.

Whitehead, V. M. Cancer treatment needs better antiemetics. *New England Journal of Medicine*, 1975, *293*, 199–200.

Winick, M. A., & Robbins, G. F. The post-mastectomy rehabilitation group program: Structure, procedure, and population demography. *American Journal of Surgery*, 1976, *132*, 599–602.

Winick, M. A., & Robbins, G. F. Physical and psychological readjustment after mastectomy: An evaluation of Memorial Hosital's PMRG program. *Cancer*, 1977, *39*, 478–486.

Witkin, M. H. Sex therapy and mastectomy. *Journal of Sex and Marital Therapy*, 1975, *1*, 290–304.

8

Diabetes Mellitus: A Cognitive–Functional Analysis of Stress*

DENNIS C. TURK
MARJORIE A. SPEERS

Introduction

We ask the reader to ignore the title of this chapter for a moment and to participate in a brief survey.

Each of the items listed below consists of two potential causes of death. The question you are to answer for each item is: Which of the following factors causes more deaths, in general, in the United States?

1. (a) Pregnancy, childbirth, and abortion or (b) diabetes
2. (a) Tuberculosis or (b) diabetes
3. (a) Leukemia or (b) diabetes
4. (a) Homicide or (b) diabetes
5. (a) Breast cancer or (b) diabetes
6. (a) Stroke or (b) diabetes
7. (a) Heart disease or (b) diabetes

In items 1–5, the correct answer is (b), diabetes. Diabetes is the tenth leading cause of death in the United States across all age groups and the sixth

*Completion of the chapter was funded by Biomedical Research Support Grant NIH5-507RR07015 and an award sponsored by the American Association of Diabetes Educators and Ames Division of Miles Laboratories.

191

leading cause of death among persons over 65 years of age (U.S. Surgeon General's Report, 1979). It is reported to be the direct cause of over 37,000 deaths in the United States annually (USDHEW, 1979). The correct answers to items 6 and 7 are (a), stroke and heart disease, respectively.

The frequencies of the causes of death were derived from vital statistics reports prepared by the National Center for Health Statistics (reported in Fischhoff, Slovic, & Lichtenstein, 1977). These statistics are based on the causes of death recorded on death certificates. Of people with diabetes, 25% have cardiovascular disease, which itself is a major cause of death. Diabetes is rarely listed as the direct cause of death when cardiovascular disease is present. Thus, although the ostensible cause of death may be cardiovascular disease, the underlying cause may be diabetes. The United States Department of Health, Education, and Welfare (1979) has acknowledged this fact and estimated that diabetes may be, at least indirectly, a cause of an additional 91,000 deaths.

Based on preliminary results reported recently (USDHEW, 1979), there are 4.8 million diagnosed diabetics in the United States with an additional 5 million undiagnosed cases. In 1978, 612,000 persons were newly diagnosed as diabetic. The incidence of diabetes, moreover, has been increasing steadily over the past 20 years (USDHEW, 1979).

In addition to the role of diabetes in mortality, it is a major cause of other serious health problems. Diabetes is the leading cause of new blindness in the United States. Diabetics are 25 times more likely than nondiabetics to become blind; approximately 5000 diabetics become blind each year (Lipsett, 1980). Neurological and vascular disease resulting from diabetes make the diabetic person 30 times more likely than a nondiabetic to suffer the loss of a limb (Lipsett, 1980). Degeneration of the kidneys is a major problem among diabetic patients; many diabetics require renal dialysis and about 50% of all insulin-dependent diabetics die from kidney failure. Patients with diabetes may suffer either severe pain or loss of tactile sensation from nerve impairment. Perinatal losses to pregnant diabetic women are 5–7 times higher than among the nondiabetic population; the rate of congenital abnormalities in the neonates of diabetic mothers is 3 times higher than the expected rate (Metzger, 1980). The range and severity of medical complications in conjunction with regular medical maintenance of the disease makes diabetes the fourth leading cause of visits to physicians.

These statistics have been catalogued to emphasize the magnitude and range of the problem of diabetes. Yet diabetes has received relatively little attention from behavioral scientists (Hamburg, Lipsett, Inoff, & Drash, 1980). Our purpose in this chapter is to describe the nature of diabetes, review the available literature on the relationship between stress and diabetes and on coping with diabetes, and to propose a model that describes the stress–diabetes association.

What Is Diabetes?

Diabetes mellitus is a chronic disease of uncertain cause, characterized by chronic hyperglycemia (i.e., high blood glucose) and other disturbances of carbohydrate and lipid metabolism, and associated with the development of vascular complications. These complications may affect specific organs such as the eye, the kidney, and the heart or be more general, affecting peripheral blood vessels and nerves.

Currently, many believe that diabetes is a heterogeneous syndrome with two distinct defects: One is characterized by an insulin deficiency involving malfunctioning beta cells in the pancreas; the other is characterized by the inability to use, or resistance to, insulin by tissue in the liver, muscle, and adipose (Arky, 1978). Some level of insulin is present in the blood (a level that may be subnormal, normal, or even elevated) when the diabetes results from the body's inability to use insulin.

The National Diabetes Data Group (1979) classifies diabetes into a number of types and subtypes. The two major types are Type I, insulin-dependent diabetes mellitus (IDDM), and Type II, non-insulin-dependent diabetes mellitus (NIDDM). Type I diabetes is characterized by the necessity of insulin injection to prevent ketosis (i.e., a breakdown in body fat) and to preserve life. Type I diabetes occurs most frequently in children and adults under 40. Patients with Type II diabetes are not ketone-prone and their blood insulin levels may be normal, depressed, or elevated. Type II diabetes occurs most frequently in individuals who are over 40 and female. Type II diabetes is further divided into two subtypes, obese and nonobese, Types IIA and IIB, respectively. It has been estimated that from 60 to 90% of Type II diabetics are obese. Type IIA diabetics may require insulin injection; however, with weight loss these individuals may maintain reasonable blood-glucose levels with proper diet or oral hypoglycemic medication. The prevalence of Type II diabetes is between 7 and 10 times greater than Type I.

Common symptoms of diabetes are excessive urination, extreme thirst, constant hunger, loss of weight, fatigue, itching, slow healing of infections or cuts, recurrent boils, blurred vision, and pain or numbness in hands and feet. Because of the insidious nature of diabetes, none or only some of these symptoms may be present at diagnosis. This absence of symptoms may account for the estimated 5 million undiagnosed diabetics noted earlier and the fact that frequently diabetes, especially Type II, is diagnosed during regular checkups rather than in response to specific symptoms.

Pathophysiology of Diabetes

The physiology of diabetes is complex, and a detailed description is beyond the scope of this chapter (see Bondy & Rosenberg, 1980; Sherwin & Felig, 1978). However, we provide a brief summary to give the reader a basic understanding of the disease process.

Insulin is a protein hormone that is secreted by the beta cells of the islets of Langerhans of the pancreas. In normal individuals the amount of insulin synthesis is regulated by the concentration of glucose in the blood. When food enters the body it is broken down in the intestines into glucose. From the intestines, glucose is absorbed into the blood stream and transported to the liver where approximately 60% of it is retained and the other 40% of it goes into general circulation. When glucose is circulated in the arteries it enters the pancreas where the glucose levels are monitored and insulin is secreted in response to increases in glucose levels.

For years, physicians have known that when insulin is not available or inappropriately used, glucose levels in the blood increase and ketosis (breakdown of fatty tissue) results. In fact, ketosis and its consequences—acidosis and coma—are often the first signs of diabetes. When glucose is not used by the cells and the blood glucose level rises, the muscles are deprived of needed energy. Fat and protein that is stored in the muscle by the action of insulin are broken down to supply energy. Protein is broken down, enters the blood stream, goes to the liver, and is converted into glucose. When fat is broken down and converted into energy, an undesirable byproduct, ketone bodies, results from the conversion. The hyperketonemia that results from severe and sustained hyperglycemia is similar to the acidic state of the body when it is starved of nutrition.

The danger of ketosis is that it will progress to dehydration and acidosis. Dehydration occurs when the glucose level in the blood is so high that it begins to "spill over" into the urine. When glucose enters the urine it causes a change in the electrolyte balance so that large amounts of water are lost from the body. If the dehydration progresses, blood volume shrinks, peripheral resistance is reduced, blood pressure falls, and renal function is impaired. The consequence can be coma and subsequent death (Bondy & Rosenberg, 1980).

At the present, there is no universal explanation of the cause(s) of diabetes. Because the pathology of diabetes varies by type, there is good reason to believe that there is probably no single etiology. Generally five factors have been implicated as possible causes: heredity (e.g., Leslie & Pyke, 1980), viral infections (e.g., Craighead, 1978), autoimmunity (e.g., Cahill & McDevitt, 1981), and psychological stress (e.g., Hinkle & Wolf, 1952a, 1952b) in Type I diabetes; prolonged obesity (e.g., Bondy & Rosenberg, 1980) and psychological stress (e.g., Hinkle & Wolf, 1952a, 1952b) in Type II diabetes. The greatest amount of interest among behavioral scientists has been directed toward the relationship between stress and both the etiology and course of diabetes. We address the relationship between stress and diabetes later in this chapter.

Adherence

Diabetes is one of several diseases in which patients or family members have increased responsibility for health care largely independent of direct medical supervision. Patients or family members must make treatment decisions based on daily clinical observations of objective (e.g., urine glucose levels) and often vague subjective symptoms (e.g., feelings of lightheadedness, sweating).

The levels of adherence to diabetic self-care regimens are notoriously low, a fact that should not be surprising in light of the many demands and complexities (including diet planning, spacing of meals, home monitoring of blood and urine, skin care, exercise). Adherence levels generally have been reported to be 48% or lower (e.g., Watkins, Williams, Martin, Hogan, & Anderson, 1967). For example, in a study of insulin-dependent diabetics (Bloom Cerkoney & Hart, 1980), fewer than 7% of the patients were judged to be completely adherent with essential behaviors (e.g., insulin administration, diet, treatment of hypoglycemia, foot care, and urine testing). Even those patients who seem to be adhering to the self-care regimen may do so in an unsatisfactory manner. The most thorough study of diabetes self-care, for example, revealed that 80% of the patients administered insulin in an unhygienic and unacceptable way; 58% administered the wrong dosage of insulin, 77% tested urine inaccurately or interpreted the results "in a manner likely to be detrimental to their treatment" (Watkins, Williams, et al., 1967, p. 453), 75% were not eating with satisfactory regularity, 75% were not eating prescribed foods, and 50% exhibited poor foot care (Watkins, Roberts, Williams, Martin, & Coyle, 1967; Watkins, Williams, et al., 1967).

Failure to adhere to diabetic self-care regimens is likely to contribute to poor metabolic control, resulting in short-term complications (e.g., hyperglycemia, hypoglycemia); nonadherence also may be associated with degenerative changes on a long-term basis. Although the relationship between poor metabolic control and degenerative changes continues to be a subject of controversy, poor control is likely to be at least one factor contributing to long-term complications. Estimates of "good" metabolic control have been reported to be 37% or fewer (e.g., Stone, 1964). We do not mean to imply that all examples of "poor" control are attributable to nonadherence; wide individual fluctuations can occur even among those who strictly adhere to the self-care regimen.

Evidence for the failure of many diabetics to adhere to self-care behaviors and of the concomitant poor control has led a number of diabetes educators to develop patient education programs that are designed to increase patients' knowledge of diabetes and the self-care regimen. Little, if any, attention has been given to the host of factors outlined by Speers and Turk (1982)—for example, patients' beliefs and motivations. The failure to consider such important factors may account for the dismal results obtained in most pa-tient-education programs (Watts, 1979).

Although many studies have shown that knowledge increases following the education program, increased knowledge does not seem to translate into satisfactory performance of self-care behaviors (e.g., Etzwiler & Robb, 1972; Hulka, Kupper, Cassel, & Mayo, 1975; Kasl, 1975). Surprisingly, Watkins, Williams, et al. (1967) reported that diabetic patients who had the highest cognitive understanding of their disease had the poorest metabolic control! Sanders, Mills, Martin, and Horne (1975) found that patients who had accu-rate information about diabetes and potential consequences of the disease *and* who believed that they could engage in some behaviors that might reduce the occurrence of complications were motivated to adhere to the diabetic self-care regimen. The sobering statistic presented by Sanders *et al.* (1975) was that only 23% of the patients with accurate knowledge *believed* in their ability to prevent complications. This lack of perceived self-control likely contributed to the large numbers of patients who failed to adhere to the therapeutic regimen. In summary, it is apparent that general knowledge alone is insufficient to produce the performance of self-care behaviors.

Stress and Diabetes

When an individual is exposed to a problem, demand, or threat (either physiological or psychological), a complex set of physiological events is set in motion. Of particular importance to diabetes is the fact that exposure to a threat, problem, or demand leads to the secretion of a number of hormones known to increase blood glucose and/or ketone levels and suppress insulin production (e.g., cortisol, catecholamines, glucagon, growth hormone).

Following episodes of acute stress, a relatively rapid reduction of the counterregulatory hormones occurs with a concomitant increase of insulin in the blood. Under conditions of prolonged, intense, or recurrent demand, it has been hypothesized that the body may deplete or resist the efforts of insulin to break down glucose in the blood, and permanent physiological changes resulting in diabetes may occur (Selye, 1956). Such permanent physiological effects have been called "diseases of adaptation" (Hinkle, Evans, & Wolf, 1951; Selye, 1956). These permanent changes may result in one of two psychophysiological defects: (a) an augmented stress response in the metabolic system, or (b) a dysfunctional metabolic system that has difficulty returning to a homeostatic state (Tarnow & Silverman, 1981–1982). In support of these psychophysiological defects, data have shown that diabetics display abnormally high levels of catecholamines both at rest and during exercise (Christensen, 1970) and increased ketone and free fatty acid (FFA) levels following catecholamine secretion (Baker, Barcai, Kaye, & Haque, 1969).

Three questions have been raised regarding the relationship between stress and diabetes: (a) Does stress have a causal role in diabetes onset? (b) Does stress affect the course of diabetes? (c) Do everyday stresses affect blood glucose levels? Studies addressing each of these questions are summarized next.

STRESS AS A CAUSAL FACTOR

Many investigations of the etiological effects of stress on diabetes have been reported; however, the data are divergent. Several authors (e.g., Hinkle & Wolf, 1952a, 1952b; Slawson, Flynn, & Kollar, 1963) have claimed that the onset of diabetes frequently occurs in response to stress, whereas other investigators have been unable to find empirical support for this contention (e.g., Crowell, 1953; Geiger, Barta, & Hubay, 1973; Koch & Molnar, 1974).

The relationship between stress and the onset of diabetes remains confused. One problem has been the reliance on stress evoked in laboratory or clinical settings, with generalization to the natural environment. The obverse of this problem is seen in the studies that have relied on major stressful life events. This latter set of studies fails to consider individual differences in evaluation of the importance of standard sets of stressful events. Although there are some reports of diabetes onset following stressful life events such as death of a spouse, there are many instances where no antecedent stressful event can be identified prior to onset of diabetes. Moreover, the relationship between precipitating events and diabetes has relied on retrospective reporting.

The answer to the question of why some people develop diabetes in response to a stressful event and others do not has been a diathesis–stress explanation. Basically, this explanation suggests that some factor, either genetically based or related to a prior illness, predisposes an individual to diabetes. Under conditions of high levels of stress, these predisposed individuals will develop diabetes (e.g., Mirsky, 1948). The diathesis–stress explanation, although intuitively appealing, has not been supported by the available data. For example, Gendel and Benjamin (1946) noted no increase in the frequency of diabetes during war-induced stress. Moreover, in the only large-scale prospective study, Cobb and Rose (1973) reported that North American air traffic controllers did not show an increased tendency to develop diabetes over a 2-year period when they were compared to a matched group of men who were employed in jobs that did not require rapid decision making, high responsibility, and high stress. The diathesis–stress explantion would have predicted some increases in the frequency of diabetes onset in both air traffic controllers and military personnel. The evidence, in general, does not support the hypothesis that stress causes diabetes onset.

EFFECTS OF MAJOR LIFE STRESSES ON THE COURSE OF DIABETES

In addition to examining the role of stress in the etiology of diabetes, investigators have sought to establish a relationship between stressful life events and episodes of diabetic decompensation (hypoglycemia and severe hyperglycemia). Beginning with the classic studies of Hinkle and Wolf (1952a, 1952b) investigators have attempted to link diabetic instability to major stressful life events (e.g., loss of a significant other, marriage, or legal problems; Bedell, Giordani, Amour, Tavormina, & Boll, 1977; Bradley, 1979b; Coddington, 1972; Grant, Kyle, Teichman, & Mendels, 1974).

Hinkle and Wolf (1952a, 1952b) interviewed a number of diabetic patients during a 3-year period in an attempt to determine the relationship between life events and fluctuations in diabetic control. Patients for whom a relationship between a specific stressful life event and diabetic control could be identified were interviewed extensively. The interview consisted of three phases: a base-line period during which general topics were discussed, the abrupt changing of topics from benign to stressful ones, and a period of support and return to general topics. Physiological indications were obtained at each of the three points during the interview.

Hinkle and Wolf reported that during the discussion of the stressful topics, diabetics showed an increase in urine output, an increase in ketones in the blood, and fluctuations in blood and urine glucose levels. During the supportive phase of the interview there was a reversal of the physiological changes with a return to base-line levels in a relatively short period. Nondiabetic subjects responded in an analogous manner; however, they differed in both the intensity of the physiological changes and the latency period required to return to base line. Thus, the nondiabetics' physiological responses were less extreme and required shorter periods to return to base line than the diabetic patients.

Baker and his colleagues (e.g., Baker, Kaye, & Haque, 1969) employed a research strategy similar to that of Hinkle and Wolf and supported a relationship between physiological responsivity and stress. They noted, particularly, that diabetic patients showed increases in FFA during the stress interview and a relatively slow return to base-line levels.

There are several problems with studies that use a discussion of stressful life events during interviews. Since relatively small subsamples of diabetic patients were selected from larger groups of patients it is impossible to tell whether the patients were representative of the entire population of diabetics. These studies often fail to report the number of patients for whom the relationship between stressful life situations and physiological responses was demonstrated. Furthermore, the subjects who are described may have had an unstable form of the disease and they may have been more reactive in general (e.g., to infection, to exercise, to dietary changes; Shima, Tanaka, Morishita, Tauri, Kumahara, & Nishikawa, 1977).

Following along the same lines as Hinkle and Wolf, several studies have attempted to induce stress by suggesting distressing topics during hypnosis. The rationale for using hypnosis is not clear but there seems to have been an expectancy on the part of the investigators that stress is more readily induced during hypnosis than during more typical stress interviews. Findings of these studies are inconsistent. For example, VandenBergh, Sussman, and Titus (1966) reported decreases in blood glucose levels of diabetics during hypnotically induced stress, whereas Pinter, Peterfy, Cleghorn, and Pattee (1967) found no changes in blood glucose levels but did note increases in FFA. Weller, Linder, Nuland, and Kline (1961) found no changes in blood glucose measures in either diabetic or nondiabetic subjects. One of the problems with these studies is the reliance on blood glucose to assess the effects of stress on physiology. These contradictory findings raise some question about the adequacy of levels of blood glucose as a measure of the impact of stress. Increases in urine output, blood ketones, and levels of FFA seem more valid dependent measures of stress response.

In all of the interview and hypnosis studies, the criteria of stressful events are not defined. For example, Hinkle and Wolf mention several examples of stressful life events that are quite varied (e.g., a difficult board of directors meeting, discussion of erotic fantasies, situations of anxiety and conflict) and are not the typical life events that are considered to be major stressors (e.g., Holmes & Rahe, 1967). Thus, it is not readily apparent whether it is objective life stress that is associated with the observed physiological changes or whether subjective evaluation of any event as stressful is related to the physiological changes observed (for example, see Lazarus, 1966; Mason, 1971; Turk, Meichenbaum, & Genest, 1983). The distinction between objective and subjective criteria of stressors is addressed in the next section.

In addition to these stress interviews and hypnosis studies, two studies have examined the relationship between stressful life events (employing the Holmes and Rahe scale, 1967) and incidence of glycosuria (glucose in urine; Bradley, 1979a; Grant *et al.*, 1974). Grant *et al.* report a nonsignificant trend for increases in glycosuria associated with an increased number of stressful life events. Bradley did not find any relationship between stressful life events and urine glucose but did find significant correlations between increases in blood glucose and the number of stressful life events.

The stressful life events approach, in general, has received a great deal of criticism (e.g., Rabkin & Struening, 1976; Sarason, Johnson, & Siegel, 1978). A particular problem with research that focuses exclusively on physiological data is that one cannot determine whether the presence of stressful life events directly affects diabetic stability or indirectly affects stability by influencing patients' adherence behavior. The latter alternative has received some support from studies reporting that up to 25% of ketoacidotic episodes may be attributed to the deliberate omission of insulin by patients (e.g., Beigelman, 1971; Cohen, Vance, Runyan, & Hurwitz, 1960).

EVERYDAY STRESSES AND THE COURSE OF DIABETES

Although there is frequent suggestion that low-intensity or everyday stress may influence physiological activity in diabetics, there are relatively few data available upon which to support this assumption; we are aware of only two studies. In an attempt to examine the destabilizing effect of habitual low-level stresses in diabetes, Baker and Barcai (1970) conducted stress interviews that included stressful topics relevant to each patient as well as more general stressful topics. Although significant elevations in FFA (100% increases) were noted when specific stressful topics were discussed, no such changes were observed when general stress topics were included.

In the second study, Bradley and Cox (1978, cited in 1979b) examined the effects of an aversive (stressful) noise on levels of blood glucose. Bradley noted that the aversive noise produced an increase in blood glucose levels in some subjects and a decrease in blood glucose levels in others. In trying to explain the contradictory findings Bradley noted that subjects with high levels of blood glucose prior to the experiment tended to show increases in blood glucose during the noise exposure, whereas subjects with low pre-experiment levels of blood glucose displayed a reduction in blood glucose in response to the laboratory stress. Thus the effect of low-intensity stress on blood glucose may be either to raise or to lower it, depending on prestressor levels.

From these data it is impossible to draw any conclusions about the destabilizing effects of everyday or low-intensity stresses. The data again raise the question of the appropriateness of the blood glucose measure as the sole physiological indicant of the effect of psychological stress on diabetes. Further, the Bradley data suggest that if blood glucose is measured in future studies, it will be necessary to examine base-line levels of blood glucose.

In general, the studies on stress and diabetes do not support the etiological role of stress. It does appear, however, that stressful events have some effect on destabilizing the course of diabetes by increasing ketones, FFA, and urine output with a much more variable effect on blood glucose levels. It is difficult to determine from the available data whether the destabilizing effects occur in all diabetic patients or specifically in those with more labile forms of the disease. Future studies are needed to address this issue as well as to clarify the role of low-intensity and everyday stresses on metabolic control.

The Role of Psychological Factors in Diabetic Decompensation

LINEAR CAUSATION MODEL

The research examining the role of psychological factors in diabetes etiology and decompensation has focused almost exclusively on the impact of psychological stress. Most of the research on the impact of psychological stress and diabetic decompensation has been based on a linear causation model whereby a stimulus, objectively defined as stressful, directly affects physiological functioning either by hormonal and autonomic stimulation or through metabolic changes. The linear causation model is not satisfactory in providing an explanation for the effect of stress on the physiological functioning of diabetics. The model is unable, for example, to account for the fact that not all diabetics will show decompensation following an identical stressful life event (e.g., job loss, divorce). Additionally, not all diabetics show physiological aberrations during stress interviews (e.g., Hinkle & Wolf, 1952a) nor do all diabetics respond with excessive physiological responses to stressful topics induced during hypnosis (e.g., Weller et al., 1961).

PSYCHOPHYSIOLOGICAL MODEL

Recently, Tarnow and Silverman (1981–1982) presented a psycho-physiological model to describe the process whereby cognitive factors that follow the presence of objectively defined stressful stimuli produce physiological reactions. Their model expands upon the linear causation model by proposing that central nervous system activity (cognitive information processing) and subsequent coping behaviors mediate the impact of the stressful stimuli. In addition, their model incorporates a feedback loop whereby decompensation may influence the stressful stimulus creating a vicious circle, with decompensation serving as an additional stress.

Within the psychophysiological model, the presence of a stressful stimulus leads to preconscious central nervous system (CNS) arousal prior to cognitive processing of the event as stressful and, subsequently, to physiological alterations or a conscious level where "the individual cognitively tries to understand, integrate, problem solve, and plan ways to cope with the stressful event. Past memories may be stimulated during this stage. The memories may themselves be stressful [Tarnow & Silverman, 1981–1982, p. 34]." Following the processing of information the individual may engage in a

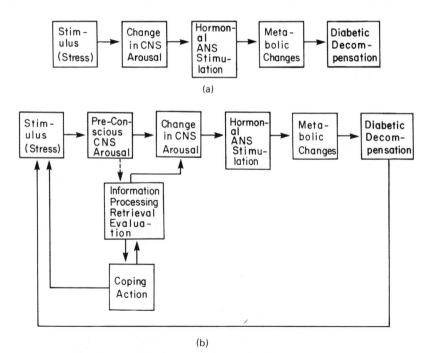

(a)

(b)

FIGURE 8.1 (a) Linear-causation and (b) psychophysiological (Tarnow & Silverman, 1981–1982) models of the effects of stress on diabetic decompensation.

coping action to influence the stressful stimulus. Figure 8.1 schematically displays the linear-causation and psychophysiological models.

Although the psychophysiological model is a significant advance over the linear-causation model, it assumes that the function of cognitive processing is exclusively reactive; the cognitive processing influences the response to the objectively defined stressor. The model fails to consider the role of cognitive factors in the initial definition of a stimulus as stressful. Stimuli may be subjectively defined as stressful or nonstressful regardless of objective criteria. The influence of subjective appraisal of stimuli may account for the individual differences in response to objectively equivalent events. A more comprehensive model of cognitive processing and the transaction between the individual and the environment is needed to understand fully the role of psychological factors in diabetes.

TRANSACTIONAL MODEL

In the linear causation and psychophysiological models, the role of stress in diabetic decompensation is based on the important assumption that stress and ultimately decompensation are responses to stimuli that are predetermined to be stressful. The linear causation model suggests that the presence of the stressful stimulus leads inevitably to a set of physiological responses characteristic of stress. The psychophysiological model suggests that the individual's response to the stressor stimulus will depend, to some extent, on how the individual processes information about the stimulus. Thus, the psychophysiological model proposes that cognitive mediation occurs between the stressor and the stress response.

An alternative model, one that we call transactional, expands the psychophysiological model by proposing two stages of cognitive processing. The transactional model that we propose is based on the work of Lazarus and his colleagues (Lazarus, 1966; Lazarus & Launier, 1978), who suggest that cognitive processing occurs in three stages—primary appraisal, secondary appraisal, and reappraisal. Primary appraisal is initiated when individuals are exposed to a stimulus. The most important outcome at this stage is the appraisal of the relevance of the stimulus that confronts the individual. During secondary appraisal available resources for coping with the stimulus are evaluated. Although secondary appraisal depends on the motivating role of primary appraisal, they may overlap rather than being sequential, as characteristics of threat and coping may occur simultaneously. It is the result of the interaction of both primary and secondary appraisal processes and the stimulus configuration that determines whether a stimulus is stressful. This relationship is not static, but rather is an ongoing transaction between the individual and the environment, with changes occurring over time. A stressful episode is not simply a circumscribed stimulus in the environment to which an individual responds (i.e., affect, cognition, somatic stimulus, or behavior) but a sequence of events and responses that changes. Reappraisal refers to feedback from changes in the person–environment transaction during the course of a stressful episode.

The transactional model we propose acknowledges the relative contributions of both psychological and physiological processes to a stress response and offers an explanation of how these two processes interrelate. Before we are able to describe the complex interaction of psychological and physiological factors, we need to elaborate the nature of the complex cognitive activity involved in information processing. Detailed explanation of the mechanics of information processing is beyond the scope of this chapter (see Anderson & Bower, 1973; Shiffrin & Schneider, 1977). To summarize the major components we need to consider the storage, encoding, and retrieval of information.

Individuals selectively abstract information from their experiences and store information in long-term memory. The information may be stored along a number of dimensions (e.g., content, function, associations). The information is encoded within a set of interrelated cognitive structures. What information is stored and how it is encoded depends upon a number of variables such as the amount and nature of affect present when the information is presented, prior experiences, beliefs, and expectations.

When an individual faces a stimulus, different idiosyncratic cognitive structures are activated against which the stimulus is compared and decisions are made concerning whether to respond and, if so, how to respond. Most of the information processing is automatic and the individual is not usually aware that it is taking place. The individual's ultimate response, psychologically and to some extent physiologically, is a result of information processing. Moreover, the outcome of the processing of information and of the psychological and physiological responses of the individual will be stored in memory and retrieved in the future. It is this complex set of processes that contribute to the determination of stress.

According to our transactional model, when an individual is confronted with a stimulus, increased autonomic nervous system (ANS) and CNS activity are initiated. The increased ANS activity serves to arouse the individual and orient him or her to the presence of the stimulus. The first stage of cognitive activity answers the question "what is it"; the answer is based upon abstracting features from the stimulus (e.g., size, location, intensity) and comparing these features to existing cognitive representations activated and retrieved from long-term memory. Figure 8.2 presents a schematic representation of the transactional model.

An example will help to clarify the processes we have been describing. When a diabetic patient performs a urine test and obtains a reading of .5%

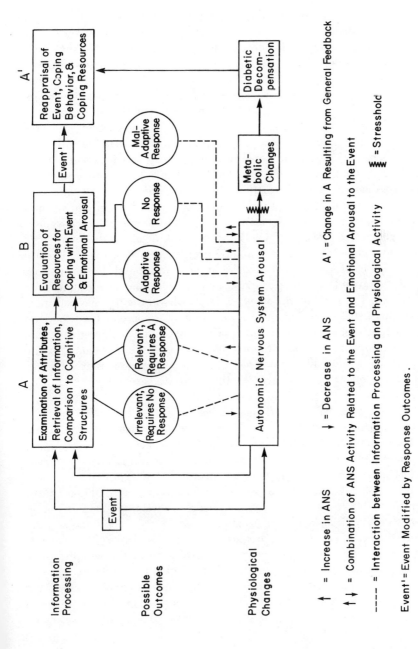

Information Processing

Possible Outcomes

Physiological Changes

A
Examination of Attributes, Retrieval of Information, Comparison to Cognitive Structures

Event

Irrelevant, Requires No Response

Relevant, Requires A Response

B
Evaluation of Resources for Coping with Event & Emotional Arousal

Event'

Adaptive Response

No Response

Mal-Adaptive Response

A'
Reappraisal of Event, Coping Behavior,& Coping Resources

Autonomic Nervous System Arousal

Meta-bolic Changes

Diabetic Decom-pensation

↟ = Increase in ANS   ↓ = Decrease in ANS   A' = Change in A Resulting from General Feedback

↟↓ = Combination of ANS Activity Related to the Event and Emotional Arousal to the Event   wwww = Stresshold

---- = Interaction between Information Processing and Physiological Activity

Event' = Event Modified by Response Outcomes.

FIGURE 8.2   Transactional model of the effects of psychological factors on diabetic decompensation.

(500 mg/dl; a moderately high level of glucose in the urine), he or she evaluates it in relation to knowledge stored in memory and retrieved in the present circumstances. Prior experiences with urine test results, knowledge of the implications of a reading of .5%, and the recall of other related information will cause the patient to evaluate the event as irrelevant (requiring no action), a major deviation from his or her usual level of urine glucose (requiring some response), or any evaluation between these two extremes. Increases in autonomic activity co-occur with the cognitive processing. As noted earlier, an increase in ANS activity from base line occurs from the awareness of the novel stimulus. In the case of the diabetic with the .5% reading there may be an additional increase in ANS activity related to the physiological change associated with hyperglycemia.

The ANS activity and information-processing activity interact with each other. For example, ANS activity related to elevated urine glucose may produce symptoms of hyperglycemia (e.g., dizziness, fatigue) that may interfere with cognitive processing. On the other hand, results of the information processing may lead to increased emotional arousal (ANS activity). To illustrate the effect of information processing on ANS arousal, let us consider some of the possible results of the information processing of a urine glucose level of .5%. The patient with labile diabetes who in the past has had spontaneous fluctuations in urine glucose without any response on his or her part may conclude that no response is necessary, and that he or she can disregard the elevated reading. If the patient reaches this conclusion, then the cognitive processing will have little direct effect on the ANS activity, although ANS activity might be influenced by the failure to respond and by further physiological decompensation.

Alternatively, a diabetic patient who has been well controlled and who rarely obtains readings as high as .5% may conclude that this reading is a serious alteration in the stability of his or her diabetes, one that requires immediate action to determine the cause and the appropriate action to bring the glucose level within the usual level of control. The appraisal of a serious threat and an indication of the worsening of his or her condition by the patient probably leads to increased emotional arousal (ANS activity).

Following the first stage of information processing, a second stage is initiated. In the second stage the individual evaluates the causes of the elevated urine glucose, the resources available for dealing with the elevated urine test, the alternatives for responding, and decides how best to respond. Again, this second stage of information processing is quite complex and depends upon stored information that must be retrieved. Information that is retrieved includes data about the effectiveness of different responses based on knowledge and past experience.

During this second stage, the individual may also process information about his or her increased autonomic activity. For example, the individual may perceive that he or she is aroused and this arousal is interfering with decisions regarding how to respond. In this case, the individual may decide that it is important to relax or slow down, and then proceed with evaluating how best to respond to the urine glucose elevation.

As a result of the information processing during the second stage, several alternatives can occur. We will consider three possibilities. The individual may become so distressed that he or she is unable to retrieve information about what to do when the urine glucose is elevated, feel that there is little he or she can do, and conclude that he or she is helpless to respond. Such an appraisal leads to a further increase in ANS activity. A second possibility is that the individual may have stored inaccurate information about how to respond to the elevated urine glucose and choose an inappropriate response—for example, drinking orange juice. This response might reduce some of the emotional arousal because the individual believes that he or she has responded appropriately. ANS activity may not be reduced, however, because of the direct physiological effect of the sugar in the orange juice. A third possible response may be to relax, look up information about how to respond to the urine-glucose elevation, and decide to retest urine and to test for ketones. The impact of the patient's behavior on resolving the problem of elevated urine glucose will be evaluated by the patient and stored in memory for future use.

Consider the individuals who either erroneously made the inappropriate response (drank the orange juice) or chose not to respond. In this case, the next urine glucose reading may be even higher (1%, 1000 mg/dl) and ketones may be present. This higher level of urine glucose and presence of ketones indicates decompensation (e.g., severe hyperglycemia). Moreover, the higher second reading may increase the emotional distress of the patient based on an appraisal of the inadequacy of his or her responding and/or worsening of stability. It is at the point where the individual decides that he or she has exhausted his or her coping resources in combination with increased physiological activity that stress results according to the transactional model.

During the time when the individual is evaluating information and choosing responses, he or she is autonomically and centrally aroused. Either during the evaluation of information or shortly thereafter the individual will respond with a stress response. Stress consists of psychological (heightened cognitive and emotional) distress and high levels of ANS and endocrine responses. Once the individual's stress threshold ("stresshold") is surpassed, a number of physiological changes are set in motion (e.g., increased catecholamine production, increased adrenocorticotropic hormone (ACTH) secretion, increased production of cortisol, increases in glucogen). These physiological changes will influence still further changes in physiological functioning including suppression of insulin, increased FFA, increased ketone bodies, and increased breakdown of glycogen. The result of these processes is diabetic decompensation and severe hyperglycemia. Following an episode of decompensation, the diabetic patient will select and abstract information about the episode and his or her responding, and store this information in memory for future use. In summary, we have tried to present a simplified explanation of an extremely complex process.

The models presented in Figures 8.1 and 8.2 differ widely in their suggestions for interventions with diabetics. The linear-causation model suggests intervening by removing stressful environmental demands; by administering antianxiety medications, biofeedback (e.g., Fowler, Budzynski, & VandenBergh, 1976), or hypnosis-assisted relaxation to reduce CNS arousal; by administering beta-adrenergic blocking medication (e.g., propranalol; Baker, Kaye, & Haque, 1969; Baker, Barcai, Kaye, & Haque, 1969) to block the peripheral manifestations of the autonomic nervous system; or by administering medication that can inhibit the production of glucagon (e.g., somatostatin; Lundback & Hansen, 1977). Thus, the model suggests treatment should focus on alleviation of stress response symptoms. The psychophysiological model suggests similar treatment of symptoms but includes modification of perceptions of coping resources.

The transactional model has important implications for intervention because it emphasizes the contributions of cognitive processes to the appraisal of information related to a stimulus as well as to the appraisal of resources for satisfactory response to both the stimulus and the individual's emotional reaction to the presence of the stimulus. The transactional model suggests that, in addition to palliation of symptoms, patients can be taught to prevent the onset of maladaptive metabolic responding by examination of maladaptive beliefs and response patterns, reappraisal of the stimulus through problem solving, and learning new coping skills to deal with environmental demands. Following from the transactional model, the cause of the symptoms (maladaptive beliefs, expectancies, evaluations), rather than the symptoms per se, become a major focus of intervention (Turk et al., 1983). Of course, physiological factors are also causes of diabetic decompensation. In these instances symptomatic treatment is essential.

Coping with Diabetes

Despite the long interest and extensive theorizing about the relationship between stress and diabetes, relatively little attention has been focused on coping with the major life changes and complications created by diabetes.

The few papers that have been published in this area have focused almost exclusively on children with diabetes and their families, even though this group consists of only about 5% of patients with diabetes.

What is perhaps most surprising is how resilient most children with diabetes seem to be. Although diabetes has a major impact on most areas of their lives (such as day-to-day interference with school and leisure time activity, threat of acute exacerbations, complex self-care regimens and increased responsibility for health care, restricted diet, and restricted activities), the majority of children and adolescents seem to be coping quite well. Most studies of children with diabetes show that they function within normal limits on standardized measures of adjustment and psychopathology (e.g., Johnson, 1980; Simonds, 1977; Sullivan, 1978; Watts, 1979). Social problems and feelings of alienation are the reported common difficulties (e.g., Delbridge, 1975; Fallstrom, 1974; Tavormina, Kastner, Slater, & Watt, 1976).

Another area in which coping with diabetes has been examined is the impact on the families of children with diabetes. Studies have reported that families with diabetic children experience more stress than control families (e.g., Crain, Sussman, & Weil, 1966; Gath, Smith, & Baum, 1980) and experience more family disruption and marital conflict (e.g., Crain et al., 1966; Koski & Kumento, 1977). Some anecdotal evidence also has been reported indicating that mothers with diabetic children are more anxious and depressed than mothers of healthy children (e.g., Stersky, 1963).

The data on the impact of diabetes on the family must be viewed with caution. When the observation of "more stress" among families with a child with diabetes is presented, it is important to ask the questions "How much more?" "Compared to what control groups?" and "How representative were the families studied?" We can consider the last question first. The studies of families with diabetic children are usually based on families that have been referred to mental health professionals. These families may not be representative of the more general population of families with a diabetic child. Results based on such studies are likely to overemphasize psychopathology. Because most studies in this area examine dysfunctional families after the development of diabetes, one cannot determine whether dysfunctional coping patterns existed in the families prior to the diagnosis. Another problem concerning the representativeness of the families relates to stability. Unstable diabetes (frequent episodes of hyperglycemia, hypoglycemia, and hospitalization) is likely to create additional stresses in families. Most studies of families fail to report the level of stability achieved by the child with diabetes. Simonds (1977) reported that families with children in good metabolic control had fewer conflicts than those in poor control or healthy peers. Thus, it is possible that the quality of control is an important factor to consider when examining the impact of diabetes on the family.

The second question posed was that of the control groups used to compare diabetic families' distress and coping. Often the control groups have been "healthy" families, those without a chronically ill child. This approach would permit examination of the problems created by the presence of a chronic disease in the family. However, if the question of interest concerns what problems are specific to diabetes and not what problems are characteristic of chronic disease in general, then more appropriate control groups would include families with a child who has a chronic disease other than diabetes (e.g., asthma).

Coping that is specific to diabetes has not been identified. Moreover, studies have focused on the global question of coping with diabetes per se, without considering specific threats and demands of living with diabetes. Little attention has been given to how families and the diabetic patients cope with specific problems of diabetes. Moreover, the state of research in this area is so rudimentary that little is known about the nature of problems as perceived by the patient or the family. What problems do patients and families regard as the most difficult to handle? What are their major concerns? Are the concerns of patients and families congruent with what the workers in the field view as the problems of diabetes? What are patients' and families' attitudes toward health care providers and diabetes? Some preliminary work has begun in addressing these questions, but at the present time little can be said with any confidence (see, e.g., Khurana & White, 1970; Laron, Galatzer, Amir, Gil, Karp, & Mimouni, 1979; Melamed & Johnson, 1981).

The first question posed of the family coping literature asked, "How much more distressed were the families with a diabetic child?" Although several studies (e.g., Crain et al., 1966; Gath et al., 1980) suggest that diabetic families are distressed and coping less adequately than controls, the percentages of distress are relatively small. For example, Gath et al. (1980) reported that 33% (25 of 76) of families were viewed as being under stress, compared to 20% of control families—a difference of only 13%. Examined in another light, the study reveals that 66% of the families with a diabetic child appeared to be coping adequately. No attention has been given to the characteristics of coping patterns of the large proportion of the families who are coping effectively (Anderson & Auslander, 1980; Turk, 1979). The same point can be made about the diabetic children themselves. Little is known about how they cope with the diversity of problems and threats posed by diabetes.

Another issue in the area of coping may be apparent to the reader. All of the studies on coping mentioned have focused on outcome measures. Minimal attention has been given to the process of coping (Koski, 1969; Tietz & Vidmar, 1972). Chronic diseases by definition extend over time and thus require continued adjustments and readjustments, appraisals and reappraisals. Longitudinal studies are necessary to explicate the coping patterns as they evolve and change during the course of the disease.

Somewhat of a surprise is the fact that, even though 95% of diabetics are adults, there is a paucity of research regarding how adult diabetics cope with the disease. We are aware of two papers that have examined the impact of diabetes on spouses of patients (Katz, 1969; Wishner & O'Brien, 1978). Neither of these provides any empirical data; they both offer only speculations about changing roles, power shifts, secondary gains, and conflicts. The nature of the problems and coping patterns of adult patients and spouses remains to be clarified.

Although it has been noted that many diabetic patients and their families seem to make satisfactory adjustment, a minority do seem to have difficulties. Inadequate data limit the suggestions that can be made regarding interventions to be employed with distressed diabetics or their families. Several approaches to assisting these patients and families to cope more effectively have been reported; however, the empirical bases for the efficacy of these approaches are thin. Several case studies have reported on the efficacy of stress-reduction techniques, attitude modification of parents (Hinkle & Wolf, 1952a), biofeedback and relaxation (e.g., Fowler et al., 1976), support groups (Tarnow, 1978), social skills training (Gross, Johnson, Wildman, & Mullett, in press), and family therapy (e.g., Minuchin, Rosman, & Baker, 1978). Well-controlled treatment research with diabetics and families of diabetics is unavailable. Perhaps the best approach to assisting diabetic patients and families is for the health care provider to begin by assessing the individual beliefs, needs, and concerns of the client and tailoring the treatment to the individual or family. This approach is described more fully in Chapter 6.

Conclusions

In this chapter we have attempted to provide a summary of what is currently known about diabetes, emphasizing the complexities of both the disease process and of living with the disease. We have focused on the behavioral science research on diabetes, noting the methodological and conceptual difficulties as well as the questions that remain unanswered. We believe that tremendous opportunities for research and treatment exist in the area of diabetes, opportunities for behavioral scientists as well as other health care professionals. Research is needed to clarify the relationship between stress and diabetes, to identify the specific problems that diabetics view as most distressing, to identify maladaptive and adaptive patterns of coping with the disease by patients as well as significant others, to increase adherence to complex self-care regimens, and to develop treatment programs that can assist in the maintenance of normal metabolic control.

To answer questions concerning the impact of stress on the course of diabetes, several types of investigations are required. To identify the association between acute stress and metabolic control, a number of diabetic patients need to be exposed to objectively identical threats. Laboratory studies of the effects of aversive noise on diabetes glucose metabolism have addressed this issue (e.g., Bradley, 1979b); however, the ecological validity of such laboratory stress studies is questionable. An alternative strategy is to identify a set of diabetic patients who are going to be exposed to a naturally occurring threat or demand (e.g., surgery, marriage) and to examine their responses prior to and following the threat.

A second type of study that is needed is one in which diabetics and their families are studied longitudinally in order to examine the association between everyday annoyances (Kanner, Coyne, Schaefer, & Lazarus, 1981) and fluctuations in metabolic control. Longitudinal studies are also appropriate for examining changing patterns of coping by diabetic patients and their families, as over the course of the disease different problems, threats, and demands are likely to arise.

We have proposed a transactional model that delineates the underlying psychological process as it relates to diabetic decompensation. The model suggests that one cause of severe hyperglycemia may be the manner in which individuals process information about novel stimuli that create threats or demands. Following from this model, patients who perceive problems erroneously, have inadequate coping resources, or fail to address both the problem and the accompanying physiological arousal are most likely to experience diabetic decompensation. To assess the validity and utility of this model, studies are required to examine the nature of both general and specific attitudes and beliefs of diabetic patients concerning all aspects of the disease process, the self-care regimens, and the nature of patients' own resources. At present there are no empirical data to support the validity of applying the transactional model specifically to diabetes; however, there is some support for the heuristic value of the transactional model in understanding the nature of stress and suggestions for stress-management training (e.g., Coyne & Holroyd, 1981; Lazarus & Launier, 1978; Meichenbaum & Turk, 1981).

We have noted the complexities of the diabetic self-care regimens and the problem of adherence. The magnitude of the problem of nonadherence underscores the need for much more research into the causes of nonadherence and ways to ameliorate the problem (Speers & Turk, 1981). One major problem in this area is that successful studies have frequently been conducted with well-educated, middle-class patients. There is a great need to examine the generalizability of results from middle-class patients to other groups with widely differing attitudes and beliefs about weight control, self-responsibility, and disease.

Throughout this chapter we have attempted to suggest a number of questions that need to be investigated. The success of our efforts will be measured by both the number and quality of future research attempts in this area.

References

Anderson, B. J., & Auslander, W. F. Research on diabetes management and the family: A critique. *Diabetes Care*, 1980, *3*, 696–702.

Anderson, J. R., & Bower, G. H. *Human associative memory*. Washington, D.C.: Hemisphere Press, 1973.

Arky, R. A. Current principles of dietary therapy of diabetes mellitus. *Medical Clinics of North America*, 1978, *62*, 655–662.

Baker, L., & Barcai, A. Psychosomatic aspects of diabetes. In O. W. Hill (Ed.), *Modern trends in psychosomatic illness* (Vol. 2). New York: Appleton-Century-Crofts, 1970.

Baker, L., Barcai, A., Kaye, R., & Haque, N. Beta adrenergic blockade and juvenile diabetes: Acute studies and long-term therapeutic trial. *Journal of Pediatrics*, 1969, *75*, 19–29.

Baker L., Kaye, R., & Haque, N. Metabolic homeostasis in juvenile diabetes mellitus. *Diabetes*, 1969, *18*, 421–427.

Bedell, J., Giordani, B., Amour, J., Tavormina, J., & Boll, T. Life stress and the psychological and medical adjustment of chronically ill children. *Journal of Psychosomatic Research*, 1977, *21*, 237–242.

Beigelman, P. M. Severe diabetic ketoacidosis (diabetic "coma"). *Diabetes*, 1971, *20*, 490–500.

Bloom Cerkoney, K. A., & Hart, L. K. The relationship between the health beliefs model and compliance of persons with diabetes mellitus. *Diabetes Care*, 1980, *3*, 594–598.

Bondy, P. K., & Rosenberg, L. E. *Metabolic control and disease* (8th ed.). Philadelphia: W. B. Saunders, 1980.

Bradley, C. Life events and the control of diabetes mellitus. *Journal of Psychosomatic Research*, 1979, *23*, 159–162. (a)

Bradley, C. Psychophysiological effects of stressful experiences and the management of diabetes mellitus. In D. J. Oborne, M. M. Gruneberg, & J. R. Eiser (Eds.), *Research in psychology and medicine* (Vol. 1). London: Academic Press, 1979. (b)

Bradley, C., & Cox, T. Stress and health. In T. Cox (Ed.), *Stress*. London: Macmillan, 1978.

Cahill, G. F., & McDevitt, H. O. Insulin-dependent diabetes mellitus. The initial lesion. *New England Journal of Medicine*, 1981, *304*, 1454–1465.

Christensen, N. J. Abnormally high plasma catecholamines at rest and during exercise in ketotic juvenile diabetics. *Scandinavian Journal of Clinical Investigation*, 1970, *26*, 343.

Cobb, S., & Rose, R. M. Hypertension, peptic ulcer and diabetes in air traffic controllers. *Journal of the American Medical Association*, 1973, *224*, 489–492.

Coddington, R. The significance of life events as etiologic factors in the diseases of children. II. A study of a normal population. *Journal of Psychosomatic Research*, 1972, *16*, 205–213.

Cohen, A. S., Vance, V. K., Runyan, J. W., & Hurwitz, D. Diabetic acidosis: An evaluation of the cause, course and therapy of 73 cases. *Annals of Internal Medicine*, 1960, *52*, 55–86.

Coyne, J. C., & Holroyd, K. Stress, coping, and illness: A transactional perspective. In T. Millon, C. Green, & R. Meagher (Eds.), *Handbook of health care clinical psychology*. New York: Plenum Press, 1982.

Craighead, J. E. Current views of the etiology of insulin-dependent diabetes mellitus. *New England Journal of Medicine*, 1978, *299*, 1439–1445.

Crain, A. J., Sussman, M. B., & Weil, W. B. Effects of a diabetic child on marital integration and related measures of family functioning. *Journal of Health and Human Behavior*, 1966, *7*, 122–127.

Crowell, D. Personality and physical disease: A test of the Dunbar hypothesis applied to diabetes mellitus and rheumatic fever. *General Psychology Monographs*, 1953, *48*, 117–153.

Delbridge, L. Educational and psychological factors in the management of diabetes in childhood. *Medical Journal of Australia*, 1975, *2*, 737–739.

Etzwiler, D. D., & Robb, J. R. Evaluation of programmed education among juvenile diabetics and their families. *Diabetes*, 1972, *21*, 967–971.

Fallstrom, K. On the personality structure in diabetic school children. *Acta Paediatrica Scandinavica*, 1974, *251*, 5–71. (Supplement)

Fischhoff, B., Slovic, P., & Lichtenstein, S. Knowing with certainty: The appropriateness of extreme confidence. *Journal of Experimental Psychology: Human Perception and Performance*, 1977, *3*, 552–564.

Fowler, J. E., Budzynski, T. H., & VandenBergh, R. L. Effects of an EMG biofeedback relaxation program on the control of diabetes. *Biofeedback and Self-Regulation*, 1976, *1*, 105–112.

Gath, A., Smith, M. A., & Baum, J. D. Emotional, behavioral and educational disorders in diabetic children. *Archives of Disorder of Children*, 1980, *55*, 371–375.

Geiger, A., Barta, L., & Hubay, M. Diabetes and mental state. *Acta Paediatrica Academica Scientifica Hungary*, 1973, *14*, 119–124.

Gendel, B. R., & Benjamin, J. E. Psychogenic factors in the etiology of diabetes. *New England Journal of Medicine*, 1946, *243*, 556–560.

Grant, I., Kyle, G. C., Teichman, A., & Mendels, J. Recent life events and diabetes in adults. *Psychosomatic Medicine*, 1974, *36*, 121–128.

Gross, A. M., Johnson, W. G., Wildman, H., & Mullett, N. Coping skills training with insulin dependent pre-adolescent diabetics. *Child Behavior Therapy*, in press.

Hamburg, B. A., Lipsett, L. F., Inoff, G. E., & Drash, A. L. (Eds.) *Behavioral and psychosocial aspects of diabetes: Proceedings of a national conference* (NIH Publication No. 80-1993). Washington, D.C.: U.S. Government Printing Office, 1980.

Hinkle, L. E., Evans, F. M., & Wolf, S. Studies in diabetes mellitus. IV. Life history of three persons with relatively mild, stable diabetes and relation of significant experiences in their lives to the onset and course of the disease. *Psychosomatic Medicine*, 1951, *13*, 193–202.

Hinkle, L. E., & Wolf, S. Importance of life stress in the course and management of diabetes mellitus. *Journal of the American Medical Association*, 1952, *148*, 513–520. (a)

Hinkle, L. E., & Wolf, S. A summary of experimental evidence relating life stress to diabetes mellitus. *Journal of Mt. Sinai Hospital*, 1952, *19*, 537–570. (b)

Holmes, T. H., & Rahe, R. H. The social readjustment rating scale. *Journal of Psychosomatic Research*, 1967, *11*, 213–218.

Hulka, B., Kupper, L. L., Cassel, J. C., & Mayo, E. Doctor–patient communication and outcome among diabetic patients. *Journal of Community Health*, 1975, *1*, 15–27.

Johnson, S. B. Psychosocial factors in juvenile diabetes: A review. *Journal of Behavioral Medicine*, 1980, *3*, 95–116.

Kanner, A. D., Coyne, J. C., Schaefer, C., & Lazarus, R. S. Comparison of two modes of stress measurement: Daily hassles and uplifts versus major life events. *Journal of Behavioral Medicine*, 1981, *4*, 1–39.

Kasl, S. V. Issues in patient adherence to health care regimens. *Journal of Human Stress*, 1975, *1*, 5–18.

Katz, A. M. Wives of diabetic men. *Menninger Clinic Bulletin*, 1969, *33*, 279–294.

Khurana, R., & White, P. Attitudes of the diabetic child and his parents toward his illness. *Postgraduate Medicine*, 1970, *48*, 72–77.

Koch, M. F., & Molnar, G. D. Psychiatric aspects of unstable diabetes. *Psychosomatic Medicine*, 1974, *36*, 57–68.

Koski, M. L. The coping process in childhood diabetes. *Acta Paediatrica Scandinavica*, 1969, *198*, 7–56. (Supplement)

Koski, M., & Kumento, A. The interrelationship between diabetic control and family life. In Z. Laron (Ed.), *Pediatric and adolescent endocrinology* (Vol. 3): *Psychological aspects of balance of diabetes in juveniles*. New York: Karger, 1977.

Laron, Z., Galatzer, A., Amir, S., Gil, R., Karp, M., & Mimouni, M. A multidisciplinary, comprehensive, ambulatory treatment for diabetes mellitus in children. *Diabetes Care*, 1979, *2*, 342–348.

Lazarus, R. S. *Psychological stress and the coping process*. New York: McGraw-Hill, 1966.

Lazarus, R. S., & Launier, R. Stress-related transactions between person and environment. In L. A. Pervin & M. Lewis (Eds.), *Perspectives in interactional psychology*. New York: Plenum Press, 1978.

Leslie, R. D. G., & Pyke, D. A. Identical twins and diabetes. In W. J. Irvine (Ed.), *Immunology of diabetes*. Edinburgh: Teriot Scientific Publications, 1980.

Lipsett, L. F. Overview of diabetes mellitus. *Behavioral Medicine Update*, 1980, *2*, 15–17.

Lundback, K., & Hansen, A. P. Diabetes mellitus and somatostatin. *Danish Medical Bulletin*, 1977, *24*, 1–7.

Mason, J. W. A re-evaluation of the concept of "nonspecificity" in stress theory. *Journal of Psychiatric Research*, 1971, *8*, 323–333.

Meichenbaum, D. H., & Turk, D. C. Stress, coping, and disease: A cognitive–behavioral perspective. In R. Neufeld (Ed.), *Stress and psychopathology*. New York: McGraw-Hill, 1982.

Melamed, B. G., & Johnson, S. B. Chronic illness: Asthma and diabetes. In E. Mash & L. Terdal (Eds.), *Assessment of childhood disorders*. New York: Guilford Press, 1981.

Metzger, B. E. Complications in pregnancy and fetal development. In B. A. Hamburg, L. F. Lipsett, G. E. Inoff, & A. L. Drash (Eds.), *Behavioral and psychosocial aspects of diabetes: Proceedings of a national conference (NIH Publication No. 80-1993)*. Washington, D.C.: U.S. Government Printing Office, 1980.

Minuchin, S., Rosman, B. L., & Baker, L. *Psychosomatic families*. Cambridge, Mass.: Harvard University Press, 1978.

Mirsky, J. A. Emotional factors in patients with diabetes mellitus. *Bulletin of the Menninger Clinic*, 1948, *12*, 187–194.

National Diabetes Data Group. Classification and diagnosis of diabetes mellitus and other categories of glucose intolerance. *Diabetes*, 1979, *28*, 1039–1057.

Pinter, E. J., Peterfy, G., Cleghorn, J. M., & Pattee, C. J. The influence of emotional stress on fat metabolism: The role of endogeneous catecholamines and the beta adrenergic receptors. *American Journal of the Medical Sciences*, 1967, *254*, 634–651.

Rabkin, J. G., & Struening, E. L. Life events, stress, and illness. *Science*, 1976, *194*, 1013–1020.

Sanders, K., Mills, J., Martin, F., & Horne, D. J. Emotional attitudes in adult insulin-dependent diabetes. *Journal of Psychosomatic Research*, 1975, *19*, 241–246.

Sarason, I. G., Johnson, J. H., & Siegel, J. M. Assessing the impact of life change: Development of the life experiences survey. *Journal of Consulting and Clinical Psychology*, 1978, *46*, 932–946.

Selye, H. *The stress of life*. New York: McGraw-Hill, 1956.

Sherwin, R., & Felig, P. Pathophysiology of diabetes mellitus. *Medical Clinics of North America*, 1978, *62*, 695–711.

Shiffrin, R. M., & Schneider, W. Controlled and automatic human information processing: II. Perceptual learning, automatic attending, and a general theory. *Psychological Review*, 1977, *84*, 127–190.

Shima, K., Tanaka, R., Morishita, S., Tauri, S., Kumahara, Y., & Nishikawa, M. Studies on the etiology of "brittle diabetes": Relationship between diabetic instability and insulinogenic reserve. *Diabetes*, 1977, *26*, 717–725.

Simonds, J. F. Psychiatric status of diabetic youth matched with a control group. *Diabetes*, 1977, *26*, 921–925.

Slawson, P. F., Flynn, W. R., & Kollar, E. J. Psychological factors associated with the onset of diabetes mellitus. *Journal of the American Medical Association*, 1963, *185*, 166–170.

Speers, M. A., & Turk, D. C. *Enhancing adherence to diabetic self-care regimens*. Paper presented at the annual convention of the Association for the Advancement of Behavior Therapy, Toronto, November, 1981.

Speers, M. A., & Turk, D. C. Diabetes self-care: Knowledge, belief, motivation, and action. *Patient Counselling and Health Education*, 1982, *3*, 144–149.

Stersky, G. Family background and state of mental health in a group of diabetic school children. *Acta Paediatrica*, 1963, *52*, 277–290.

Stone, D. B. A study of the incidence and causes of poor control in patients with diabetes mellitus. *The American Journal of the Medical Sciences*, 1964, *241*, 436–441.

Sullivan, B. J. Self-esteem and depression in adolescent diabetic girls. *Diabetic Care*, 1978, *1*, 18–22.

Tarnow, J. D. The psychological implication of the diagnosis of juvenile diabetes on the child and family. *Psychosomatics*, 1978, *19*, 487–491.

Tarnow, J. D., & Silverman, S. W. The psychophysiologic aspects of stress in juvenile diabetes mellitus. *International Journal of Psychiatry in Medicine*, 1981–1982, 11, 25–44.

Tavormina, J. B., Kastner, L. S., Slater, P. M., & Watt, S. L. Chronically ill children: A psychologically and emotionally deviant population? *Journal of Abnormal Child Psychology*, 1976, *4*, 99–110.

Tchobroutsky, G. Relation of diabetes control to development of microvascular complications. *Diabetologia*, 1978, *15*, 143–152.

Tietz, W., & Vidmar, J. T. The impact of coping styles on the control of juvenile diabetes. *Psychiatry in Medicine*, 1972, *3*, 67–74.

Turk, D. C. Factors influencing the adaptive process with chronic illness. In I. G. Sarason & C. D. Spielberger (Eds.), *Stress and anxiety* (Vol. 6). Washington, D. C.: Hemisphere, 1979.

Turk, D. C., Meichenbaum, D. H., & Genest, M. *Pain and behavioral medicine: Theory, research, and a clinical guide*. New York: Guilford Press, 1983.

U.S. Department of Health, Education, and Welfare. *Diabetes data compiled 1977* (NIH Publication No. 79-1468). Washington, D.C.: U.S. Government Printing Office, 1979.

U. S. Surgeon General's Report. *Healthy people*. (DHEW (PHS) Publication No. 79-55071). Washington, D.C.: U.S. Government Printing Office, 1979.

VandenBergh, R. L., Sussman, K. E., & Titus, C. C. Effects of hypnotically induced acute emotional stress on carbohydrate and lipid metabolism in patients with diabetes mellitus. *Psychosomatic Medicine*, 1966, *28*, 382–390.

Watkins, J. D., Roberts, D. E., Williams, T. F., Martin, D. A., & Coyle, I. V. Observations of medication errors made by diabetic patients in the home. *Diabetes*, 1967, *16*, 882–885.

Watkins, J. D., Williams, T. F., Martin, D. A., Hogan, M. D., & Anderson, E. A study of diabetic patients at home. *American Journal of Public Health*, 1967, *57*, 452–459.

Watts, F. N. Behavioral aspects of management of diabetes mellitus: Education, self-care and metabolic control. *Behaviour Research and Therapy*, 1979, *18*, 171–180.

Weller, C., Linder, M., Nuland, W., & Kline, M. V. The effects of hypnotically induced emotions on continuous, uninterrupted blood glucose measurements. *Psychosomatics*, 1961, *2*, 375–378.

Wishner, W. J., & O'Brien, M. D. Diabetes and the family. *Medical Clinics of North America*, 1978, *62*, 849–856.

9

Coping with Obesity*

MARGRET K. STRAW

Introduction

Fifteen years ago, with the advent of behavior therapy, it appeared that a major breakthrough had occurred in the long-term treatment of obesity. Early positive results prompted an explosion of treatment outcome investigations, most of which viewed the disorder very simplistically. Obesity often was defined as being synonymous with overweight, and nonclinical populations usually were studied. It was presumed that most obese patients overate and that returning patients' eating patterns to "normal" would cause weight loss to occur. Exercise was recognized as important, but was rarely included as a major focus of treatment. Physiological factors that might influence obesity generally were not assessed; if assessed, they were used primarily for screening purposes.

Recently, behavioral researchers have approached obesity with greater sophistication and respect for the difficulty of successfully treating the disorder. Perhaps the most significant change has been the recognition that obesity is a very complex disorder. It has been acknowledged that variability in patients' responses to treatment is the norm (Wilson, 1980) and that physiological factors often are crucial to patients' ability to lose weight (Rodin, 1982). Relapse is so common that one author has suggested that obesity should be viewed as simply "in remission" following a weight loss (Haber, 1980).

*Preparation of this chapter was supported in part by Grant R01 AM 27333 from the National Institute of Arthritis, Diabetes, Digestive and Kidney Diseases.

COPING WITH
CHRONIC DISEASE
219

Our new recognition of the problems inherent in obesity treatment has had a number of benefits. It has forced the behavior therapist to combine his or her talents with those of other health professionals to assess and treat the disorder adequately. It has prompted research efforts that have included more sophisticated assessment tools (Rogers, Mahoney, Mahoney, Straw, & Kenigsberg, 1980) and have asked more appropriate questions. Most importantly, it has forced us to recognize obesity as a chronic disease that requires sophisticated maintenance planning and that must be followed up over a period of years rather than of weeks.

This chapter is designed to provide an overview of the prevalence, chronicity, and costs of obesity. Emphasis is on recent developments in the field and on an understanding of why obesity may be resistant to treatment. The chapter also focuses on treatment, maintenance of weight loss, and the clinical issues raised by the fairly modest changes that generally are produced by behavioral treatments. Finally, future directions for research and treatment are discussed.

PREVALENCE OF OBESITY

The Task Force on the Definitions, Criteria and Prevalence of Obesity from the Fogarty International Conference on Obesity concluded that there is a virtual "epidemic of obesity" and related medical problems in the United States (Sims, 1980). Data obtained in the U.S. Health and Nutrition Examination Study, 1971–1974, indicated that 14% of adult men and almost 24% of adult women are at least 20% overweight; an additional 18% of men and 12.6% of women are 10% overweight. Among various subpopulations, these figures are even higher. For example, 49% of black women below poverty level are obese (Bray, 1980a).

This evidence strongly suggests that the prevalence of obesity is high. There also is some evidence that the prevalence of obesity among males gradually has been increasing. Sims (1980) noted that the average weight of military inductees has been steadily increasing in recent years. Successive cohorts of the Framingham study (Kannel & Gordon, 1980) also have increased in mean weight. In the Seven Countries study (Keys, 1970), the United States was tied with Italy for the highest percentage of men who were 10% or more overweight; twice as many U.S. men, compared to Italian men, actually were obese.

NATURAL HISTORY OF OBESITY

In the case of the individual who is developing normally, the percentage of body fat reaches a childhood peak at about 1 year of age, declines slightly throughout childhood, and then increases dramatically at puberty, especially among females (Forbes, 1980; Garn & Clark, 1976). As the adolescent moves into early adulthood, body fat declines slightly again, leveling off at about 15 to 20% for males and 20 to 25% for females (Salans, 1980).

Unfortunately, some individuals deviate from this pattern early in life. Children who become overweight at a young age tend to diverge progressively from the normal pattern of development, especially at adolescence when they gain dramatically. There is good reason to believe that most of these overweight children will never reach and maintain a normal weight. Studies have shown that as many as 80% of children who were overweight between the ages of 10 and 13 were overweight adults 20 years later (Abraham & Nordsieck, 1960). Even weight status in infancy predicts adult weight. Among infants whose weight was above the 75th percentile sometime during the first 6 months of life and who had one overweight parent, 51% become overweight adults (Charney, Goodman, McBride, Lyon, & Pratt, 1976).

For other individuals, weight gain becomes a problem for the first time in adulthood. Data suggest that the prevalence of obesity increases with age, at least through middle age and probably through old age (Salans, 1980). Weight gains in adulthood may be associated with many factors including pregnancy (Salans, 1980), lack of exercise (Thompson, Jarvie, Lahey, & Cureton, 1982), poor eating habits, and cultural factors (Stunkard, 1980). Regardless of its cause, once obesity has occurred it usually is a chronic condition. According to Bray, "the percentage of patients maintaining long-term weight loss after a course of treatment is small, ranging from 5–25 percent [1980a, p. 12]." The following section highlights several factors that seem to contribute to the maintenance of obesity.

FACTORS CONTRIBUTING TO OBESITY

Family History

Many sources of data converge to indicate that obesity runs in families. For example, in the Ten State Nutrition Study, family history data were available for thousands of spouses, parent–child pairs, and sibling pairs (Garn & Clark, 1976). The obesity status of children was directly related to the status of their parents. Children with two obese parents were the fattest, as assessed by triceps skinfolds; by age 17, they were three times fatter than children of two lean parents. Even the presence of one obese parent, regardless of sex, led to a greater tendency toward obesity in the child. The fatness level of sibling pairs was also related. If one child in a two-child family was identified as obese, there was a 40% chance that his or her sibling also was obese. In a three-child family in which one child was obese, there was an 80% chance that at least one of the other children was obese.

These and other data (e.g., Hartz, Giefer, & Rimm, 1977) have shown clearly that obesity tends to occur in certain families. However, the degree to which family obesity is attributable to genetic or environmental factors is not known. In a brief review of genetics and obesity, Foch and McClearn (1980) concluded that there is clearly a heritable component to obesity. In fact, some twin studies have produced heritability indexes as high as .7 to .9. However, several adoption studies have suggested that there is a strong environmental component to the familial trend toward obesity as well. For example, Hartz *et al.* (1977) concluded that at least one-third of the variance in obesity status was attributable to environmental factors such as food preferences, eating patterns, and activity habits within the family. In the final analysis, regardless of whether children primarily are biologically and genetically predisposed or environmentally trained for the development of obesity, there exists a strong familial link to obesity. This family tie proba-bly produces a significant drive toward maintenance of the obese state among adults and the production of obese offspring.

Social and Cultural Factors

Social and cultural factors also have been linked to obesity status. Epi-demiological studies indicate that socioeconomic status (SES) is positively correlated with obesity in childhood. Among adults, this trend continues for men, but not for women. Low-SES women are considerably heavier than their high-SES counterparts (Garn & Clark, 1976; Lowenstein, 1978). Racial differences in the prevalence of obesity also have been noted. With SES held constant, white males tend to be heavier than blacks at all ages. White females are heavier than black females in childhood, but the trend reverses among adults; thus, black females constitute one of the heaviest subpopula-tions in this country (Bray, 1980a; Garn & Clark, 1976). Indeed, the rate of obesity among black females makes them the highest risk group for a num-ber of chronic diseases associated with obesity (Lowenstein, 1978). In sum-mary, obesity is clearly related to social and cultural factors. The exact nature of the influence of these factors is not known, but it generally is presumed that differing norms within various populations pressure some to remain thin and allow others to become overweight.

Adipose Cellularity

Systematic studies of the development of adipose tissue have shed some light on the development and maintenance of obesity. Through develop-ments in microscopic and automated techniques, laboratories can now assess the size and number of adipocytes (fat cells). It appears that human infants add to their fat stores during the first year of life by increasing the size of fat cells (Lukert, 1982; Sjöström, 1980). The growth of adipose tissue throughout childhood and adolescence involves both an increase in cell size and in cell number. Thereafter, it appears that growth in adipose tissue is initially associated with an increase in cell size; if cell size becomes excessive, new adipose tissue is generated through an increase in the number of cells (Sjöström, 1980). The exact mechanism by which adipose tissue growth is triggered is not yet understood.

Moderate obesity usually is explained primarily by adipose cell hypertrophy (large cell size). In cases of severe or morbid obesity, both hypertrophy and the hyperplasia (large cell numbers) are seen. When the individual with both hypertrophy and hyperplasia attempts to lose weight, the fat cell size decreases, but the cell number does not. Thus, these patients generally do not reach a normal weight while dieting and they relapse more quickly and severely than those with only hypertrophy (Bosello, Ostuzzi, Rossi, Armellini, Cigolini, Micciolo, & Scuro, 1980). In one study (Sjöström, 1980), 80% of the variance in degree of patient weight reduction was explained by the number of fat cells and metabolic rate prior to weight reduction. Maintenance of weight loss was more difficult to explain, but 29% of the variance was accounted for by the number of fat cells (Sjöström, 1980).

In summary, the number of adipose cells found in obese individuals may determine their ability to lose weight and to maintain that loss. This finding suggests that early intervention, before extreme hyperplasia begins, is one of the most promising approaches to obesity. Even among those with hyperplasia, weight control efforts may be important to prevent further weight gains and increased health risks (Salans, 1980).

Metabolic Factors

Rodin (1982) summarized the impact of metabolic factors on obesity as follows: "it . . . seems clear that our metabolic machinery is devised in such a way that the fatter we are, the fatter we are primed to become [p. 34]." There are two major factors that seem to contribute to the obese individual's fat-making capabilities. First, many obese persons are hyperinsulinemic. Indirectly, a higher basal insulin level may promote overeating because it is associated with increased hunger. More directly, excessive levels of insulin promote extremely efficient fat storage. Second, obese individuals have large fat cells, which have been shown to have a greater capability for producing and storing fat (Lukert, 1982; Rodin, 1982).

The obese individual who has been a chronic dieter may be in double jeopardy. In response to severe caloric restriction, basal metabolic rate may decrease by as much as 15 to 30% (Wooley, Wooley, & Dyrenforth, 1979). This adaptation appears to occur more rapidly and more severely with successive diets. Moreover, when the dieter attempts to return to a maintenance calorie level, he or she may regain weight rapidly because the metabolic rate of chronic dieters remains temporarily depressed (Wooley, Wooley, & Dyrenforth, 1980).

Regardless of the genetic and environmental causes of obesity, once an individual has become obese there may be a number of potent factors operating to maintain that obese state. Certainly the eating habits, activity patterns, and social patterns of a lifetime are difficult to change on a permanent basis. Beyond the difficulty in promoting behavior change, even among motivated adults, physiological factors make weight losses extremely difficult to achieve. For example, changes in adipose cellularity produced during periods of rapid weight gain appear to reduce weight losses. Additionally, the metabolism of the obese individual seems often to all too successfully defend excess body fat.

COSTS OF OBESITY

Emotional

The current evidence suggests that obese persons do not suffer a higher incidence of emotional or personality disorders than do the nonobese (Leon, 1982; Leon & Roth, 1977). However, among the subpopulation of obese people who are active in weight-reduction programs, there have been reports of nonassertiveness, depression, anxiety, body-image disturbance, and "addictive personality" (Leon, 1982).

The only emotional chracteristic that has repeatedly been associated with obesity is low self-concept. For example, in a study of children in the 3rd, 5th, 8th, and 11th grades, the obese group had a lower self-concept than normal-weight children. No differences existed in either social or personality adjustment (Sallade, 1973). In a study comparing obese, normal weight, and a handicapped control group of cleft palate children, the obese had lower levels of self-esteem and self-confidence than did either of the other groups (Brantley & Clifford, 1979). Relatively low self-image levels also have been found in a college-age obese population (Popkess, 1981) and among adults seeking treatment (Leon, 1982).

Social

In examining the social costs of obesity, one will not find it difficult to understand why a negative self-image among obese persons is relatively common. There is a strong consensus in both the theoretical and empirical literature that the obese are discriminated against and socially stigmatized (Allon, 1982; Tobias & Gordon, 1980). Theoretically, this stigmatization occurs because the obese, unlike other handicapped populations, are held responsible for their problem. Because of this attribution of responsibility, obesity is viewed as a moral or character defect rather than a handicap (DeJong, 1980).

As anyone with a vivid memory of elementary school knows, stigmatization begins at an early age. Children asked to rank order pictures of normal, obese, and handicapped children according to how much they expected to like the pictured child consistently placed the obese child in one of the lowest ranks (Goodman, Richardson, Dornbusch, & Hastorf, 1963). When asked to characterize obese children, subjects labeled them as weak, selfish, and dirty (Lerner & Korn, 1972). Adolescents characterized the obese as self-indulgent and lazy (DeJong, 1980).

College students and adults follow in this trend, ranking pictures of obese as least preferred (Lerner, 1969; Maddox, Back, & Liederman, 1968). Even among health professionals involved in obesity treatment, the obese are viewed as self-indulgent (Maiman, Wang, Becker, Finlay, & Simonson, 1979), weak-willed, ugly, and awkward (Maddox & Liederman, 1969).

Negative attitudes toward the obese tend to be manifested behaviorally as discrimination. In a now-classic study, college admission rates were examined in relationship to obesity. Although obese high school seniors applied to as many schools and had academic records comparable to normal weight students, a significantly higher proportion of nonobese students actually were admitted to college (Canning & Mayer, 1966). The postgraduate experiences of individuals also have been related to obesity. In a naturalistic study, letters requesting advice on graduate school and career options were sent to public administrators together with resumés and photographs. Helping rate, defined as the percentage of responses to the initial inquiry, was lower if the letter writer were obese (25%) than if she were normal weight (57%) or if she enclosed no photograph (64%). Of the advice received on graduate school prospects, 70% of the letters returned to the obese writers were negative, compared to about 20% for the nonobese writers. The advice on jobs was similar, with 70% negative for the obese writers and about 30% negative for the nonobese writers (Benson, Severs, Tatgenhorst, & Loddengaard, 1980). In summary, the evidence indicates that obese persons generally are viewed negatively by others. Negative attitudes regarding the obese may result in educational or occupational discrimination against them.

Physical

Obesity has been implicated as a contributory factor in several chronic diseases (e.g., diabetes, hypertension) and has been closely linked with a variety of other disorders. A particularly high association has been found between obesity and diabetes. A cross-cultural study showed that the prevalence of diabetes and obesity was correlated at .89 (Bray, 1979). Studies conducted in the United States indicate that the risk of diabetes increases dramatically and consistently with increasing obesity (Bray, 1979; Rimm & White, 1980). Similarly, hypertension has been shown to increase dramatically with obesity. Among extremely obese individuals, as many as 65% may be hypertensive (Drenick, 1979). Obesity also has been found to be closely associated with increases in endometrial carcinoma (Bray, 1980a), atherosclerotic disease (Kannel, Gordon, & Castelli, 1979; Stamler, 1979), gall bladder disease (Lewis, 1979), and arthritis (Silberberg, 1979). Moreover, there is evidence that obesity increases the risks inherent in surgery, anesthesia, and childbearing (Bray, 1980a; Drenick, 1979).

In addition to the relationship between obesity and chronic disease, there also appears to be an association between obesity and early mortality. In an epidemiological study based on 750,000 insured and noninsured individuals who were followed from 1959 to 1972, Lew and Garfinkel (1979) noted an increase in mortality of 46% in those 30 to 39% overweight and of 87% among those 40% or more overweight. This mortality pattern was virtually identical to that found in the Build and Blood Pressure study (Society of Actuaries, 1959). The major factor contributing to the excessive mortality among the obese was coronary disease. The impact of obesity status on mortality was most significant among those 40 to 50 years of age.

SUMMARY

It is clear that obesity is a fairly common condition in the United States. The relative contributions of genetic and environmental factors to the onset of obesity are not presently established. However, once obesity manifests itself, whether early in life or in adulthood, it is chronic in nature. A variety of familial, sociocultural, and physiological factors combine to promote maintenance of excess weight and to mitigate strongly against successful weight loss. Thus, the chronically obese are caught in an unfortunate trap that has significant emotional, social, and health implications. The obese individual is likely to suffer from low self-esteem, derogation, and possibly discrimination. With increasing levels of obesity, he or she also will be at significant risk for chronic disease or early death. Given the health-related correlates of obesity, it seems crucial to find effective treatment options for those who choose to lose weight. The remainder of this chapter is devoted to a review of the literature concerning treatment outcome and factors affecting maintenance of weight losses and to a discussion of the clinical implications of the literature.

Obesity Treatment

An examination of the weight-loss advertisements in the printed media suggests that the range of options for the treatment of obesity is limited only by the imagination. However, the number of treatments that have been systematically evaluated in the medical, dietary, and psychological literature is limited. The present discussion includes brief descriptions and evaluations of several of the most common nonbehavioral treatments, beginning with those associated with low health risks and progressing to the high-risk options. It then focuses, in more detail, on the efficacy of behavioral treatments and on the long-term maintenance of weight loss.

DIETARY TREATMENT

The first treatment choice of most obese individuals is the reducing diet. Although multiple variations of the reducing diet are marketed each year, the low-calorie balanced diet and low-carbohydrate diet are most commonly used (Munves, 1980). For an excellent overview and evaluation of both new and standard diets, see *Consumer Guide's Rating the Diets* (Berland & the editors of *Consumer Guide*, 1979).

Although this represents the most common approach to weight loss, diets do not produce large or long-term weight losses. In a review of nine dietary studies conducted between 1966 and 1977, Wing and Jeffery (1979) found that the average weight loss was 18.4 lb in about 10 weeks. Several of the reviewed studies included follow-up data; at 32 weeks, the average patient had regained 3.9 lb. Additional information on dietary treatment can be obtained through nutrition education comparison groups studied in the behavioral treatment literature. Weight losses ranged from 5 to 12 lb in three such programs lasting 8–16 weeks. At follow-ups conducted 7–9 months after termination of treatment, the average loss since pretest ranged from 2.5 to 7.5 lb (Collins, Wilson, & Rothblum, 1980; Gormally & Rardin, 1981; Paulsen, Lutz, McReynolds, & Kohrs, 1976).

In summary, dietary treatments produce modest weight losses with relatively few side effects. Maintenance of those losses following termination of treatment is problematic. It is probably safe to assume that nutrition education and dietary restriction are necessary, but not sufficient, conditions for producing lasting weight loss.

ANORECTIC DRUGS

The prescription of anorectic drugs is probably the most widely used obesity treatment procedure other than dietary restriction. In one survey of

American general practitioners, 78% reported prescribing diet pills to patients trying to lose weight (Lasagna, 1973).

Most anorectic drugs are chemical derivatives of phenylethylamine which is thought to act on various neurotransmitter systems within the brain to reduce appetite. The drugs have a true pharmacological effect; experimental studies have demonstrated that both hunger ratings and food intake are inversely related to dosage of the anorectics. Additionally, they produce increased locomotor activity and subjective feelings of arousal that may increase energy expenditure (Bray & Greenway, 1976).

The efficacy of the anorectics was evaluated by the Food and Drug Administration in a series of over 200 double-blind experiments lasting for periods of from 3 to 20 weeks. Those patients receiving appetite suppressants lost about .5 lb more per week than did patients receiving placebos (Scoville, 1973). A more recent review of 62 studies using anorectics indicated that the average loss during 10.9 weeks of treatment was 11.2 lb. Three of those studies included follow-up assessments at 1 month following termination of treatment; subjects had, on average, regained 2.9 lb from their posttest weight (Wing & Jeffery, 1979). Long-term follow-ups of drug-treatment comparison groups have become available in several behavioral studies. Losses during treatment with anorectic drugs ranged from an average of 12.5 to 32 lb in 16 to 26 weeks. At the 1-year follow-up, however, losses from pretreatment weights averaged between 1.75 and 14 lb (Brownell & Stunkard, 1981; Craighead, Stunkard, & O'Brien, 1981; Öst & Götestam, 1976). Thus, although anorectic drugs produce some benefit during treatment, the losses achieved with medication are not well maintained.

FASTS AND MODIFIED FASTS

Fasts produce the most dramatic results of the noninvasive weight loss procedures. Two major fast options are available. The total fast eliminates all caloric intake, and is usually undertaken on an inpatient basis. The modified fast provides protein, carbohydrate, vitamins, and minerals in a 400- to 600-Cal daily supplement; it generally is administered on an outpatient basis.

The complete fast has a very high patient-compliance rate and produces weight losses of as much as a pound per day (Drenick, Swendserd, Blahd, & Tuttle, 1964). However, the procedure has several significant drawbacks. First, the cost has been estimated at over $400/lb, making it an impractical weight loss procedure for most patients (Bray, 1978). Second, a substantial portion of the weight lost early in the fast is derived from body protein (Van Itallie, 1980a, 1980b). Medical complications of complete fasts may include arthritis, renal uric acid calculi, hypotensive episodes, electrolyte imbalance, and cardiovascular disturbance.

The modified fast has a lower patient compliance rate because it is conducted on an outpatient basis. However, for those who follow the regimen, weight loss is rapid and clinically significant. Weight losses usually average 3 to 4.5 lb/week (Van Itallie, 1980a). Indeed, Genuth, Vertes, and Hazelton (1978) reported that 75% of their modified fast patients lost at least 40 lb. The supplement provided on the modified fast was designed to protect body protein and to decrease risks such as ketosis, hyperuricemia, and other clinical side effects associated with a complete fast (Van Itallie, 1980a). Nonetheless, medical complications including sudden death have been reported (Isner, Sours, Paris, Ferrans, & Roberts, 1979).

Although the short-term results of fasts are quite promising, maintenance has been problematic. Gries, Berger, and Berchtold (1978) reported that, at 2 years, 21% of their patients weighed more than they had at pretest, 45% had regained most but not all of the weight they had lost, and 34% had maintained weight loss. Genuth *et al.* (1978) reported that of 47 successful patients contacted 22 months after treatment, only 9% had maintained 90% or more of their weight loss; 56% had regained at least half of the original weight lost.

SURGICAL INTERVENTIONS

Intestinal Bypass

One of the major surgical interventions for treating obesity is the intestinal (jejunoileal) bypass, pioneered by Payne (Payne, DeWind, Schwab, & Kern, 1973) and by Scott (Scott, Sandstead, Brill, & Younger, 1971). The procedure involves surgically bypassing most of the small intestine so that 10–14 in. of jejunum and 2–12 in. of ileum, including the ileocecal valve, are left intact (Chlouverakis, 1975). The remainder of the intestine, as much as 18 ft., is left within the abdomen in case side effects necessitate surgical resection (Bray, 1980b; Heydman, 1974).

The bypass operation was developed on the assumption that reduction of the surface area of the small intestine would ensure that not all available nutrients would be absorbed and that weight loss would occur automatically. In fact, about 450 Cal/day are lost to malabsorption (Bray, 1980a). However, as much as 75% of the weight loss produced by the jejunoileal bypass is attributable not to malabsorption but to caloric restriction (Bray, 1980b). Several studies have indicated that patients spontaneously reduce intake by as much as 1500–2000 Cal/day following surgery (Bray, Barry, Benfield, Castelnuovo-Tedesco, & Rodin, 1976; Pilkington, Gazet, Ang, Harrison, Kilby, Walker-Smith, France, & Wood, 1976). This reduction is probably due to abdominal discomfort, diarrhea, and flatulence associated with food intake following surgery.

The jejunoileal bypass is recommended for only a carefully screened group of patients. Generally, preoperative weight must be 100% above ideal and resistant to other treatments. Patients are usually between ages 15 and 50 and free of significant diseases that would increase operative risk (Fikri & Cassella, 1974).

The results of bypass surgery surpass all other obesity treatments. Most patients lose 30–48% of their preoperative weight (Fikri & Cassella, 1974). A typical loss at 1 year is 95 lb (Fikri & Cassella, 1974; O'Leary, 1976), with weight stabilizing 18–30 months following surgery. Beyond the substantial weight loss, there are a number of other benefits of bypass surgery. Patients tend to experience improvements in mood, body image, and self-concept (Quaade & Members of the Danish Obesity Group, 1978; Solow, Silberfarb, & Swift, 1978). In addition, a variety of risk factors tend to decrease, including blood pressure, hyperlipidemia, and hyperinsulinemia (O'Leary, 1976). However, even with bypass surgery, weight loss may not be totally maintained. For example, a follow-up assessment at 78 months following surgery showed that patients had regained an average of 19 lb from their lowest postoperative weight (Solow et al., 1978). The weight increase following bypass surgery may occur due to intestinal adaptation; that is, the intestines have been shown to eventually restore surface area for absorption both by elongation and increase in diameter (Hallberg, 1978).

Unfortunately, there are significant health-related risks involved with the bypass procedure. In a review of data on more than 2500 patients, Bray (1980b) concluded that the mortality rate was approximately 3%. The mortality rate varied considerably among the studies; rates of over 10% were reported in some series. Among the many nonfatal side effects associated with bypass surgery, diarrhea is the most common. During the first 6 weeks following surgery, patients have 8–20 liquid stools/day; by 6 months, the occurrence of liquid stools ranges from 2 to 6/day. The diarrhea may result in electrolyte imbalance as well as vitamin and mineral deficiencies. Less frequent but more serious complications include wound infection, liver disease, bacterial overgrowth, renal failure, and arthritis.

Gastric Bypass

The gastric bypass, developed by Mason in 1966 (Mason & Ito, 1967), involves surgically reducing the size of the stomach. A 50-ml stomach pouch is separated from the remaining stomach by sutures or staples. The pouch empties directly into the jejunum through a small stoma (6–12 mm; Bray, 1980a). The reduced volume of the stomach produces satiety following a small meal; should a patient overeat, the resulting stomach discomfort and vomiting generally insure that the pattern is not repeated with any regularity. Thus, weight loss occurs because of reduction in food intake. A poorly motivated patient, however, can "outeat" the bypass through consumption of small amounts of very high-calorie food and through excessive intake of high-calorie liquids.

The gastric bypass is generally restricted to patients at least twice their ideal weight. Weight losses with the technique are similar to those achieved with intestinal bypass. In one series of 700 patients, an average of 30% of initial body weight (55% of excess weight) was lost in 1 year (Halmi, 1980). Bray's (1980a) review indicated that in more than one-third of the cases, weight losses exceeded 110 lb; however, in another third losses were less than 55 lb. The other benefits of the surgery are similar to those of the intestinal bypass, including improvement in psychosocial adjustment, especially self-image, and a reduction in medical risk factors.

The health-related risks associated with gastric bypass are less severe than those associated with intestinal bypass. Although the overall mortality rates of gastric bypass surgery are about 3% (identical to those of intestinal bypass), they have decreased to less than 1% in recent years. Those at greatest risk are patients over age 50, whose mortality rate has been as high as 8% in the month following surgery (Halmi, 1980). The side effects of gastric bypass primarily include vomiting and stomach pain. The most serious complication is anastomotic leak, which can result in peritonitis.

In summary, both the intestinal and gastric bypass surgeries produce rapid weight loss, due mainly to reduced food intake. Both surgical procedures also produce improvements in psychosocial functioning and in various health-related risk factors. However, the intestinal bypass surgery is associated with a high risk of mortality and a number of serious side effects including liver damage. Because the number of identified problems stemming from the procedure of jejunoileal bypass has increased since its introduction, the long-range effects may well prove to be more harmful than sustained obesity. Gastric bypass, on the other hand, presents relatively fewer risks to the patient. However, lack of substantial weight loss occurs more frequently with the gastric bypass because the poorly motivated, noncompliant patient can "outeat" the bypass.

BEHAVIOR THERAPY

Behavioral treatments for obesity have been available for over 15 years. Although the components of the behavioral treatment package vary somewhat across clinics, most current programs include self-monitoring, nutrition and exercise counseling, stimulus control, eating-style change, and contracting or self-reward. Additional components such as problem solving, cognitive restructuring, relaxation training, and assertiveness training are frequently included. Although popular in the early 1970s, aversive techniques such as covert sensitization and aversive conditioning are rarely used in contemporary clinics.

The results found across behavioral programs and across time have been remarkably consistent. Jeffery and his colleagues (Jeffery, Vender, & Wing, 1978) reviewed 21 behavioral studies conducted between 1969 and 1974. On average, patients lost 11.5 lb regardless of the client population or length of treatment. A second review, covering 48 published behavior therapy studies performed from 1966 to 1977, showed an average weight loss of 11.2 lb (Wing & Jeffery, 1979). A more recent review, based on 95 behavioral studies published or presented between 1972 and 1979, found an average loss of 9.0 lb (Stuart, Mitchell, & Jensen, 1981).

It might be expected that the relatively recent behavioral studies would produce better weight losses than those included in previous reviews because the designs of the more recent studies have incorporated the strengths of earlier investigations. Table 9.1 contains information on 28 studies published between 1978 and June 1982. All articles examining the effectiveness of behavioral treatments that could be located through computer literature searches, various abstracts, and current journals were included. The median length of treatment was 10 weeks, with an average weight loss across studies of 11.0 lb. Thus, more recent research has produced results that are highly consistent with earlier studies.

Several factors in recent studies seemed to be associated with above-average mean weight losses. First, studies that included the heaviest patients obtained the best results. A mean weight loss of 15.2 lb was reported in studies ($N = 8$) that included patients with average weights of over 200 lb. Mean losses of 9.4 and 9.8 lb were found in studies with subjects in the 180 to 200 ($N = 10$) and the under-180-lb ($N = 8$) ranges, respectively. The second factor associated with above-average weight loss was the length of the treatment program. The investigations that included treatments lasting 15 weeks or longer found average losses of 17.1 lb ($N = 6$), compared to losses of 9.4 lb for both programs 10–14 weeks ($N = 11$) in length and less than 10 weeks ($N = 11$) in length. The final factor associated with above-average weight loss was spouse involvement. The five studies that employed couples therapy reported average weight losses of 15.2 lb, somewhat better results than those obtained in individual therapy programs.

Despite these more successful treatment investigations, the magnitude of the losses reported among the studies is fairly modest considering that the average patient entered treatment at 189.3 lb. Initially, behavioral researchers believed that patients would continue to lose weight following the termination of treatment and would eventually achieve clinically significant levels of weight reduction. In an effort to investigate the long-term impact of treatment, a number of studies have been published that contain data collected at least 9 months following termination of treatment. Table 9.2 summarizes 26 studies that provide follow-up information. Again, these studies were identified through computerized literature searches, use of abstracts, and examination of current journals.

An examination of the studies listed in Table 9.2 suggests that, on the average, subjects maintained virtually all of their treatment weight losses. The average weight gain during the follow-up period was only .25/lb. However, some of those studies had relatively high attrition rates during the follow-up period. The studies characterized by high attrition (over 20%) reported an average loss during the follow-up period of almost 4 lb, suggesting that a disproportionately high number of relapsers were lost to follow-up. A more conservative estimate of maintenance can be obtained by examining only those studies with less than 20% attrition. In those 20 studies, an average of about 92% of the treatment weight loss was maintained; on average, subjects gained 1.3 lb from posttest to follow-up. Only 8 of the 20 low-attrition studies showed a mean loss during the follow-up period. Thus, assumptions concerning continued weight loss following termination of treatment have not proven accurate. However, the level of maintenance achieved at about 1 year compares quite favorably with that of other treatment procedures.

It is difficult to evaluate data regarding maintenance following 1-year posttreatment periods because of the high attrition rate from posttest to 18 months or more. However, the average percentage of treatment loss maintained in the 5 long-term studies with follow-up periods of 18 months or more and attrition rates under 20% was about 62%. If all 10 studies with long-term follow-ups are examined, regardless of attrition rate, an average of about 98% of the initial weight losses were maintained. Again, the low-attrition studies probably represent a more realistic evaluation of long-term maintenance.

A number of studies summarized in Table 9.2 utilized special maintenance procedures, such as booster sessions or contingency contracts, that were designed to facilitate continued weight loss. An examination of the studies with low attrition rates (i.e., less than 20%) shows that those studies with special maintenance procedures fared only slightly better than those with no planned maintenance. On average, those with continuing contact during the follow-up period maintained 99% of their treatment weight losses, compared to 88% maintenance for those with no booster procedures. From a cost–benefit point of view, this slight increase in weight loss maintenance may not justify the time and expense involved in providing additional services. It certainly suggests that we have not yet identified the important elements of a potent maintenance procedure.

TABLE 9.1
Behavioral Treatment Studies (1978–1982)

Author	Treatment	Treatment length (wk)[a]
Beneke & Paulsen (1979)	Behavior therapy with continuous maintenance	20
	Behavior therapy with gradual withdrawal	
Brownell, Heckerman, & Westlake (1978)	Behavior therapy, group	10
	Behavior therapy, manual and minimal contact	
Brownell, Heckerman, & Westlake (1979)	Behavior therapy	10
Brownell, Heckerman, Westlake, Hayes, & Monti (1978)	Behavior therapy with Cooperative spouse, couples training	10
	Cooperative spouse, patient alone	
	Noncooperative spouse, patient alone	
Brownell & Stunkard (1981)	Behavior therapy with Cooperative spouse, couples treatment	16
	Cooperative spouse, patient alone	
	Uncooperative spouse, patient alone	
	Drug adjunct	
	No drug	
	Total	
Chapman & Jeffrey (1978)	Behavioral package	7
	Behavioral package and goal setting	
	Behavioral package, goal setting, and self-reward	
Collins, Wilson, & Rothblum (1980)	Cognitive therapy	8
	Behavior therapy	
	Cognitive and behavior therapy	
	Nutrition and exercise	

N^b	% Attrition[c]	M original weight (lb)	M weight loss (lb)	M loss across behavioral treatments[a,d]
	25.0	180.2		17.2
58			17.3	
53			17.2	
29	—	194.4		4.8
			7.4	
			2.2	
98	33.3	202.0	11.0	11.0
	0	207.8		15.0
9			19.5	
9			14.8	
11			11.5	
112	9.6			18.7
		208.3	19.8	
		207.7	17.4	
		197.6	18.9	
		218.0	23.8	
		195.8	15.6	
		204.4	18.7	
19	6.9	—	4.0	5.4
18			7.5	
17			4.7	
13	21.7	—	5.5	8.6
12			10.5	
12			10.1	
10			4.9	

(*continued*)

TABLE 9.1 (*Continued*)

Author	Treatment	Treatment length (wk)[a]

Craighead, Stunkard, & O'Brien (1981)	Behavior therapy
	Pharmaco-
	   therapy
	Combined behavior therapy and
	   pharmacotherapy
	Doctor's office
	   medication
	Waiting-list
	   control
		26

Dahlkoetter, Callahan, & Linton (1979)	Behavior therapy with focus on
	   Exercise
	   Eating habits
	   Exercise and eating habits
	Delayed treatment control
		8

Foreyt, Mitchell, Garner, Gee, Scott, & Gotto (1982)	Behavior therapy	8

Fremouw & Zitter (1978)	Behavior therapy,
	   patient alone
	Behavior therapy,
	   couples
		6

Gormally & Rardin (1981)	Behavior therapy Nutrition education	16
Gormally, Rardin, & Black (1980)	Behavior therapy	16

Hall, Bass, & Monroe (1978)	Behavior therapy with
	   Continuing contact
	      maintenance
	   Monitoring, minimum contact
	      maintenance
	   Minimal contact
	      maintenance
		10

Jeffery, Vender, & Wing (1978)	Behavior therapy
	   Males
	   Females
		20

Jeffery & Wing (1979)	Behavior therapy
	   and additional personal contact
	Behavior therapy and
	   additional phone contact
	Behavior therapy with
	   no additional contact
		6

N^b	% Attrition^c	M original weight (lb)	M weight loss (lb)	M loss across behavioral treatments^{a,d}
32	11.1	201.5	24.0	28.1
25		210.3	31.9	
23		215.8	33.7	
6		180.8	13.2	
10		205.8	+2.9	
	0	169.3		8.8
11			6.1	
11			7.0	
11			13.3	
11			1.2	
590	20.7	192.3	10.7	10.7
	0			10.3
13		185.4	9.1	
11		171.2	11.8	
53	11.0	176.4	17.3	17.3
47			14.2	
35	9.2	176.9	12.1	12.1
	10.7			7.9
24		195.8	8.4	
25		187.7	7.2	
23		196.0	8.0	
	—		12.8	12.8
16		257.0		
72		209.0		
	2.2			7.8
12		164.7	8.7	
10		164.2	10.1	
13		158.1	5.3	

(continued)

TABLE 9.1   (*Continued*)

Author	Treatment	Treatment length (wk)[a]
Johnson, Stalonas, Christ, & Pock (1979)	Behavior therapy	10
Loro, Fisher, & Levenkron (1979)	Situational engineering Eating behavior control Behavioral problem solving	6
Mahoney, Rogers, Straw, & Mahoney (1977); Rogers, Mahoney, Mahoney, & Straw (1980)	Cognitive behavior therapy with Maximal contact Minimal contact	26
Miller & Sims (1981)	Intensive behavior therapy	4
Pearce, LeBow, & Orchard (1981)	Behavior therapy with Couples training Wives alone with cooperative spouse Wives alone with nonparticipating spouse Alternative treatment Delayed treatment control	10
Rodriguez & Sandler (1981)	Monitoring and contracting Monitoring only Attention placebo	10
Rosenthal, Allen, & Winter (1980)	Behavior therapy with No husband involvement Partial husband involvement Husband involvement	8
Saccone & Israel (1978)	No treatment Behavior therapy with Monitoring weight Monitoring behavior	9

N^b	% Attrition[c]	M original weight (lb)	M weight loss (lb)	M loss across behavioral treatments[a,d]
54	12.9	185.0	9.7	9.7
	25.5			8.0
17		174.1	6.2	
17		171.4	8.4	
17		166.9	9.4	
	19.6	202.5		8.3
24			8.6	
21			7.9	
67	—	204.4	17.2	17.2
	0	—		11.7
14			14.3	
13			9.5	
14			11.2	
14			3.6	
14			.5	
	—			6.7
5		194.0	9.5	
5		217.6	3.8	
5		179.9	2.4	
	13.9			9.3
12		170.1	6.7	
12		173.0	10.9	
13		162.8	10.3	
5	37.5	182.6	+4.0	6.9
6	0	162.5	5.1	
8	0	185.6	3.7	

(continued)

TABLE 9.1   *(Continued)*

Author	Treatment	Treatment length (wk)[a]
	Therapeutic reinforcement for weight loss	
	Therapeutic reinforcement for behavior change	
	Significant-other reinforcement for weight loss	
	Significant-other reinforcement for behavior change	
Schreiber, Schauble, Epting, & Skovholt (1979)	Behavior therapy	8
Stalonas, Johnson, & Christ (1978)	Behavior therapy with Exercise and contingencies Exercise Contingencies Behavior therapy only	10
Straw (1979; 1980)	Cognitive behavior therapy	12
Straw & Terre (1983)	Group-standard behavior therapy Individual-standard behavior therapy Individual-individualized behavior therapy	10
Wing & Epstein (1981)	Behavior therapy with Moderate caloric restriction Small caloric restriction Large caloric restriction	10

[a]Entries in this column apply to all treatments used in the study cited.
[b]N based on number of subjects available at posttest.

Because of the relatively poor results of booster procedures, several studies have attempted to identify differences between weight-loss maintainers and relapsers. It has been found consistently that the successful maintainer is an individual who monitors body weight regularly (Gormally & Rardin, 1981; Levitz, Jordan, LeBow, & Coopersmith, 1980), exercises regularly (Gormally & Rardin, 1981; Gormally, Rardin, & Black, 1980; Levitz *et al.*, 1980; Miller & Sims, 1981), and monitors food intake at least occasionally (Gormally & Rardin, 1981; Levitz *et al.*, 1980). The results of some investigations have shown that maintainers *(a)* use various cognitive skills including

N^b	% Attrition[c]	M original weight (lb)	M weight loss (lb)	M loss across behavioral treatments[a,d]
8	0	174.4	5.3	
7	0	180.8	6.9	
8	0	170.9	7.6	
7	0	175.4	13.0	
33	32.6	162.2	8.6	8.6
	0	181.1		10.7
10			9.5	
10			13.1	
12			10.0	
12			10.3	
24	11.1	198.8	6.8	6.8
	14.3			8.1
14		187.8	7.3	
14		191.2	9.3	
14		188.4	7.8	
	8.3			10.9
11		208.0	10.7	
10		204.0	8.9	
12		210.4	12.7	

[c]Entries in this column apply to all treatments used in the study cited, except for the Saccone & Israel (1978) study.

[d]M loss across treatments is weighted by number of subjects in each treatment condition.

problem solving (Gormally & Rardin, 1981) and cognitive restructuring (Miller & Sims, 1981); (b) show relatively less eating in response to life stress (Gormally et al., 1980); and (c) regularly use available support systems (Stuart & Guire, 1978). These findings suggest that an optimal maintenance program might provide some structure that encourages regular self-monitoring of weight, a facility for exercise with other individuals who are trying to lose weight or maintain a loss, and special coping or problem-solving work with persons under unusual life stress on an as-needed basis.

In summary, behavioral treatment programs consistently produce modest

TABLE 9.2

Behavioral Studies with at Least 9 Months Follow-Up

		Treatment	
		M weight loss[a]	
Author	Procedures	(lb)	N[b]
Ashby & Wilson (1977)	Behavior therapy	9.3	71
Beneke & Paulsen (1979)	Behavior therapy	17.3	111
Beneke, Paulsen, McReynolds, Lutz, & Kohrs (1978)	Behavior therapy package	16.1	21
	Stimulus control	18.5	20
Brightwell (1976)	Behavior therapy	18.7	6
Brownell & Stunkard (1981)	Behavior therapy with Cooperative spouse, couples treatment	19.8	36
	Cooperative spouse, patient alone	17.4	36
	Uncooperative spouse, patient alone	18.9	40
	Drug adjunct	23.8	69
	No drug	15.6	43
	Total	18.7	112
Craighead, Stunkard, & O'Brien (1981)	Waiting-list control	+2.9	10
	Pharmacotherapy and support	31.9	25
	Combined behavior therapy and pharmaco-therapy	33.7	23
	Behavior therapy	24.0	32
	Doctor's office medication	13.2	6
Foreyt, Mitchell, Garner, Gee, Scott, & Gotto (1982)	Behavior therapy	10.7	590

	Follow-up		
		M weight loss[a]	
Maintenance procedures	Length (mo)	(lb)	N[b]
Behavior therapy, every 2 wk	12[c]	5.9	13
Behavior therapy, every 4 wk		9.5	15
Nonspecific support, every 2 wk		9.3	14
Nonspecific support, every 4 wk		8.1	15
Weigh-ins every 3 mo		8.1	14
Monthly meetings	12	17.1	71
Meetings at 6 and 12 mo	18	13.7	68
None	12	12.8	20
	18	8.4	18
None	12	13.9	17
	18	15.4	15
None	12	16.4	6
Meetings every 2 mo for a year	12		
		9.9	33
		9.0	36
		9.2	39
		10.3	40
		8.8	68
		9.2	108
	12	—	—
Booster sessions		19.1	13
No booster sessions		8.8	12
Booster sessions		9.7	11
No booster sessions		10.3	12
Booster sessions		21.1	16
No booster sessions		18.5	15
No data available		—	—
None	12	12.8	590

TABLE 9.2 (*Continued*)

Author	Procedures	M weight loss[a] (lb)	N[b]
Götestam (1979); Öst & Götestam (1976)	Behavior therapy	20.7	11
	Fenfluramine	12.5	11
	Waiting-list control	7.7	11
Hall, Bass, & Monroe (1978)	Behavior therapy	8.0	72
Hautzinger (1980)	Behavior therapy	15.2	31
Israel & Saccone (1979); Saccone & Israel (1978)	No treatment	+4.0	5
	Behavior therapy and Monitoring weight	5.1	6
	Monitoring behavior	3.7	8
	Therapist reinforcement for weight loss	5.3	8
	Therapist reinforcement for behavior change	6.9	7
	Significant-other reinforcement for weight loss	7.6	8
	Significant-other reinforcement for behavior change	13.0	7
Jeffery, Vender, & Wing (1978)	Behavior therapy	12.8	88
Johnson, Stalonas, Christ, & Pock (1979)	Behavior therapy	9.7	54
Kingsley & Wilson (1977)	Group behavior therapy	11.4	13
	Individual behavior therapy	12.4	12
	Social pressure	6.7	11
	Group behavior therapy	11.6	13
	Individual behavior therapy	12.0	12
	Social pressure	6.7	11
Levitz, Jordan, LeBow, & Coopersmith (1980)	Behavior therapy	26.5	154[e]

	Follow-up	M weight loss[a]	
Maintenance procedures	Length (mo)	(lb)	N[b]
None	12	10.1	11
None	18	4.4	11
None	12	1.8	11
None	12	5.3	11
Minimum contact	10.5	2.3	19
Monitoring and minimal contact		7.3	23
Continued contact (biweekly)		8.6	21
None	36	24.9	21
None	12	—	—
		2.5	6
		1.3	7
		*	5
		8.0	7
		*	6
		10.4	7
None	12–18	13.5	88
Financial contingency for weight loss for 2 mo	12	14.3	32[d]
No booster sessions	12[c]	13.7	10
No booster sessions		.3	11
No booster sessions		6.9	10
Booster sessions		12.1	13
Booster sessions		9.0	11
Booster sessions		11.1	10
None	12–60	15.5	154

(continued)

TABLE 9.2   (*Continued*)

Author	Procedures	M weight loss[a] (lb)	N[b]
Mahoney & Mahoney (1976)	Cognitive behavior therapy	9.0	13
Mahoney, Rogers, Straw, & Mahoney (1977); Rogers, Mahoney, Mahoney, & Straw (1980)	Cognitive behavior therapy with Minimal contact, every 3 wk	7.9	21
	Maximal contact, every wk	8.6	24
Miller & Sims (1981)	Intensive behavior therapy	17.2	67
Paulsen, Lutz, McReynolds, & Kohrs (1976)	Behavior therapy	6.6	43[c]
	Food exchange	4.8	
	Delayed treatment control	.2	
Pearce, LeBow, & Orchard (1981)	Behavior therapy with Cooperative spouse, couples treatment	14.3	14
	Cooperative spouse, wife alone	9.5	13
	Nonparticipating spouse, wife alone	11.2	14
	Alternative treatment	3.6	14
	Delayed treatment control	.5	14
Rosenthal, Allen, & Winter (1980)	Behavior therapy with Husband involvement	10.3	13
	Partial husband involvement	10.9	12
	No husband involvement	6.7	12
Schreiber, Schauble, Epting, & Skovolt (1979)	Behavior therapy	8.6	33
Stalonas, Johnson, & Christ (1978)	Behavior therapy with Exercise and contingencies	9.5	10
	Exercise	13.1	10
	Contingencies	10.0	12
	Behavior therapy only	10.3	12

average losses, about 92% of which are maintained at 1-year posttreatment periods. However, the use of averages obscures the fact that a substantial subgroup of obese individuals are not responsive to behavioral programs; furthermore, of those who are initially successful, a substantial number relapse. It is not possible at present to identify individuals who are likely to

| | Follow-up | | |
| Maintenance procedures | Length (mo) | M weight loss[a] | |
		(lb)	N[b]
Gradual phase-out for 1 yr	12	17.1	7
	18	20.4	5
	24	18.1	7
Maintenance planning and phase-out for both groups	18	5.9	39
None	12	29.2	62
None	9[c]	4.6	37
		2.4	
None	12		
		18.2	12
		4.8	12
		12.4	12
		.7	12
		—	—
	36		
None, combined husband involvement		9.6	11
None, no husband involvement		8.0	9
None	18	11.5	20
None	12		
		13.1	10
		16.3	9
		11.4	10
		5.2	12

(continued)

lose weight successfully (Weiss, 1977). Nonetheless, pretreatment cognitions (Mahoney et al., 1977), self-reinforcement style (Rozensky & Bellack, 1976), and previous successes at weight loss (Gormally et al., 1980) have all been identified in various investigations as potential predictors of success. It has not yet been possible either to successfully individualize treatment pro-

TABLE 9.2   (*Continued*)

	Treatment		
		M weight loss[a]	
Author	Procedures	(lb)	*N*[b]
Straw (1979; 1980)	Cognitive behavior therapy	6.8	24
Straw & Terre (1983)	Group-standard behavior therapy	7.3	14
	Individual-standard behavior therapy	9.3	14
	Individual-individualized behavior therapy	7.8	14
Stunkard & Penick (1979)	Behavior therapy	22.2	15
	Traditional treatment	16.5	17

[a] *M* weight loss is calculated from available data if it is not reported by the authors. Asterisk indicates attrition was high enough that calculations would be misleading.
[b] *N* is based on number of subjects completing treatment or providing follow-up data.

cedures to meet the needs of a wide range of patients or to develop very potent maintenance procedures. Considering the current limitations of behavioral treatments, the final section of this chapter suggests directions for future research and treatment efforts.

Future Directions

TREATMENT

Given that current behavioral treatment programs are only moderately effective, it is important to identify factors that might improve their success rates. First, as noted earlier, the length of the treatment program seems to be related to outcome. Thus, long-term treatments should probably be the norm rather than the rare exception. A second change in service delivery

| | Follow-up | | |
| Maintenance procedures | Length (mo) | M weight loss[a] | |
		(lb)	N[b]
None	27	7.1	21
	9		
Individual problem solving		11.0	5
Weigh-ins only		11.4	8
Individual problem solving		13.8	5
Weigh-ins only		+2.0	8
Individual problem solving		16.6	6
Weigh-ins only		6.9	8
None	12	27.7	13
None	18	11.6	13
None	12	26.6	15
None	18	12.1	13

[c]Applies to all maintenance procedures used in the study cited.
[d]Last 22 subjects had not reached 12-month follow-up.
[e]Only successful subjects were followed.

that might improve outcome would entail an increase in the frequency of patient contact in the early stages of treatment. Although it has not been frequently studied, Jeffery and Wing (1979) found that the addition of two telephone contacts per week to a regular weekly meeting almost doubled the rate of weight loss among their subjects. Third, two components of the treatment package itself that seem especially important to emphasize are exercise and spouse involvement; both have improved treatment outcomes and should positively impact patients' maintenance efforts. Finally, and perhaps most importantly, some degree of individualization of treatment should be investigated as a means of reducing the interindividual variability often seen in response to behavioral treatments. Treatment should focus not only on idiosyncratic behavioral and psychological problems, but also on social, cultural, and physiological factors that may influence an individual's ability to lose weight. Interdisciplinary work involving psychologists, nutritionists, physicians, and exercise physiologists may be needed to design appropriate treatment programs for some persons.

MAINTENANCE

Because continued weight loss following the termination of formal treatment is needed to produce clinically significant weight losses for most patients, it is clear that our maintenance procedures should be more fully developed. The group booster meetings, which have been tested on a number of occasions, do not add significantly to maintenance. One alternative, individual problem-solving sessions, seems to show promise as a maintenance strategy; however, the use of these sessions requires further study and development (Straw & Terre, 1983). Given the evidence that regular monitoring and exercise are important to maintenance, another alternative that should be evaluated is the development of ongoing maintenance clinics that provide exercise programs, regular monitoring, and group support. These clinics might also be able to provide individual problem-solving sessions to patients on an as-needed basis. Finally, a factor clearly associated with relapse is life stress, which often results in an increase in emotional eating and a simultaneous decrease in attendance at clinic meetings. Including Marlatt and Gordon's (1979) relapse prevention procedures may improve maintenance under these circumstances. These procedures are designed to help patients identify high-risk situations and to use problem-solving strategies in those situations. If a patient fails to cope and regains some weight, the cognitive skills emphasized in relapse prevention help patients to reinterpret the relapse less negatively and to develop plans for reinstituting their weight loss program.

PREVENTION

Because it is difficult to successfully treat obesity on a long-term basis, one of the highest priorities for future research and for service delivery should be the development of effective prevention strategies. At the level of primary prevention, a wide variety of interventions are available and should be systematically evaluated. At minimum, basic information on nutrition, exercise, and weight control should be readily accessible for the average individual. At the local level, health professionals and educators can work to see that adequate nutrition, health, and physical education are provided through schools and community agencies, and that adequate exercise facilities are available to community members. It is important for health professionals and others to urge their elected officials to provide continuing financial support not only for school based programs, but also for community-based nutrition programs, food industry regulation, and demonstration projects such as the Stanford Heart Disease Project (Maccoby, Farquhar, Wood, & Alexander, 1977). Persons within the private sector may also play a role in prevention through the development of quality weight-control products and services. Finally, the media are in the unique position of being able to provide health-related information and programming that will reach millions of people. For example, the cable television network devoted entirely to health programming may have a very positive impact on prevention of obesity. At this point, it is not clear which, if any, of the interventions noted above will be useful in the effort to prevent obesity. However, they have significant potential and need to be systematically evaluated.

At the secondary prevention level, there are several high-risk populations that might benefit from early intervention. For example, overweight children might benefit from treatment prior to the development of severe obesity or hyperplasia. (See Brownell and Stunkard, 1980; Coates, Perry, Killen, and Slinkard, 1981; and Coates and Thoresen, 1978 for reviews of behavioral treatment of childhood obesity.) Some form of treatment also may be warranted for mildly overweight adults who have shown significant weight gains within the last 6–12 months, because that population is probably at risk of gradually developing more severe weight problems. In short, it may be that the greatest successes in dealing with obesity will be found in interventions for high-risk populations before the development of chronic problems.

THE CHRONICALLY OBESE

It is realistic to expect that, despite efforts to prevent or treat obesity, there will always be a substantial number of people who remain obese. There are a variety of psychological, cultural, and physical factors that perpetuate obesity. As noted earlier, once hyperplasia develops it may be virtually impossible for an individual to attain a "normal" weight. In addition, for some individuals the costs in terms of time, deprivation, and effort may outweigh the benefits of weight loss.

The chronically obese who do not desire or who are unable to achieve weight loss probably constitute one of the greatest underserved populations in this country. A variety of services would be helpful for the chronically obese. First, maintenance counseling might be of significant benefit in helping moderately obese patients avoid the health risks of extreme obesity. For any obese patient, it would be beneficial to avoid the risks of the "yo-yo syndrome." Second, support groups are needed for the chronically obese. One such organization, the National Association to Aid Fat Americans, Inc. (NAAFA), provides a network of support in the face of discrimination and the constant pressure to diet. Although the primary goal of NAAFA is to help improve the self-concepts of overweight people, it also provides needed services and information such as directories of unprejudiced physicians, lists of sources for large clothes, and ideas on coping with problems encountered with travel (Allon, 1982). Third, exercise facilities and classes designed specially for obese individuals are needed. Better physical condition might counteract some of the problems associated with obesity such as hypertension, diabetes, and even low self-concept. Overweight individuals are likely to become discouraged and drop out of exercise programs that do not take into account their limitations of flexibility and endurance. In short, as with all other chronic diseases, we need to provide services other than treatment that might allow patients to cope more effectively with problems associated with their disorder.

SUMMARY

A number of issues in obesity management must be addressed. Perhaps the most promising direction for future efforts is research on prevention of obesity. A reasonable starting place for this effort is the development and evaluation of community, school, and media interventions and of early treatments for high-risk patients. For already obese individuals, more potent treatments are needed. Longer, more intensive, and more individualized treatments should be evaluated. Given the high relapse rate following even successful treatment, effective maintenance programming is also needed. An examination of the maintenance literature suggests that this programming should focus on relapse prevention and physical activity. Finally, for those with intractable obesity, quality health promotion and support services should be developed and evaluated.

References

Abraham, S., & Nordsieck, M. Relationship of excess weight in children and adults. *Public Health Reports*, 1960, *75*, 263–273.

Allon, N. The stigma of overweight in everyday life. In B. B. Wolman (Ed.), *Psychological aspects of obesity*. New York: Van Nostrand Reinhold, 1982.

Ashby, W. A., & Wilson, G. T. Behavior therapy for obesity: Booster sessions and long-term maintenance of weight loss. *Behaviour Research and Therapy*, 1977, *15*, 451–463.

Beneke, W. M., & Paulsen, B. K. Long-term efficacy of a behavior modification weight loss program: A comparison of two follow-up maintenance strategies. *Behavior Therapy*, 1979, *10*, 8–13.

Beneke, W. M., Paulsen, B., McReynolds, W. T., Lutz, R. N., & Kohrs, M. B. Long term results of two behavior modification weight loss programs using nutritionists as therapists. *Behavior Therapy*, 1978, *9*, 501–507.

Benson, P. L., Severs, D., Tatgenhorst, J., & Loddengaard, N. The social costs of obesity: A non-reactive field study. *Social Behavior and Personality*, 1980, *8*, 91–96.

Berland, T. and the Editors of *Consumer Guide. Rating the diets*. New York: Beekman House, 1979

Bosello, O., Ostuzzi, R., Rossi, F. A., Armellini, F., Cigolini, M., Micciolo, R., & Scuro, L. A. Adipose tissue cellularity and weight reduction forecasting. *The American Journal of Clinical Nutrition*, 1980, *33*, 776–782.

Brantley, H. T., & Clifford, E. Cognitive, self-concept, and body image measures of normal, cleft palate, and obese adolescents. *Cleft Palate Journal*, 1979, *16*, 177–182.

Bray, G. A. To treat or not to treat—that is the question? In G. A. Bray (Ed.), *Advances in obesity research II*. London: Newman, 1978.

Bray, G. A. Diabetes mellitus and obesity. In M. Mancini, B. Lewis, & F. Contaldo (Eds.), *Medical complications of obesity*. New York: Academic Press, 1979.

Bray, G. A. (Ed.). *Obesity in America* (DHEW Publication No. [NIH]80-359). Washington, D.C.: U.S. Government Printing Office, 1980. (a)

Bray, G. A. Jejunoileal bypass, jaw wiring, and vagotomy for massive obesity. In A. J. Stunkard (Ed.), *Obesity*. Philadelphia: W. B. Saunders, 1980. (b)

Bray, G. A., Barry, R. E., Benfield, J. R., Castelnuovo-Tedesco, P., & Rodin, J. Intestinal bypass surgery for obesity decreases food intake and taste preferences. *American Journal of Clinical Nutrition*, 1976, *29*, 779–783.

Bray, G. A., & Greenway, F. L. Pharmacological approaches to treating the obese patient. *Clinics in Endocrinology and Metabolism*, 1976, *5*, 455–479.

Brightwell, D. R. One year follow-up of obese subjects treated with behavior therapy. *Diseases of the Nervous System*, 1976, *37*, 593–594.

Brownell, K. D., Heckerman, C. L., & Westlake, R. J. Therapist and group contact as variables in the behavioral treatment of obesity. *Journal of Consulting and Clinical Psychology*, 1978, *46*, 593–594.

Brownell, K. D., Heckerman, C. L., & Westlake, R. J. The behavioral control of obesity: A descriptive analysis of a large-scale program. *Journal of Clinical Psychology*, 1979, *35*, 864–869.

Brownell, K. D., Heckerman, C. L., Westlake, R. J., Hayes, S. C., & Monti, P. M. The effect of couples training and partner cooperativeness in the behavioral treatment of obesity. *Behaviour Research and Therapy*, 1978, *16*, 323–333.

Brownell, K. D., & Stunkard, A. J. Behavioral treatment for obese children and adolescents. In A. J. Stunkard (Ed.), *Obesity*, Philadelphia: W. B. Saunders, 1980.

Brownell, K. D., & Stunkard, A. J. Couples training, pharmacotherapy, and behavior therapy in the treatment of obesity. *Archives of General Psychiatry*, 1981, *38*, 1224–1229.

Canning, H., & Mayer, J. Obesity—its possible effects on college acceptance. *New England Journal of Medicine*, 1966, *275*, 1172–1174.

Chapman, S. L., & Jeffrey, D. B. Situational management, standard setting, and self-reward in a behavior modification weight loss program. *Journal of Consulting and Clinical Psychology*, 1978, *46*, 1588–1589.

Charney, M., Goodman, H. C., McBride, M., Lyon, B., & Pratt, R. Childhood antecedents of adult obesity: Do chubby infants become obese adults? *New England Journal of Medicine*, 1976, *295*, 6–9.

Chlouverakis, C. Dietary and medical treatments of obesity: An evaluative review. *Addictive Behaviors*, 1975, *1*, 3–21.

Coates, T. J., Perry, C., Killen, J., & Slinkard, L. A. Primary prevention of cardiovascular disease in children and adolescents. In C. K. Prokop & L. A. Bradley (Eds.), *Medical psychology: Contributions to behavioral medicine*. New York: Academic Press, 1981.

Coates, T. J., & Thoresen, C. E. Treating obesity in children and adults: A public health problem. *American Journal of Public Health*, 1978, *68*, 143–151.

Collins, R. L., Wilson, G. T., & Rothblum, E. *The comparative efficacy of cognitive and behavioral approaches in weight reduction.* Paper presented at the meeting of the Association for Advancement of Behavior Therapy, New York, November 1980.

Craighead, L. W., Stunkard, A. J., & O'Brien, R. M. Behavior therapy and pharmacotherapy for obesity. *Archives of General Psychiatry,* 1981, *38,* 763–768.

Dahlkoetter, J., Callahan, E. J., & Linton, J. Obesity and the unbalanced energy equation: Exercise vs. eating habit change. *Journal of Consulting and Clinical Psychology,* 1979, *47,* 898–905.

DeJong, W. The stigma of obesity: The consequences of naive assumptions concerning the cause of physical deviance. *Journal of Health and Social behavior,* 1980, *21,* 75–87.

Drenick, E. J. Definition and health consequences of morbid obesity. *Surgery Clinics of North America,* 1979, *59,* 963–976.

Drenick, E. J., Swendserd, M. E., Blahd, W. H., & Tuttle, S. G. Prolonged starvation as a treatment for severe obesity. *Journal of the American Medical Association,* 1964, *187,* 100–105.

Fikri, E., & Cassella, R. R. Jejunoileal bypass for massive obesity. *Annals of Surgery,* 1974, *179,* 460–464.

Foch, T. T., & McClearn, G. E. Genetics, body weight, and obesity. In A. J. Stunkard (Ed.), *Obesity.* Philadelphia: W. B. Saunders, 1980.

Forbes, G. B. Body composition and the natural history of fatness. In G. A. Bray (Ed.), *Obesity in America* (DHEW Publication No. [NIH]80-359). Washington, D.C.: U.S. Government Printing Office, 1980.

Foreyt, J. P., Mitchell, R. E., Garner, D. T., Gee, M., Scott, L. W., & Gotto, A. M. Behavioral treatment of obesity: Results and limitations. *Behavior Therapy,* 1982, *13,* 153–161.

Fremouw, W. J., & Zitter, R. E. *Individual and couple behavioral contracting for weight reduction and maintenance.* Paper presented at the meeting of the Association for Advancement of Behavior Therapy, Chicago, November 1978.

Garn, S. M., & Clark, D. C. Trends in fatness and the origins of obesity. *Pediatrics,* 1976, *57,* 433–456.

Genuth, S. M., Vertes, V., & Hazelton, I. Supplemented fasting in the treatment of obesity. In G. A. Bray (Ed.), *Advances in obesity research II.* London: Newman, 1978.

Goodman, N., Richardson, S. A., Dornbusch, S., & Hastorf A. H. Variant reactions to physical disabilities. *American Sociological Review,* 1963, *28,* 429–435.

Gormally, J., & Rardin, D. Weight loss and maintenance and changes in diet and exercise for behavioral counseling and nutrition education. *Journal of Counseling Psychology,* 1981, *28,* 295–304.

Gormally, J., Rardin, D., & Black, S. Correlates of successful response to a behavioral weight control clinic. *Journal of Counseling Psychology,* 1980, *27,* 179–191.

Götestam, K. G. A three year follow-up of a behavioral treatment for obesity. *Addictive Behaviors,* 1979, *4,* 179–183.

Gries, F. A., Berger, M., & Berchtold, P. Clinical results with starvation and semistarvation. In G. A. Bray (Ed.), *Advances in obesity research II.* London: Newman, 1978.

Haber, S. Effective treatment of obesity produces remission, not cure. *International Journal of Obesity,* 1980, *4,* 265–267.

Hall, S. M., Bass, A., & Monroe, J. Continued contact and monitoring as follow-up strategies: A long-term study of obesity treatment. *Addictive Behaviors,* 1978, *3,* 139–147.

Hallberg, D. Surgical problems with intestinal bypass for obesity. In G. A. Bray (Ed.), *Advances in obesity research II.* London: Newman, 1978.

Halmi, K. Gastric bypass for massive obesity. In A. J. Stunkard (Ed.), *Obesity.* Philadelphia: W. B. Saunders, 1980.

Hartz, A., Giefer, E., & Rimm, A. A. Relative importance of the effect of family environment and heredity on obesity. *Annals of Human Genetics*, 1977, *41*, 185–193.

Hautzinger, M. Three year follow-up data in overweight treatment. *Journal of Clinical Psychology*, 1980, *36*, 530–533.

Heydman, A. H. Intestinal bypass for obesity. *American Journal of Nursing*, 1974, *74*, 1102–1104.

Isner, J. M., Sours, H. E., Paris, A. L., Ferrans, V. J., & Roberts, W. C. Sudden, unexpected death in avid dieters using the liquid-protein-modified-fast diet: Observations in 17 patients and the role of the prolonged QT interval. *Circulation*, 1979, *60*, 1401–1412.

Israel, A. C., & Saccone, A. J. Follow-up of effects of choice of mediator and target of reinforcement on weight loss. *Behavior Therapy*, 1979, *10*, 260–265.

Jeffery, R. W., Vender, M., & Wing, R. R. Weight loss and behavior change one year after behavioral treatment for obesity. *Journal of Consulting and Clinical Psychology*, 1978, *46*, 368–369.

Jeffery, R. W., & Wing, R. R. Frequency of therapist contact in the treatment of obesity. *Behavior Therapy*, 1979, *10*, 186–192.

Johnson, W. G., Stalonas, P. M., Christ, M., & Pock, S. R. The development and evaluation of a behavioral weight reduction program. *International Journal of Obesity*, 1979, *3*, 229–238.

Kannel, W. B., & Gordon, T. Physiological and medical concomitants of obesity: The Framingham Study. In G. A. Bray (Ed.), *Obesity in America* (DHEW Publication No. [NIH]80-359). Washington, D.C.: U.S. Government Printing Office, 1980.

Kannel, W., Gordon, T., & Castelli, W. Obesity, lipids, and glucose intolerance: The Framingham Study. *American Journal of Clinical Nutrition*, 1979, *32*, 1238–1245.

Keys, A. (Ed.). Coronary heart disease in seven countries. *Circulation*, 1970, *41*, I1–I211.

Kingsley, R. G., & Wilson, G. T. Behavior therapy for obesity: A comparative investigation of long-term efficacy. *Journal of Consulting and Clinical Psychology*, 1977, *45*, 288–298.

Lasagna, L. Attitudes toward appetite suppressants: A survey of U.S. physicians. *Journal of the American Medical Association*, 1973, *225*, 44–48.

Leon, G. R. Personality and behavioral correlates of obesity. In B. B. Wolman (Ed.), *Psychological aspects of obesity: A handbook*. New York: Van Nostrand Reinhold, 1982.

Leon, G. R., & Roth, L. Obesity: Psychological causes, correlations, and speculations. *Psychological Bulletin*, 1977, *84*, 117–139.

Lerner, R. M. Some female stereotypes of male body build–behavior relations. *Perceptual and Motor Skills*, 1969, *28*, 363–366.

Lerner, R. M., & Korn, S. J. The development of body-build stereotypes in males. *Child Development*, 1972, *43*, 908–920.

Levitz, L. S., Jordan, H. A., LeBow, M. D., & Coopersmith, M. L. Weight loss five years after behavioral treatment. In R. C. Hawkins (Chair), *Maintenance of weight loss in behavioral treatment programs*. Symposium presented at the meeting of the American Psychological Association, Montreal, August 1980.

Lew, E. A., & Garfinkel, L. Variations in mortality by weight among 750,000 men and women. *Journal of Chronic Diseases*, 1979, *32*, 563–576.

Lewis, B. Gallstone disease, obesity and lipoprotein metabolism. In M. Mancini, B. Lewis, & F. Contaldo (Eds.), *Medical complications of obesity*. New York: Academic Press, 1979.

Loro, A. D., Fisher, E. B., & Levenkron, J. C. Comparison of established and innovative weight-reduction treatment procedures. *Journal of Applied Behavior Analysis*, 1979, *12*, 141–155.

Lowenstein, F. W. Some preliminary findings from the first health and nutrition survey in the USA relating to leanness and obesity in adults. *Bibliotheca Nutrition et Dieta*, 1978, *26*, 154–158.

Lukert, B. Biology of obesity. In B. B. Wolman (Ed.), *Psychological aspects of obesity: A handbook.* New York: Van Nostrand Reinhold, 1982.

Maccoby, N., Farquhar, J. W., Wood, P. D., & Alexander, J. K. Reducing the risk of cardiovascular disease. *Journal of Community Health,* 1977, *3,* 100–114.

Maddox, G. L., Back, K. W., & Liederman, V. R. Overweight as social deviance and disability. *Journal of Health and Social Behavior,* 1968, *9,* 287–298.

Maddox, G. L., & Liederman, V. R. Overweight as a social disability with medical implications. *Journal of Medical Education,* 1969, *44,* 210–220.

Mahoney, M. J., & Mahoney, B. K. Treatment of obesity: A clinical exploration. In B. J. Williams, S. Martin, & J. P. Foreyt (Eds.), *Obesity: Behavioral approaches to dietary management.* New York: Brunner/Mazel, 1976.

Mahoney, B. K., Rogers, T., Straw, M., & Mahoney, M. J. *Results and implications of a problem-solving treatment program for obesity.* Paper presented at the meeting of the Association for Advancement of Behavior Therapy, Atlanta, December 1977.

Maiman, L. A., Wang, V. L., Becker, M. H., Finlay, J., & Simonson, M. Attitudes toward obesity and the obese among professionals. *Journal of the American Dietetic Association,* 1979, *74,* 331–336.

Marlatt, G. A., & Gordon, J. R. Determinants of relapse: Implications for the maintenance of behavior change. In P. O. Davidson & S. M. Davidson (Eds.), *Behavioral medicine: Changing health lifestyles.* New York: Brunner/Mazel, 1979.

Mason, E. E., & Ito, C. Gastric bypass in obesity. *Surgical Clinics of North America,* 1967, *47,* 1345–1351.

Miller, P. M., & Sims, K. L. Evaluation and component analysis of a comprehensive weight control program. *International Journal of Obesity,* 1981, *5,* 57–65.

Munves, E. Managing the diet. In A. J. Stunkard (Ed.), *Obesity.* Philadelphia: W. B. Saunders, 1980.

O'Leary, J. P. An appraisal of the status of small bowel bypass in the treatment of morbid obesity. *Clinics in Endocrinology and Metabolism,* 1976, *5,* 481–502.

Öst, L., & Götestam, K. G. Behavioral and pharmacological treatments for obesity: An experimental comparison. *Addictive Behaviors,* 1976, *1,* 331–338.

Paulsen, B. K., Lutz, R. N., McReynolds, W. T., & Kohrs, M. B. Behavior therapy for weight control: Long-term results of two programs with nutritionists as therapists. *American Journal of Clinical Nutrition,* 1976, *29,* 880–888.

Payne, J. H., DeWind, L., Schwab, C. E., & Kern, W. H. Surgical treatment of morbid obesity. *Archives of Surgery,* 1973, *106,* 432–437.

Pearce, J. W., LeBow, M. D., & Orchard, J. Role of spouse involvement in the behavioral treatment of overweight women. *Journal of Consulting and Clinical Psychology,* 1981, *49,* 236–244.

Pilkington, T. R. E., Gazet, J-C., Ang, L., Harrison, M., Kilby, A., Walker-Smith, J. A., France, N. E., & Wood, G. B. S. Explanations for weight loss after ileo-jejunal bypass for gross obesity. *British Medical Journal,* 1976, *1,* 1504–1505.

Popkess, S. A. Assessment scales for determining the cognitive–behavioral repertoire of the obese subject. *Western Journal of Nursing Research,* 1981, *3,* 199–215.

Quaade, F., & Members of the Danish Obesity Group. Intestinal bypass for severe obesity: A randomized trial. In G. A. Bray (Ed.), *Advances in obesity research II.* London: Newman, 1978.

Rimm, A. A., & White, P. L. Obesity: Its risks and hazards. In G. A. Bray (Ed.), *Obesity in America* (DHEW Publication No. [NIH]80-359). Washington, D.C.: U.S. Government Printing Office, 1980.

Rodin, J. Obesity: Why the losing battle? In B. B. Wolman (Ed.), *Psychological aspects of obesity: A handbook.* New York: Van Nostrand Reinhold, 1982.

Rodriguez, L., & Sandler, J. The treatment of adult obesity through direct manipulation of specific eating behaviors. *Journal of Behavior Therapy and Experimental Psychiatry*, 1981, *12*, 159–162.

Rogers, T., Mahoney, B. K., Mahoney, M. J., & Straw, M. K. *Two-year follow-up results of a problem solving treatment program for obesity*. Paper presented at the meeting of the Association for Advancement of Behavior Therapy, New York, November 1980.

Rogers, T., Mahoney, M. J., Mahoney, B. K., Straw, M. K., & Kenigsberg, M. I. Clinical assessment of obesity: An empirical evaluation of diverse techniques. *Behavioral Assessment*, 1980, *2*, 161–181.

Rosenthal, B., Allen, G. J., & Winter, C. Husband involvement in the behavioral treatment of overweight women: Initial effects and long-term follow-up. *International Journal of Obesity*, 1980, *4*, 165–173.

Rozensky, R. H., & Bellack, A. S. Individual differences in self-reinforcement style and performance in self- and therapist-controlled weight reduction programs. *Behaviour Research and Therapy*, 1976, *14*, 357–364.

Saccone, A. J., & Israel, A. C. Effects of experimenter versus significant other-controlled reinforcement and the choice of target behavior on weight control. *Behavior Therapy*, 1978, *9*, 271–278.

Salans, L. B. Natural history of obesity. In G. A. Bray (Ed.), *Obesity in America* (DHEW Publication No. [NIH]80-359). Washington, D.C.: U.S. Government Printing Office, 1980.

Sallade, J. A comparison of the psychological adjustment of obese vs. non-obese children. *Journal of Psychosomatic Research*, 1973, *17*, 89–96.

Schreiber, F. M., Schauble, P. G., Epting, F. R., & Skovholt, T. M. Predicting successful weight loss after treatment. *Journal of Clinical Psychology*, 1979, *35*, 851–854.

Scott, H. W., Jr., Sandstead, H. H., Brill, A. B., & Younger, R. K. Experience with a new technique of intestinal bypass in the treatment of morbid obesity. *Annals of Surgery*, 1971, *174*, 560–572.

Scoville, B. A. Review of amphetamine-like drugs by the Food and Drug Administration. In G. A. Bray (Ed.), *Obesity in perspective* (DHEW Publication No. [NIH]75-708). Washington, D.C.: U.S. Government Printing Office, 1973.

Silberberg, R. Obesity and osteoarthrosis. In M. Mancini, B. Lewis, & F. Contaldo (Eds.), *Medical complications of obesity*. New York: Academic Press, 1979.

Sims, E. A. H. Definitions, criteria, and prevalence of obesity. In G. A. Bray (Ed.), *Obesity in America* (DHEW Publication No. [NIH]80-359). Washington, D.C.: U.S. Government Printing Office, 1980.

Sjöström, L. Fat cells and body weight. In A. J. Stunkard (Ed.), *Obesity*. Philadelphia: W. B. Saunders, 1980.

Society of Actuaries. *Build and blood pressure study, 1959*. Chicago: Author, 1959.

Solow, C., Silberfarb, P. M., & Swift, K. Psychological and behavioral consequences of intestinal bypass. In G. A. Bray (Ed.), *Advances in obesity research II*. London: Newman, 1978.

Stalonas, P. M., Jr., Johnson, W. G., & Christ, M. Behavior modification for obesity: The evaluation of exercise, contingency management, and program adherence. *Journal of Consulting and Clinical Psychology*, 1978, *46*, 463–469.

Stamler, J. Overweight, hypertension, hypercholesterolemia and coronary heart disease. In M. Mancini, B. Lewis, & F. Contaldo (Eds.), *Medical complications of obesity*. New York: Academic Press, 1979.

Straw, M. K. *Evaluation of a brief cognitive–behavioral treatment for obesity*. Paper presented at the meeting of the Association for Advancement of Behavior Therapy, San Francisco, December 1979.

Straw, M. K. Evaluation of a brief cognitive–behavioral treatment for obesity (Doctoral dissertation, The Pennsylvania State University, 1979). *Dissertation Abstracts International,* 1980, *40,* 466B. (University Microfilms No. 7915741)

Straw, M. K., & Terre, L. An evaluation of individualized behavioral obesity treatment and maintenance strategies. *Behavior Therapy,* 1983, *14,* 255–266.

Stuart, R. B., & Guire, K. Some correlates of the maintenance of weight lost through behavior modification. *International Journal of Obesity,* 1978, *2,* 127–137.

Stuart, R. B., Mitchell, C., & Jensen, J. A. Therapeutic options in the management of obesity. In C. K. Prokop & L. A. Bradley (Eds.), *Medical Psychology: Contributions to behavioral medicine.* New York: Academic Press, 1981.

Stunkard, A. J. The social environment and the control of obesity. In A. J. Stunkard (Ed.), *Obesity.* Philadelphia: W. B. Saunders, 1980.

Stunkard, A. J., & Penick, S. B. Behavior modification in the treatment of obesity. *Archives of General Psychiatry,* 1979, *36,* 801–806.

Thompson, J. K., Jarvie, G. J., Lahey, B. B., & Cureton, K. J. Exercise and obesity: Etiology, physiology, and intervention. *Psychological Bulletin,* 1982, *91,* 55–79.

Tobias, A. L., & Gordon, J. B. Social consequences of obesity. *Journal of the American Dietetic Association,* 1980, *76,* 338–342.

Van Itallie, T. B. Conservative approaches to treatment. In G. A. Bray (Ed.), *Obesity in America* (DHEW Publication No. [NIH]80-359). Washington, D.C.: U.S. Government Printing Office, 1980. (a)

Van Itallie, T. B. Dietary approaches to the treatment of obesity. In A. J. Stunkard (Ed.), *Obesity.* Philadelphia: W. B. Saunders, 1980. (b)

Weiss, A. R. Characteristics of successful weight reducers: A brief review of predictor variables. *Addictive Behaviors,* 1977, *2,* 193–201.

Wilson, G. T. Behavior modification and the treatment of obesity. In A. J. Stunkard (Ed.), *Obesity.* Philadelphia: W. B. Saunders, 1980.

Wing, R. R., & Epstein, L. H. Prescribed level of caloric restriction in behavioral weight loss programs. *Addictive Behaviors,* 1981, *6,* 139–144.

Wing, R. R., & Jeffery, R. W. Outpatient treatments of obesity: A comparison of methodology and clinical results. *International Journal of Obesity,* 1979, *3,* 261–279.

Wooley, S. C., Wooley, O. W., & Dyrenforth, S. R. Theoretical, practical, and social issues in the behavioral treatments of obesity. *Journal of Applied Behavior Analysis,* 1979, *12,* 3–25.

Wooley, S. C., Wooley, O. W., & Dyrenforth, S. The case against radical interventions. *American Journal of Clinical Nutrition,* 1980, *33,* 465–471.

10

Coping with Epilepsy

BONNIE J. KAPLAN
ALLEN R. WYLER

Historical Review

The disorder of epilepsy often evokes an emotional response that differs significantly from the reaction to other chronic illnesses, primarily because of the stigma associated with it. We have all experienced sympathy and understanding, or perhaps pity and sorrow, for the individual who has a chronic disorder such as diabetes or cancer or a neurologic disorder such as stroke. Yet for hundreds of years the epileptic has been shackled with the social stigma of evoking horror and fear from the public.

The awareness of epilepsy is ancient. Some Stone Age cave paintings in France are believed to display skull trephination (the drilling of holes) as a treatment of epilepsy (O'Leary & Goldring, 1976). Certainly by 2000 B.C. epilepsy was well known: an Akkadian text describes an attack and attributes it to the god Sin (Temkin, 1971). In ancient Greece, epilepsy was believed to be caused by the gods and was referred to as the *sacred disease.* One of the oldest theories for the etiology of epilepsy attributes it to possession by the devil. Probably because of the dominant theory of satanic possession, for centuries epileptics were treated as untouchables in many cultures. Religious superstitions and the fear of witchcraft have resulted in countless epileptics over the centuries becoming social outcasts. The early treatments themselves have been frightening; epileptics have been subjected to attempted cure by the use of ground skull bone, human blood, and religious incantations (O'Leary & Goldring, 1976).

Not until the seventeenth century was the cerebral origin of epilepsy recognized; even then, superstitions persisted. An American medical text published in the early nineteenth century suggested that disappointments in love affairs often led to epilepsy and that the treatment should include "swallowing the heart of a rattlesnake, sleeping over a cow's stable, or being passed three times through the crotch of a forked hickory tree that had been wedged open [O'Leary & Goldring, 1976, p. 28]." Actually, the belief that the brain was the source of epilepsy was not fully confirmed until Hans Berger first recorded the human electroencephalogram (EEG) in 1929.

In addition to the centuries of ignorant treatment, the epileptic patient also has had to deal with the surprisingly slow development of pharmacological therapy. For many years, there were no anticonvulsants to replace rattlesnake hearts, peonies, or mistletoe. In 1857 the use of bromides was introduced, but it was not until 1938 that phenytoin (Dilantin) was first available.

In summary, those coping with the chronic disease of epilepsy have been burdened by centuries of ignorance and a lack of useful medical intervention. Perhaps no other disorder in history (except possibly leprosy) has resulted in such profound rejection and ostracism. The next section of this chapter presents a summary of the social and economic ramifications of this chronic disorder. Following that is an overview of current research on pharmacological, surgical, and behavioral treatments of epilepsy. A subsequent section of this chapter focuses on several controversies surrounding epilepsy, including issues in the area of mental health and neuropsychological function. Because social rejection has been such a major problem for the epileptic, an overview of social support systems is also provided. Finally, we review acceptable procedures to be followed when witnessing a major motor seizure.

Social and Economic Ramifications

For many chronic diseases, the major handicap is the necessity of regular monitoring and frequent medical attention. Although this can be a difficulty for some epileptics, for many it is a relatively minor problem compared to the other limitations presented by their disorder. One of the greatest problems for many individuals with epilepsy is the difficulty in obtaining a driver's license. In most U.S. states and Canadian provinces now an individual must be seizure-free for at least 1 year in order to qualify for a driver's license (Epilepsy Foundation of America, 1976). In addition to the obvious social inconvenience that this presents, particularly for people living in cities with limited mass transit, the lack of a driver's license sometimes results in decreased job opportunities. In addition, for teenagers, the absence of a car can put restrictions on social interactions such as dating. This can be particularly upsetting to youngsters who are already handicapped with a chronic disorder that sets them apart.

Epileptics who are taking anticonvulsants are also somewhat restricted in another aspect of social interaction—social drinking. Many anticonvulsants have a synergistic effect with alcohol, so epileptics have to watch their alcohol consumption very carefully. Ironically, even though many epileptics do not drink at all because of their anticonvulsants, they are occasionally mistakenly thought to be drunk if the drug levels in their serum reach a toxic level. The behavioral symptoms of excessive anticonvulsant medication can sometimes be misinterpreted as drunkenness. This can happen even to individuals who are taking the appropriate quantity of anticonvulsants, but perhaps take some other medication that alters the metabolism of the anticonvulsant. For instance, aspirin will cause decreased binding of phenytoin (Dilantin), thereby increasing the amount that reaches the brain. Hence, a person taking a normal dose of phenytoin might appear inebriated if aspirin has been ingested simultaneously.

Another problem faced by many epileptics is that some employers discriminate against them out of ignorance and fear. In reality, most types of work are quite safe even for individuals whose seizures are not adequately controlled by medication. Nonetheless, countless jobs are made unavailable to epileptics if the employers know about the disorder. Many people conceal their epilepsy when applying for jobs. This, of course, should not be encouraged, for several reasons. First, it is unwise to obtain a job on false pretenses because discovery of the disorder may well lead to the loss of the job on grounds of deception. Second, in the event that a seizure occurs, it is best if an employer has been warned about the possibility and also educated as to how to deal with it (see "What To Do for a Seizure").

In addition to employer discrimination, which is largely due to ignorance, there are other forms of discrimination confronting epileptics. Various forms of insurance, such as life and health insurance, legally discriminate against individuals with chronic disorders such as epilepsy. Premiums can be more expensive, and the ability to obtain comprehensive insurance can be restricted.

One of the other social ramifications of epilepsy is manifested when an epileptic woman becomes pregnant. Not only will the cost of her pregnancy be greater because of the increased requirements for medical supervision during gestation, but she will also face the uncertainties surrounding the potentially teratogenic effects of her anticonvulsant medications and her seizures. This is an unresolved issue (see "Controversial Issues"), and it is no comfort to the pregnant woman that science is unable to help her assess the potential risk of either factor for her fetus.

Diagnosis

We must first establish a clear definition of epilepsy. The diagnosis of epilepsy does not speak to etiology or pathophysiology, but only to the fact that the patient suffers paroxysmal, chronic, recurrent seizures. Hence, not every patient who has had a seizure is an epileptic. For example, acute illnesses such as meningitis, uremia, and other metabolic problems may disturb brain function to the extent that a seizure occurs. Thus, the first step in diagnosis is to determine whether the patient has an acute toxic or metabolic problem that has caused a seizure or whether the patient has chronic recurrent seizures. Once this has been established, the diagnosis is based on several sequential steps.

First, a detailed history is obtained, concentrating on such things as perinatal trauma, febrile seizures, meningitis, head trauma, and so on. Second, a complete physical examination is performed, including a detailed neurologic examination. This is followed by routine laboratory tests including a complete blood count (CBC) and assessment of serum electrolytes including calcium, creatinine, and blood urea nitrogen (BUN). At this juncture, if acute metabolic processes have been ruled out, the diagnosis of epilepsy can be made if there is confirming evidence of epileptiform activity on an EEG. The patient is typically given both an awake and an asleep (induced by chloral hydrate) EEG. If these EEGs are negative for epileptiform abnormalities, they may be repeated at weekly intervals until three complete awake and asleep EEGs have been obtained. If none of the EEGs shows evidence of epileptiform abnormalities, the diagnosis needs reconsideration.

The next step in the evaluation is to determine the etiology of the seizure disorder. Although the majority of seizure disorders will not have concomitant structural central nervous system (CNS) lesions, a thorough evaluation of the intracranial contents must be made to exclude such things as arteriovenous malformations (AVM) and, most importantly, brain tumors. Even for patients who apparently have had seizures since an early age, a slow-growing glioma must be excluded. The examination that supplies the most information with the least risk to the patient is a computerized tomographic brain scan (CT scan) with and without contrast enhancement. It should be reiterated that the CT scan does not help make the diagnosis; it only helps to clarify the etiology.

Because the diagnosis of epilepsy does not designate a specific etiology or a pathology, epilepsy has been difficult to classify; hence the famous British neurologist Hughlings Jackson coined the term *the epilepsies* to underscore the complexities of the clinical phenomenon. The International League Against Epilepsy has been struggling with a comprehensive understandable classification for the myriad of seizure manifestations. As of 1969, the classification listed in Table 10.1 was in use; however, a new classification has been proposed (Commission of Classification and Terminology, 1981).

An important point to emphasize here is that an accurate diagnosis is absolutely necessary, because some seizures may be clinically similar yet should be treated with different medications. For example, true petit mal (absence) is best treated with ethosuximide (Zarontin), whereas complex partial seizures with a similar loss of consciousness are best treated with phenytoin. All too often a child is thought to have petit mal seizures and is incorrectly treated until at adolescence the seizure secondarily generalizes (becomes grand mal; see Table 10.1), and then the appropriate medication is given. Since it is a clinical observation that seizures beget seizures, one

TABLE 10.1
The International Classification of the Epilepsies[a]

I. Partial seizures or seizures beginning locally
   A. Partial seizures with elementary symptomatology
      1. With motor symptoms (e.g., focal motor, Jacksonian)
      2. With sensory symptoms
      3. With autonomic symptoms
   B. Partial seizures with complex symptomatology (temporal lobe, psychomotor)
      1. With impaired consciousness alone
      2. With cognitive symptomatology
      3. With affective symptomatology
      4. With psychosensory symptomatology
      5. With psychomotor symptomatology (automatisms)
   C. Partial seizures secondarily generalized

II. Generalized seizures, bilateral symmetrical seizures, or seizures without local onset
   A. Absences (petit mal)
   B. Bilateral massive epileptic myoclonus
   C. Infantile spasms
   D. Clonic seizures
   E. Tonic seizures
   F. Tonic–clonic seizures (grand mal)
   G. Atonic seizures
   H. Akinetic seizures

III. Unilateral or predominantly unilateral seizures
     Same as group II except that the clinical signs are restricted principally, if not exclusively, to one side

IV. Unclassified epileptic seizures (due to incomplete data)

[a]From Gastaut (1969).

wonders if the epilepsy of such a child might never have progressed if the correct drug had been prescribed initially.

Types of Treatment

PHARMACOLOGICAL TREATMENT

The history of the pharmacological treatment of epilepsy is long and colorful. The first potentially effective anticonvulsant recognized and widely used was bromine; however, its effectiveness, as gauged by modern clinical trials, has never been substantiated. The next development was the use of the barbiturates, but their use has always been plagued by the side effects of sedation. It was not until 1938 that Merritt and Putman discovered phenytoin in a search among nonsedative structural relatives of phenobarbital. Today, phenytoin is the anticonvulsant standard against which all others are compared for effectiveness. Since 1938 several other anticonvulsants have come and gone. The major clinically useful ones are listed in Table 10.2 (see Kooi, Tucker, & Marshall, 1978 for explanations of clinical seizure types).

Phenytoin (Dilantin), mephenytoin (Mesantoin), primidone (Mysoline), carbamazepine (Tegretol), ethosuximide (Zarontin), and valproic acid (Depakene) are the major primary anticonvulsants that are most popular today. Primary anticonvulsants are the drugs with the greatest antiepileptic potency. Secondary anticonvulsants have less effectiveness when used alone but can potentiate a primary anticonvulsant when used in combination. The secondary anticonvulsants are drugs that are primarily in the benzodiazepine group, such as Valium, Clonopin, and Tranxene. With the exception of

TABLE 10.2
Major Anticonvulsant Medications

Anticonvulsant medication[a]	Type of seizure for which medication is indicated
Phenytoin (Dilantin)	All types except true petit mal
Mephenytoin (Mesantoin)	All types except true petit mal
Primidone (Mysoline)	Primary generalized
Phenobarbital	Primary generalized
Carbamazepine (Tegretol)	Complex partial seizures
Ethosuximide (Zarontin)	Petit mal (absence)
Valproic acid (Depakene)	Primary generalized
Clonazepin (Clonopin)	Primary generalized

[a]Brand name, in parentheses, follows generic name.

Clonopin, which is sometimes indicated as a primary drug for some generalized seizure disorders, the secondary anticonvulsants are given only as supplements to the primary anticonvulsants.

There are several general principles that guide the choice of drug management. Generally, seizure control is attempted with the use of one primary anticonvulsant brought into therapeutic ranges as determined by blood serum levels. Most anticonvulsants induce the liver to increase the drug's breakdown and, therefore, what may originally be a therapeutic dosage may not be so 3 months later. If one anticonvulsant does not achieve seizure control, the drug dosage is tapered off and a second primary anticonvulsant is tried. For additional information the reader is referred to *Goodman and Gilman's The Pharmacological Basis of Therapeutics* (Gilman, Goodman, & Gilman, 1980).

SURGICAL TREATMENT

Regardless of how aggressive medical management is, there will always be some patients who fail to achieve seizure control with drugs. The definition of what constitutes adequate seizure control is relative. For an airline pilot, one seizure a year is a disaster because it will remove that individual's source of livelihood. For a severely retarded, institutionalized patient, four seizures a week may be of no significance to that patient's life. Therefore, if the seizures severely encumber the person's life and if the epileptic focus is within a region of brain that can be removed without incurring an unacceptable neurological deficit, surgical excision of the epileptogenic focus is a viable therapeutic option. With increasing skills in diagnosis and in defining the true extent of epileptogenic foci, the results of surgical excision are typically as follows: 30% of the patients become seizure-free, 50% of the patients have a significant reduction in seizures (greater than 60% reduction), and 20% of patients do not have their seizures significantly decreased. The mortality rate of this operation is less than 1%. However, it should be emphasized that this type of surgery is highly specialized and should not be done outside of epilepsy treatment centers that have surgeons specially trained for this procedure. It is estimated that 20–30% of epileptics are medically intractable, leading them to seek further treatment to control their seizures. Since epilepsy occurs in 1% to 2% of the population, this yields approximately 400,000 medically intractable epileptics in the United States. Because the large majority of these epileptics suffer complex partial seizures (especially of temporal lobe origin), the number of surgical candidates is great. However, at most only 200–300 operations for epilepsy are done in North America yearly, so it is apparent this approach is underutilized.

The results of other surgical approaches such as splitting the corpus callosum and stereotactic thalomotomy have been much less encouraging and still remain controversial. However, stereotactic thalomotomy is quite promising if more basic research can clarify which subthalamic target sites are best suited for various seizure disorders.

BEHAVIORAL TREATMENT

Any review of behavioral approaches to epilepsy must recognize the unique and excellent reports of both Efron and Forster. Efron (1956, 1957) reported an unusual case of a woman with epilepsy whom he treated by classically conditioning the inhibition of the seizures, pairing the sight of a bracelet with an olfactory stimulus (odor of jasmine). In spite of the beautiful documentation of this case, there appears to be no replication of this method anywhere in the literature. However, that patient was quite unusual in that the olfactory stimulus could abort her seizures during the aura.

Forster (1969, 1972) has reported on a method of extinction which he has found useful in the rarer "reflex" epilepsies. His technique, which he calls conditioned reflex therapy, involves repeated presentations of a sensory stimulus similar to the one that evokes seizures until the patient habituates to it. This approach has been successful in treating a wide variety of sensory-precipitated reflex seizures.

Although the articles by Efron and Forster are historically interesting, more recent developments in behavioral management have followed different pathways. By far the majority of current reports using behavioral approaches to seizure management fall into two categories: behavior management and EEG biofeedback.

Behavior Management

By the term *behavior management* we mean to include the entire variety of behavior modification procedures (e.g., positive and negative reinforcement, time out) and also self-management procedures (e.g., relaxation therapy). Within the subcategory of behavior modification procedures, the majority of published literature can at best be described as flimsy. Probably the greatest failing of these reports is the inappropriate way in which the term *epilepsy* is used. For instance, Gardner's report (1967) of reducing "psychogenic" seizures with a behavioral protocol is of little relevance since the patient was probably exhibiting temper tantrums (a term the author erroneously used interchangeably with seizures) and did not suffer from epilepsy. Wright's report (1973) of using electroshock to punish self-induced seizures simply demonstrates that it is possible to alter hand-waving behavior in a 5-year-old retarded boy by using a punishment paradigm. Other examples are equally unimpressive in terms of demonstrating antiepileptic properties of behavioral approaches (Adams, Klinge, & Keizer, 1973). In summary, the majority of behavior modification reports in the literature contribute little to the development of significant behavior management methods for seizure control. Unfortunately, uncritical reviews of this subject (e.g., Mostofsky & Balaschak, 1977) have been more concerned with categorization of these reports than with evaluating their importance for epilepsy.

Within the subcategory of self-management procedures, we include those articles that address the relationship between arousal–anxiety and seizure occurrence. Hippocrates noted that the spread of a (Jacksonian) seizure could be aborted by applying a tourniquet to the affected limb. Many patients report that becoming engrossed in some particular activity may abort a seizure if they are able to detect its onset at a sufficiently early stage. Zlutnick, Mayville, and Moffat (1975) reported using a punishment paradigm to alter seizure frequencies in five schoolchildren. The "punishment" consisted of grabbing the child when preseizure behavior was detected, shouting "No!" very loudly, and shaking the child. The obvious effect of such intervention was to alert the child, which is a much more plausible explanation of reduced seizures than is the idea of punishment.

The other side of the arousal–seizure relationship is reflected in the use of relaxation therapy. Although statistics are not available to indicate how often patients' seizure frequencies are positively correlated with anxiety levels, most clinicians know this to be a very common report, particularly in temporal lobe epileptics. There are a few articles in which relaxation has been shown to be positively correlated with decreased seizure frequency. Ince (1976) reported a well-documented case of a 12-year-old boy who was very fearful of having seizures in front of his friends and classmates. Systematic desensitization was used in five therapy sessions to reduce the boy's anxiety to stimulus-hierarchy items. After apparent success, continued relaxation procedures were introduced to attempt to reduce his seizure frequency. Complete success was reported, and at 9-month follow-up the child was reportedly still seizure-free. This report is an interesting example of how relaxation training may prove very useful, particularly when anxiety is known to be a problem in that individual.

Our goal here is to put the behavior management approaches into perspective, but not to belittle them. Therapists working with patients who have poorly controlled seizures may want to try a behavior modification, alerting, or relaxing protocol for certain individuals. However, in the majority of noninstitutionalized, nonretarded patients, the discovery of these techniques will probably have occurred without the assistance of any therapist. The person with a clear aura will have figured out a variety of maneuvers that sometimes abort an impending seizure, and the anxious patient with temporal lobe seizures will know the importance of leading a more relaxing life. People in the health professions who are helping patients cope with the chronic disease of epilepsy should be familiar with behavioral approaches, but also should not have exaggerated expectations of the magnitude of their significance.

EEG Feedback Training

Since the first report in 1972 by Sterman and Friar, research in the area of EEG feedback training has progressed very little toward defining its realistic value for controlling seizures in epileptics. Although there had been earlier research using operant and feedback techniques (e.g., Stevens, 1962), subsequent EEG feedback research was stimulated by Sterman and Friar's report that seizures decreased in a woman who underwent training sessions to increase 12–15 c/sec EEG activity. An interesting aspect of the reports published since Sterman's original study is a consensus that the techniques have benefited many of the subjects (Cott, Pavlovski, & Black, 1979; Dubinsky, 1980; Finley, 1976; Kaplan, 1975; Kuhlman, 1978; Lubar & Bahler, 1976; Sterman, Macdonald, & Stone, 1974; Wyler, Lockard, Ward, & Finch, 1976). Why then is the clinical value of EEG feedback training still uncertain?

One reason for the lack of certainty about clinical value is the lack of knowledge about the mechanism responsible for decreased seizures in patients who undergo such treatment. Another reason is that even in clinical drug trials of anticonvulsants there is always a significant number of patients who initially show improvement but later revert to base-line seizure frequencies. Therefore, the possibility of placebo effect cannot be eliminated from some of the biofeedback reports, especially in view of the favorable publicity that biofeedback has received in the popular press (see Kuhlman & Kaplan, 1979 for a review). Finally, even though this technique may be effective in helping a certain percentage of epileptics, the group most likely to benefit cannot yet be prospectively identified. Even if this last problem can be rectified, the cost–benefit ratio of EEG feedback (discussed in "The Issue of Cost Effectiveness") would need careful analysis before it could be endorsed by the parties responsible for paying for treatment.

In spite of these many problems, the situation is not bleak. Some excellent reports have continued to add significantly to the understanding of EEG feedback training (e.g., Lubar, Shabsin, Natelson, Holder, Whitsett, Pamplin, & Krulikowski, 1981; Sterman & Macdonald, 1978; Wyler, Robbins, & Dodrill, 1979). One of the largest obstacles faced by such researchers is that they must attempt to answer general questions about the behavioral treatment of epilepsy from studies involving nonrepresentative samples of epileptics. The people with epilepsy who are referred to biofeedback studies are inevitably the people with the most serious, difficult-to-control seizures.

Underlying Mechanism of Biofeedback Improvements in Seizure Control. The work that stimulated the case report by Sterman and Friar focused on an EEG rhythm, well recognized in the cat brain, called the sensorimotor rhythm (SMR). Feline SMR is approximately 12–14 c/sec, is best recorded over sensorimotor cortex during immobility, and is probably analogous to the human mu rhythm (Brazier, 1963; Kaplan, 1979; Roth, Sterman, & Clemente, 1967; Wyrwicka & Sterman, 1968). Although SMR training in cats may be associated with the inhibition of drug-induced seizures, this relationship is still being explored in humans. The central controversy seems to focus on two possible explanations for decreased seizure incidence in humans who undergo EEG feedback training.

The first explanation is, of course, the SMR model initially proposed by Sterman and his colleagues. They claimed that 12–14 c/sec activity in humans is comparable to feline SMR and is associated with sleep spindles, which are of approximately the same frequency. More recently, they have demonstrated changes in sleep EEGs of epileptics who have undergone EEG feedback training for several different frequency ranges (Sterman & Shouse, 1980). Interestingly, the EEG changes they documented were not specific to the SMR range as proposed by their model. On the other hand, the EEG changes that occurred indicate EEG feedback training is correlated with a shift in the EEG towards patterns that can best be described as more "normal." The best therapeutic benefit, and also the most significant sleep–EEG changes, were found during periods of training for both the SMR range (12–15 c/sec) and for higher frequency activity (18–23 c/sec). The interpretation of the results is more complicated, however, because Sterman and Shouse demonstrated that only changes in the SMR range were correlated with decreased seizures.

We must also note that another recent sleep study found contradictory results. Whitsett, Lubar, Holder, Pamplin, and Shabsin (1982) analyzed sleep EEGs in epileptics who had undergone EEG feedback training. They found no correlation between amount of 12–15 c/sec activity and seizure frequency. On the other hand, they found that decreased seizure frequency was related to decreases in 3–7 c/sec activity, and also to increases in 8–11 c/sec activity. All of these changes were found in Stage 2 sleep, and in some ways are more congruent with the theory that has been proposed as an alternative to the SMR model.

This second explanation for the therapeutic response has been called the *normalization hypothesis* (Kaplan, 1975; Kuhlman & Kaplan, 1979; Wyler *et al.*, 1976). The main premise of this theory is that there is no specific frequency range of the EEG with uniquely anticonvulsant properties, but rather that any of several changes in EEG activity (increased dominant frequency, decreased paroxysmal and slow activity) could account for improved clinical condition. For example, Cott *et al.* (1979) reported that reinforcement of SMR-range activity was not a necessary or sufficient condition for improved seizure control in epileptics. An unpublished thesis (Dubinsky, 1980) that included reinforcement for non-SMR-range activity has provided additional support for the normalization hypothesis. Hence, many reports have shown clinical improvement in controlling seizures when epileptics are trained to augment a variety of EEG activities that are not specific to the SMR spindle.

However, the line between these two differing theories has become blurred. Sterman and Shouse (1980) refer to "sensorimotor EEG [p. 558]" rather than the SMR, indicating a more global concern with any EEG activity recorded from sensorimotor cortex. They summarize their findings as suggesting a "normalization of EEG characteristics [p. 574]," again indicative of a broadening of their viewpoint. These statements probably signify a healthy reevaluation of this field of research, associated with a likelihood that progress will now be more rapid in the effort to understand the underlying mechanism responsible for EEG feedback-associated clinical improvements.

There has been surprisingly little animal work that directly addresses the mechanisms of feedback-induced changes in seizure discharge. Sterman and his colleagues have directed the majority of their animal studies toward determining the CNS events and pathways that contribute to the generation of SMR, rather than determining its alleged anticonvulsant effect.

Wyler and his colleagues have used a monkey model of epilepsy to study, on a single-cell level, two questions directly relevant to this topic (see Wyler, 1980 for a review). First they asked whether CNS activity can be operantly conditioned independently of somatic activity. Their data indicate that for the sensorimotor cortex (the cortical region presumed responsible for SMR spindles), monkeys modulate the firing rates and patterns of single neurons predominantly by manipulating the activity of peripheral muscle spindles. The muscle spindles, in turn, provide proprioceptive feedback to neurons in the sensorimotor cortex, which modulates the central neurons' firing. Hence, when cats or humans increase 12–15 c/sec activity during EEG feedback, they probably succeed by "unloading" muscle spindles (and therefore appear motionless and relaxed) rather than by directly increasing cortical inhibition. The second question asked by Wyler *et al.* was whether operant control of single neurons results in a decrease in the neurons' epileptogenicity. On a single-unit basis it does not appear that the operant task per se decreases single-unit epileptic abnormalities. Rather, the attention to the task is associated with only a transient normalization of neuronal firing; that is, epileptic single-neuron abnormalities decrease only as the monkey attends to the operant task and revert back as the monkey becomes inattentive. In light of these data it becomes even more difficult to understand how EEG feedback can be directly influencing the epileptogenicity of the brain.

The Issue of Cost Effectiveness. One issue not often considered is whether biofeedback will ever be a significant adjunct to pharmacologic therapy. The first few years of research using feedback training focused on whether or not anyone could, in fact, be helped with this method. The clinical literature reviewed previously suggests that there are indeed some epileptics who have benefited from this form of therapy. The question is, how much? And was it worth the effort?

The researchers studying EEG feedback training, most of whom are experimental psychologists, have rarely presumed that biofeedback would ever replace either anticonvulsant medications or surgery. The question usually addressed is whether biofeedback can be a useful supplement for those 15% or so of epileptics whose seizures are inadequately controlled with the more traditional methods. Most epileptics who have participated in EEG feedback training studies have received at least 25 hours of intensive one-to-one treatment from a psychologist or highly trained technician. Expensive equipment has been required during the training sessions, and computer analysis of the EEG has been a costly factor also. A significant portion of these costs is due to the "treatment" still being in a development phase. If and when it can be tried in a clinical setting, without detailed EEG analysis, and particularly with home practice units (as Sterman and his colleagues have tried), then perhaps EEG feedback training can be a worthwhile adjunctive treatment.

This discussion can only call attention to the cost–benefit issue, but cannot provide any definitive statement as a conclusion. There are still too many factors whose costs and benefits cannot yet be assessed. For instance, how significant are the long-term benefits of EEG feedback training? Also, it should be noted that in recent years there has been a tremendous increase in research and clinical availability of new anticonvulsant drugs. It may be many years before anyone can determine whether behavioral approaches to seizure control, relative to the development of the traditional approaches (medication and surgery), have been worth the effort.

Prevention

From the previous discussion it should be apparent that coping with the chronic disorder of epilepsy will continue to be an issue for many years. Pharmacological, surgical, and behavioral treatments continue to be developed, but the complexity of seizure disorders makes it unlikely that any miraculous cure will be found in the near future. One reason a panacea is not likely to be discovered is that epilepsy is not a single, unitary disorder. There are many causes and many types of epilepsies.

Bergamini, Bergamosco, Benna, & Gilli (1977) reported on a series of almost 2000 epileptic patients and concluded that the etiology of the seizure disorder was identifiable in only 44% of those individuals, but that the causes in many of those cases can, in fact, be prevented. Grass (1980) discusses three causes of epilepsy that are preventable: head injury, inadequate perinatal care, and lack of immunization. As she points out, posttraumatic epilepsy is a tremendous problem: for males, the incidence of head injury is particularly high—286 per 100,000. Roughly 5% of those who suffer head injury will develop seizures (Jennett, 1975). There is a growing literature to support the argument that prophylactic administration of phenytoin in therapeutic doses will decrease the chance of posttraumatic epilepsy in patients with severe head injuries. Servít and Musil (1981) demonstrated that the incidence of late posttraumatic epilepsy was 25% in a control group and 2.1% in the prophylactically treated group that were each followed for periods of 8 to 13 years.

Another preventable source of epilepsy is poor perinatal care. CNS infections such as encephalitis or meningitis are believed to be the third most common cause of epilepsy in childhood (Grass, 1980). Not only in developing countries, where such perinatal infections are very high, but also in North America, an unnecessary number of children experience neonatal meningitis. Of all newborn infants in the United States, .5% are estimated to experience neonatal meningitis, and almost a third of those develop seizures (Grass, 1980).

That many cases of childhood epilepsy are preventable is suggested by epidemiological data reported from the New Haven area (Shamansky & Glaser, 1979). Even when factors such as race, age, and sex were held constant, there was increased risk apparent in lower socioeconomic classes. Such an increased risk is probably attributable to factors such as nutrition, perinatal health care, and premature births.

Adequate medical care, immunization, and reduction of head injuries would not eliminate epilepsy, but they would significantly decrease its occurrence. Increased use of motorcycle helmets and other forms of accident prevention are necessary to reduce posttraumatic epilepsy. Most medical investigation is devoted to the treatment of epilepsy, and most social– psychological investigation is devoted to coping with epilepsy as a chronic disease. In the meantime, the prevention of seizure disorders through such channels as safety legislation and improved perinatal care should not be overlooked.

Controversial Issues

There are several topics involving epilepsy, particularly those concerned with behavior problems, that are controversial. This section is intended to provide an overview of several of these, describing the reasons they are sensitive.

MENTAL HEALTH AND EPILEPSY

When discussing psychological problems and epilepsy, one is torn between two different points of view. On the one hand one wants to emphasize, as part of public education regarding seizure disorders, the fact that the vast majority of epileptics lead entirely normal, unrestricted lives. On the other hand one wants to be sensitive to that minority (usually estimated at 15 to 20%) whose lives are still significantly restricted by their seizures in spite of optimal medical therapy. Because it is the minority of epileptics who are "handicapped" in the usual sense of the word, one is reluctant to over-emphasize the adjustment problems, psychological disturbances, and frank psychoses that may be associated with severe seizure disorders. In addition, as both epilepsy and mental health problems have a modestly high incidence, it is not too unlikely that a certain percentage of patients with epilepsy will also suffer from a psychiatric disease purely by chance rather than by a causal association. Thus, the fear of affecting the public image of epilepsy should not prevent the thorough scientific inquiry into the relationship between mental health and seizures.

Even in people whose seizures are controlled, problems of adjustment may occur after the diagnosis of epilepsy has been made. After optimal medical care has been obtained, counseling and psychotherapy can be useful to epileptics who have other problems (Max, 1980): (a) the individual may still live in fear of an attack occurring in public, since that possibility remains even for the individual whose seizures have been entirely controlled for many years; or (b) there may be a fear of rejection by individuals or work associates once the diagnosis is public because of the stigma associated historically with the disorder. These kinds of problems are not entirely unique to epilepsy. In some ways they characterize the sorts of fears common in any individual who has to adjust to a chronic illness, particularly if there are symptoms that are episodic in nature.

Thus, counseling in some form is often desirable for a person newly diagnosed as epileptic. A large portion of such counseling is often a matter of providing information about epilepsy because in most cases, unless the family has dealt with seizures in a friend or relative, their knowledge of the disorder may be minimal. Much of this information may be provided by the medical-care providers (family physician, neurologist, nurse, or clinic staff), and often the family may be referred to a social agency, epilepsy foundation, or other counselor for additional help. The extent of need for long-term assistance with adjustment must be assessed by the counselors. Some factors commonly encountered in newly diagnosed situations include overprotectiveness by parents of a child with epilepsy, fear of rejection by friends, and attempts at secrecy because of those fears of rejection. Issues relating to feelings of competence are typical, and in families dealing with childhood epilepsy there are many aspects of parenting that can become sources of conflict (Ziegler, 1981). In all cases, informed and sensitive counseling can be very important.

PSYCHOSIS, AGGRESSION, AND EPILEPSY

Most investigators would probably agree on two factors regarding the relationship between psychosis and epilepsy: (a) those individuals who are epileptic make up a very tiny proportion of the population of psychotics; and (b) further investigation of the relationship between psychosis and epilepsy will probably contribute more to our understanding of brain function and the organic basis of psychosis than to any real knowledge or new treatment forms for epilepsy.

Some investigators have noticed a statistically significant, though small, relationship between seizures and psychoses. There are data indicating that the appearance of a psychosis following successful surgical removal of a temporal lobe for psychomotor epilepsy occurs with an incidence greater than would be predicted by chance (Stevens, 1980; Taylor, 1975). However, this aspect of epilepsy remains extremely controversial and will probably not be resolved in the near future. The topic has been reviewed objectively by Stevens (1975).

The relationship between aggression and seizures has a long history of controversy. Occasionally epilepsy has been used as an argument in court in defense of an individual accused of a violent crime. Media attention in such cases may lead the public to think mistakenly that it is an accepted belief that crimes can be caused by epileptic seizures. Even popular novels have been written propagating the view that intentional, directed violence can result from epileptic seizures.

In 1980 an international workshop was held to examine the relationship between aggression and epilepsy (Delgado-Escueta, Mattson, King, Goldensohn, Spiegel, Madsen, Crandall, Dreifuss, & Porter, 1981). The results of the workshop were in agreement with several previous reports (e.g., Rodin, 1973) that concluded that aggressive acts during psychomotor seizures were generally random, undirected movements, such as flailing out or resisting restraint. However, a sequence of organized movements directed toward a specific purpose is not feasible as part of epileptic automatisms. The workshop also concluded that "committing murder or manslaughter during random and unsustained psychomotor automatisms [p. 715]" was nearly impossible.

In all likelihood, we can dispense with the notion that epileptic seizures can themselves be the cause of directed violence. However, this does not answer a secondary issue of whether violence is more likely to occur in individuals who also experience psychomotor seizures. As Pincus (1980) asks, is violent *interictal* behavior more prevalent among such individuals? Although there are no scientific data to support such a proposal, several discussions have been published that, on the basis of clinical experience, address this possibility (Lewis, 1975; Pincus, 1980) and also suggest a neural mechanism to account for the possibility that temporal lobe epileptics may be more emotionally labile than others (Bear & Fedio, 1977; Hermann & Chhabria, 1980). As Lewis admits, however, the theory of interictal explosiveness in epileptics is still based on "clinical lore." One attempt to address the issue quantitatively (Hermann, Schwartz, Whitman, & Karnes, 1980) found no clear support for the notion of increased aggression in temporal lobe epilepsy.

NEUROPSYCHOLOGICAL FUNCTION

Determining whether an intellectually impaired epileptic is impaired as a result of interictal epileptiform activity, anticonvulsant medication, underlying brain dysfunction associated with the cause of seizures, or whether the individual would have been impaired even without epilepsy, is a mammoth task. Nevertheless, several investigators have begun to sort out these variables. Overall, the majority of people with epilepsy are not intellectually handicapped. The population of epileptics typically involved in neuropsychological research tends to be a selected one—namely, those patients who require frequent, ongoing medical evaluation, and/or whose epilepsy is severe enough that the patient is referred to a regional epilepsy center. These are the centers in which the majority of studies have been done, which may provide a subtle bias in results.

Dodrill (1978) reported the development of a specialized neuropsychological battery designed specifically for the evaluation of seizure patients. In addition to the usual cognitive functions, the tests examine behaviors associated with specific anatomical areas in an attempt to assess functional deficits that may be attributable to localized structural damage. In particular, tests that examine abilities most typically impaired in persons with epilepsy have been included in the battery. His initial results from 172 epileptics seemed disheartening: fewer than 25% were functioning in the normal range of mental ability. However, his patient sample was from an epilepsy center and therefore does not represent the average epileptic population. Perhaps more important than the knowledge that neuropsychological functions may be impaired in patients with uncontrolled seizures is the need to determine the mechanism responsible for that impairment. Attempts to address this issue have often tried to isolate the impairments that might be attributable to anticonvulsant medication.

Cognitive Function and Anticonvulsants

The role of anticonvulsant drugs in accounting for cognitive impairments has been a sensitive and controversial issue. Obviously, it would be disturbing to discover that the medications being prescribed for seizure disorders were capable of doing more harm than good. One way in which this question can be addressed is to correlate serum concentrations with intellectual function in patients with high seizure frequencies and also in patients with low seizure frequencies, to try to distinguish seizure-induced (or neurological damage-induced) dysfunction from drug-induced dysfunction. Using this approach, Reynolds and Travers (1974) reported that in both populations high serum concentrations of phenobarbital and/or phenytoin were related to intellectual deterioration.

In one study comparing intellectual functioning on two different anticonvulsants (phenytoin and carbamazepine) a within-subject crossover design was employed (Dodrill & Troupin, 1977). Switching to carbamazepine resulted in significant improvement on cognitive tests.

There have been other reports of impairment associated with high serum phenytoin levels (Dodrill, 1975; Trimble & Corbett, 1980; Trimble, Thompson, & Huppert, 1980), but the data on phenobarbital are less consistent. However, in one recent study that compared fairly specific effects of phenobarbital on short-term and long-term memory, a clear effect was seen on the former and not the latter (MacLeod, Dekaban, & Hunt, 1978). Comparisons in this study were made in 19 epileptic patients on both medium and high therapeutic levels of phenobarbital. The short-term memory performance was significantly impaired only in patients receiving the higher dose, suggesting the importance of seeking therapeutic, but not toxic, drug dosages for patients.

In summary, although there are large individual differences in reaction to anticonvulsants, some of them may be more likely to affect cognitive function than others. It is emphasized, however, that these data are collected from epileptics whose seizures are not controlled, and not from the majority of epileptics who function with no handicap from their disorder.

Cognitive Function and EEG Abnormalities

Some of Dodrill's data have indicated a relationship between epileptiform discharges in the EEG and neuropsychological impairment (Dodrill & Wilkus, 1976, 1978). In one sample of 90 patients including 32 who had no interictal discharges, 27 whose discharges occurred at a rate of less than once a minute, and 31 whose epileptiform discharges occurred more frequently than 1 per minute, significant dysfunction on half of the psychological variables was associated with increased frequency of epileptiform discharges. In addition, the individuals whose discharges were categorized as generalized were more significantly impaired than those with focal discharges or those with none at all.

In summary, definitive answers to these sensitive issues involving mental health, aggression, psychopathology, and neuropsychological function are not yet available. As we have emphasized, these issues are of little significance for the largest proportion of persons with epilepsy (probably at least 80%), because their seizures are controlled and their lives have been adjusted to cope with this chronic disorder. For the minority, continued research will be necessary to provide further clues into the relationship between their brain dysfunction and potential neuropsychological problems.

TERATOGENICITY OF SEIZURES AND ANTICONVULSANTS

One final issue that must be dealt with is the potential problem of pregnancy. Only a few years ago several states in the United States still prevented persons with epilepsy from marrying; this anachronistic law has now been removed in all jurisdictions. But in a recent survey of physicians in Australia (Beran, Jennings, & Read, 1981), 7% of the sample was still "undecided" about whether marriage was wise. In addition, 15% agreed with the statement, "It may be unwise for people with epilepsy to have children."

In a general questionnaire of this sort, the reasoning behind the individual answers is impossible to determine. Very few causes of epilepsy are genetically determined. Perhaps some of those 15% were thinking of the occasional severely handicapped person who requires special care and would be unable to care for an infant. Or perhaps they were thinking of possible teratogenicity of seizures or anticonvulsants. For almost 20 years, research has been accumulating that indicates children born to epileptic mothers have an increased risk of cleft lip and palate. Recently, one study reported this increased risk in children with either epileptic mothers or epileptic fathers (Friis, 1979). This would seem to suggest that the seizures per se, and not the fetal exposure to anticonvulsants, might be responsible for the increased risk, particularly as some of the epileptic parents were not taking medication.

Probably the largest study reported so far was performed by a group of 11 institutions in Japan (Nakane and coauthors, 1980). Their results were from 902 cases of pregnancy, focusing only on epileptic mothers and not on fathers. In addition to data regarding medications and pregnancy outcome, Nakane et al. recorded the occurrence of seizures during pregnancy (present in 44% of the medicated and 50% of the unmedicated women). They found fetal malformations to be lowest in women who were unmedicated and who had no seizures during pregnancy; the highest rate of malformations was in women who were medicated and who did have seizures during pregnancy. However, it is important to note that the number of medications being used was a significant variable, the incidence of malformations being particularly high in women who were taking three or more anticonvulsants during the first trimester of pregnancy. Although many articles have appeared describing a fetal hydantoin syndrome and a fetal barbiturate syndrome, the collaborative Japanese study implicated trimethadione as posing the largest risk to the fetus. When women taking trimethadione were excluded from the sample, the difference between the medicated and unmedicated groups was much less.

The problem in treating a woman with an uncontrolled seizure disorder during the first trimester of pregnancy is that the data are still not sufficiently clear to balance which of two risk factors is greater for her: having seizures on relatively low doses of anticonvulsants, or having no seizures on relatively higher dosages. In addition, other factors regarding her family history and her own pregnancy history may be very relevant in determining her potential risk for giving birth to a child with congenital malformations (Nakane et al., 1980). Finally, most women have not adequately planned ahead. The majority find they are pregnant only after the first trimester (the highest-risk phase) is well underway. At present, there are no data on which to base a minimal error decision when planning a pregnancy other than to make sure the prospective mother is monitored carefully by a physician knowledgeable in the treatment of epilepsy.

Social Support Systems

By the year 2000, the world population will probably reach 6 billion. With a conservative estimate of the prevalence of epilepsy (1%), this means that there will be approximately 60 million persons with epilepsy at that time

(Grass, 1980). In addition to the types of treatment and prevention already described, another very important issue concerns the development and improvement of social and support services.

For many years the International League Against Epilepsy has brought together physicians and scientists concerned with this disorder. Although there is no international organization of lay associations, most regions in North America have organizations that are part of either the Epilepsy Foundation of America or Epilepsy Canada. The local chapters of these lay associations typically concentrate on providing support services for epileptics and their families and also on educating the public. That these services are needed is obvious. Using the frequently cited 80% figure as an estimate of the proportion of individuals whose lives are not significantly handicapped by the disorder, one can still project 12 million people by the turn of the century who will require significant assistance in adjusting to living with epilepsy. However, a more relevant way of looking at the social need is to remember that the primary adjustment obstacle for many epileptics is lack of public knowledge about epilepsy. The unfortunate social stigma still associated with seizure disorders can produce significant adjustment problems for the epileptic. Hence, when considering the existing need for the work of lay associations, one must consider the entire population of 6 billion as being the target for social programs, and not just the individuals and families who must deal with epilepsy directly.

Consequently, the dissemination of information is a high priority of the Epilepsy Foundation of America and Epilepsy Canada. The newsletters produced by the Epilepsy Foundation of America in the United States and by many local chapters often provide capsule comments on a variety of topics: developments in medical research that are relevant to epilepsy, legislation being considered on both local and federal levels that may have relevance to epilepsy, and activities by local chapters to educate the public and improve the lot of individuals with seizures. Public service announcements, television commercials, school presentations, and media coverage every year during National Epilepsy Week are all very important attempts to remove ignorance and historical prejudices.

Counseling when the diagnosis of epilepsy first occurs can be one of the most effective means of decreasing later psychosocial problems. Children with epilepsy are particularly likely to experience overprotectiveness and overindulgence during childhood, resulting in later adjustment problems (Ziegler, 1981). Early counseling can help parents dispel fears and myths about epilepsy, can assist them in avoiding the pitfalls of overprotection, and can also teach them ways in which to disclose information regarding their child's disorder that will not reinforce those fears and myths.

In addition to counseling, dissemination of information, and public education, lay associations often provide a valuable service with employment programs. A survey of patients in Norway (Løyning, 1980) indicated that only 50% of the men and 25% of the women were employed, compared to 77% and 49% respectively in the total population.

It is impossible to overemphasize the importance of public education in improving the lives of persons with epilepsy. A psychiatrist writing about the procedures of psychotherapy for epileptic patients (Max, 1980) emphasized that the first step in individual psychotherapy is the understanding of the "ancient and practically unchanged social and moral prejudices of the disorder [p. 179]." Perhaps it is essential to understand the impact of these ancient prejudices on each individual person, but the viewpoint of the social support agencies, of course, is that it is even more important to change those prejudices.

What to Do for a Seizure

If you happen to witness a partial seizure or a petit mal absence, it is unlikely that you will feel any need to provide assistance. In partial seizures there is usually no loss of consciousness, and in petit mal seizures the loss of consciousness is very brief. It is when people witness a generalized tonic–clonic (grand mal) seizure that they feel compelled to help, sometimes to the detriment of the epileptic. This section is intended to provide information on what to expect during such a seizure and also on what to do.

A generalized tonic–clonic seizure consists of several phases. Sometimes the first manifestation of the seizure is a shrill outcry caused by contraction of the respiratory muscles and the resultant expulsion of air. The tonic phase is often very brief and consists of a stiffening of the body. The clonic phase consists of muscular spasms encompassing the whole body. Incontinence, salivation, and gutteral sounds may accompany the clonic spasms. As the spasms decrease and the seizure ends, the person may be quite groggy and unresponsive to questions, or may fall asleep.

Many people do not realize how ill-prepared they are to help a person having a tonic–clonic seizure until the moment they are abruptly confronted with the situation. Many well-meaning individuals have inserted all manner of items into the mouths of epileptics in the midst of seizures, mistakenly thinking that this was a helpful act. In reality, there is very little that a bystander *can* do other than follow simple rules. It may be some comfort to the observer to know that almost all seizures are self-limiting and that what is required of the bystander is mainly patience, and protecting the epileptic from good samaritans.

1. *Protect the person from injury.* The worst injuries incurred during seizures are head injuries from falling. If possible, try to protect the person's head (if she has fallen) by putting some sort of padding (e.g., a coat) between the head and the ground.

2. *Do not put anything in the mouth.* It is anatomically impossible to swallow one's tongue! If the individual appears to be salivating a great deal, it can be helpful to turn her on her side so that the saliva is not aspirated and the airway is not obstructed.

3. *Do not restrain the person.* Rather than trying to hold her down, it is best to remove any objects you fear might injure the person during the seizure. Remember that the epileptic is not conscious during a generalized seizure, so if you try to restrain her, you may be accidentally harmed in some way yourself.

4. *If the seizure continues for more than 5 minutes, call an ambulance.* If it does not last that long, just sit with the person as she is coming out of the seizure and wait till she fully regains consciousness before assisting her home. It is common for people to desire sleep after a generalized seizure. Also it is common for some people to be mildly disoriented for several minutes after regaining consciousness.

Notice that most of the points above are commonsense items. Protect the person from self-injury, and do not put anything in the mouth. Patience and simple concern will be more than adequate in most cases.

References

Adams, K. M., Klinge, V., & Keizer, T. W. The extinction of a self-injurious behavior in an epileptic child. *Behaviour Research and Therapy*, 1973, *11*, 351–356.

Bear, D., & Fedio, P. Quantitative analysis of interictal behavior in temporal lobe epilepsy. *Archives of Neurology*, 1977, *34*, 454–469.

Beran, R. G., Jennings, V. R., & Read, T. Doctors' perspectives of epilepsy. *Epilepsia*, 1981, *22*, 397–406.

Bergamini, L., Bergamosco, B., Benna, T., & Gilli, M. Acquired etiological factors in 1,785 epileptic subjects: Clinical–anamnestic research. *Epilepsia*, 1977, *18*, 437–444.

Brazier, M. A. B. The problem of periodicity in the electroencephalogram: Studies in the cat. *Electroencephalography and clinical Neurophysiology*, 1963, *15*, 287–298.

Commission of Classification and Terminology of the International League Against Epilepsy. Proposal for Revised Clinical and Electroencephalographic Classification of Epileptic Seizures. *Epilepsia*, 1981, *22*, 489–501.

Cott, A., Pavloski, R. P., & Black, A. H. Reducing epileptic seizures through operant conditioning of central nervous system activity: Procedural variables. *Science*, 1979, *203*, 73–75.

Delgado-Escueta, A. V., Mattson, R. H., King, L., Goldensohn, E. S., Spiegel, H., Madsen, J., Crandall, P., Dreifuss, F., & Porter, R. J. The nature of aggression during epileptic seizures. *New England Journal of Medicine*, 1981, *305*, 711–716.

Dodrill, C. B. Diphenylhydantoin serum levels, toxicity, and neuropsychological performance in patients with epilepsy. *Epilepsia*, 1975, *16*, 593–600.

Dodrill, C. B. A neuropsychological battery for epilepsy. *Epilepsia*, 1978, *19*, 611–623.

Dodrill, C. B., & Troupin, A. S. Psychotropic effects of carbamazepine in epilepsy: A double-blind comparison with phenytoin. *Neurology* 1977, *27*, 1023–1028.

Dodrill, C. B., & Wilkus, R. J. Neuropsychological correlates of the electroencephalogram in epileptics: II. The waking posterior rhythm and its interaction with epileptiform activity. *Epilepsia*, 1976, *17*, 101–109.

Dodrill, C. B., & Wilkus, R. J. Neuropsychological correlates of the electroencephalogram in epileptics: III. Generalized nonepileptiform abnormalities. *Epilepsia*, 1978, *18*, 553–562.

Dubinsky, B. *The effects of high versus low amplitude training of 9–13 hertz EEG activity on the seizure rate of refractory epileptics.* Unpublished master's thesis, University of Central Florida, 1980.

Efron, R. The effect of olfactory stimuli in arresting uncinate fits. *Brain*, 1956, *79*, 267–281.

Efron, R. Conditioned inhibition of uncinate fits. *Brain*, 1957, *80*, 251–262.

Epilepsy Foundation of America. *The legal rights of persons with epilepsy.* Washington, D.C.: Author, 1976.

Finley, W. W. Effects of sham feedback following successful SMR training in an epileptic: Follow-up study. *Biofeedback and Self-Regulation*, 1976, *1*, 227–236.

Forster, F. M. Conditional reflexes and sensory-evoked epilepsy: The nature of the therapeutic process. *Conditional Reflex*, 1969, *4*, 103–114.

Forster, F. M. The classification and conditioning treatment of the reflex epilepsies. *International Journal of Neurology*, 1972, *9*, 73–86.

Friis, M. L. Epilepsy among parents of children with facial clefts. *Epilepsia*, 1979, *20*, 69–76.

Gardner, J. E. Behavior therapy treatment approach to a psychogenic seizure case. *Journal of Consulting Psychology*, 1967, *31*, 209–212.

Gastaut, H. Classification of the epilepsies. *Epilepsia* (supplement), 1969, *10*, 514–521.

Gilman, A. G., Goodman, L. S., & Gilman, A. (Eds.). *Goodman and Gilman's the pharmacological basis of therapeutics* (6th ed.). New York: Macmillan, 1980.

Grass, E. R. Prevention of epilepsy world-wide. In J. A. Wada & J. K. Penry (Eds.), *Advances in Epileptology: Xth Epilepsy International Symposium.* New York: Raven Press, 1980.

Hermann, B. P., & Chhabria, S. Interictal psychopathology in patients with ictal fear: Examples of sensory–limbic hyperconnection? *Archives of Neurology*, 1980, *37*, 667–668.

Hermann, B. P., Schwartz, M. S., Whitman, S., & Karnes, W. E. Aggression and epilepsy: Seizure-type comparisons and high-risk variables. *Epilepsia*, 1980, *22*, 691–698.

Ince, L. P. The use of relaxation training and a conditioned stimulus in the elimination of epileptic seizures in a child: A case study. *Journal of Behavior Therapy and Experimental Psychiatry*, 1976, *7*, 39–42.

Jennett, W. B. *Epilepsy after non-missile head injuries.* Chicago: Yearbook, 1975.

Kaplan, B. J. Biofeedback in epileptics: Equivocal relationship of reinforced EEG frequency to seizure reduction. *Epilepsia*, 1975, *16*, 477–485.

Kaplan, B. J. Morphological evidence that feline SMR and human mu are analogous rhythms. *Brain Research Bulletin*, 1979, *4*, 431–433.

Kooi, K. A., Tucker, R. P., & Marshall, R. E. *Fundamentals of electroencephalography* (2nd ed.). Hagerstown, Md.: Harper & Row, 1978.

Kuhlman, W. N. EEG feedback training of epileptic patients: Clinical and electroencephalographic analysis. *Electroencephalography and clinical Neurophysiology*, 1978, *45*, 699–710.

Kuhlman, W. N., & Kaplan, B. J. Clinical applications of EEG feedback training. In R. Gatchel & K. Price (Eds.), *Clinical applications of biofeedback: Appraisal and status.* New York: Pergamon Press, 1979.

Lewis, J. A. Violence and epilepsy. *Journal of the American Medical Association*, 1975, *232*, 1165–1167.

Løyning, Y. Comprehensive care. In J. A. Wada & J. K. Penry (Eds.), *Advances in Epileptology: Xth Epilepsy International Symposium*. New York: Raven Press, 1980.

Lubar, J. F., & Bahler, W. W. Behavioral management of epileptic seizures following EEG biofeedback training of the sensorimotor rhythm. *Biofeedback and Self-Regulation*, 1976, *1*, 77–104.

Lubar, J. F., Shabsin, H. S., Natelson, S. E., Holder, G. S., Whitsett, S. F., Pamplin, W. E., & Krulikowski, D. I. EEG operant conditioning in intractable epileptics. *Archives of Neurology*, 1981, *38*, 700–704.

MacLeod, C. M., Dekaban, A. S., & Hunt, E. Memory impairment in epileptic patients: Selective effects of phenobarbital concentration. *Science*, 1978, *202*, 1102–1104.

Max, G. Psychotherapy with epileptic patients. In R. Canger, F. Angeleri, & J. K. Penry (Eds.), *Advances in Epileptology: XIth Epilepsy International Symposium*. New York: Raven Press, 1980.

Mostofsky, D. I., & Balaschak, B. A. Psychobiological control of seizures. *Psychological Bulletin*, 1977, *84*, 723–750.

Nakane, Y., Okuma, T., Takahashi, R., Sato, Y., Wada, T., Sato, T., Fukushima, Y., Kumashiro, H., Ono, T., Takahashi, T., Aoki, Y., Kazamatsuri, H., Inami, M., Komai, S., Seino, M., Miyakoshi, M., Tanimura, T., Hazama, H., Kawahara, R., Otsuki, S., Hosokawa, K., Inanaga, K., Nakazawa, Y., & Yamamoto, K. Multi-institutional study on the teratogenicity and fetal toxicity of antiepileptic drugs: A report of a collaborative study group in Japan. *Epilepsia*, 1980, *21*, 663–680.

O'Leary, J. L., & Goldring, S. *Science and epilepsy: Neuroscience gains in epilepsy research*. New York: Raven Press, 1976.

Pincus, J. H. Can violence be a manifestation of epilepsy? *Neurology*, 1980, *30*, 304–307.

Reynolds, E. H., & Travers, R. Serum anticonvulsant concentrations in epileptic patients with mental symptoms. *British Journal of Psychiatry*, 1974, *124*, 440–445.

Rodin, E. A. Psychomotor epilepsy and aggressive behavior. *Archives of General Psychiatry*, 1973, *28*, 210–213.

Roth, S. R., Sterman, M. B., & Clemente, C. D. Comparison of EEG correlates of reinforcement, internal inhibition, and sleep. *Electroencephalography and clinical Neurophysiology*, 1967, *23*, 509–520.

Servít, Z., & Musil, F. Prophylactic treatment of posttraumatic epilepsy: Results of a long-range follow-up in Czechoslovakia. *Epilepsia*, 1981, *22*, 315–320.

Shamansky, S. L., & Glaser, G. H. Socioeconomic characteristics of childhood seizure disorders in the New Haven area: An epidemiological study. *Epilepsia*, 1979, *20*, 457–474.

Sterman, M. B., & Friar, L. Suppression of seizures in an epileptic following sensorimotor EEG feedback training. *Electroencephalography and clinical Neurophysiology*, 1972, *33*, 89–95.

Sterman, M. B., & Macdonald, L. R. Effects of central cortical EEG feedback training on seizure incidence in poorly controlled epileptics. *Epilepsia*, 1978, *19*, 207–222.

Sterman, M. B., Macdonald, L. R., & Stone, R. K. Biofeedback training of the sensorimotor EEG rhythm in man: Effects on epilepsy. *Epilepsia*, 1974, *15*, 395–416.

Sterman, M. B., & Shouse, M. N. Quantitative analysis of training, sleeping EEG and clinical response to EEG operant conditioning in epileptics. *Electroencephalography and clinical Neurophysiology*, 1980, *49*, 558–576.

Stevens, J. R. Endogenous conditioning to abnormal cerebral transients in man. *Science*, 1962, *137*, 974–976.

Stevens, J. R. Complex partial seizures (psychomotor epilepsy): Interictal manifestations. In J. K. Penry & D. D. Daly (Eds.), *Complex partial seizures*. New York: Raven Press, 1975.

Stevens, J. R. Biologic background of psychoses in epilepsy. In R. Canger, F. Angeleri, & J. K. Penry (Eds.), *Advances in Epileptology: XIth Epilepsy International Symposium*. New York: Raven Press, 1980.

Taylor, D. C. Factors influencing the occurrence of schizophrenia-like psychosis in patients with temporal lobe epilepsy. *Psychological Medicine*, 1975, 5, 249–254.

Temkin, O., *The falling sickness: A history of epilepsy from the Greeks to the beginnings of modern neurology* (2nd ed.). Baltimore: The Johns Hopkins Press, 1971.

Trimble, M., & Corbett, J. Anticonvulsant drugs and cognitive function. In J. A. Wada & J. K. Penry (Eds.), *Advances in Epileptology: Xth Epilepsy International Symposium*. New York: Raven Press, 1980.

Trimble, M. R., Thompson, P. J. & Huppert, F. Anticonvulsant drugs and cognitive abilities. In R. Canger, F. Angeleri, & J. K. Penry (Eds.), *Advances in Epileptology: XIth Epilepsy International Symposium*. New York: Raven Press, 1980.

Whitsett, S. F., Lubar, J. F., Holder, G. S., Pamplin, W. E., & Shabsin, H. S. A double-blind investigation of the relationship between seizure activity and the sleep EEG following EEG biofeedback training. *Biofeedback and Self-Regulation*, 1982, 7, 193–209.

Wolf, P. Psychic disorders in epilepsy. In R. Canger, F. Angeleri, & J. K. Penry (Eds.), *Advances in Epileptology: XIth Epilepsy International Symposium*. New York: Raven Press, 1980.

Wright, L. Aversive conditioning of self-induced seizures. *Behavior Therapy*, 1973, 4, 712–713.

Wyler, A. R. Operant control of CNS activity. In J. S. Lockard, & A. A. Ward, Jr. (Eds.), *Epilepsy: A window to brain mechanisms*. New York: Raven Press, 1980.

Wyler, A. R., Lockard, J. S., Ward, A. A., & Finch, C. A. Conditioned EEG desynchronization and seizure occurrence in patients. *Electroencephalography and clinical Neurophysiology*, 1976, 41, 501–512.

Wyler, A. R., Robbins, C. A., & Dodrill, C. B. EEG operant conditioning for control of epilepsy. *Epilepsia*, 1979, 20, 279–286.

Wyrwicka, W., & Sterman, M. B. Instrumental conditioning of sensorimotor cortex EEG spindles in the waking cat. *Physiology and Behavior*, 1968, 3, 703–707.

Ziegler, R. G. Impairments of control and competence in epileptic children and their families. *Epilepsia*, 1981, 22, 339–346.

Zlutnick, S. I., Mayville, W. J., & Moffat, S. Behavioral control of seizure disorders: The interruption of chained behavior. In R. C. Katz & S. I. Zlutnick (Eds.), *Behavior therapy and health care: Principles and application*. Elmsford, N.Y.: Pergamon Press, 1975.

11

Spinal Cord Injuries

BERNARD S. BRUCKER

Introduction

The term *spinal cord injury* refers to a concussion, compression, laceration, or transection of the spinal cord that results in loss of neurologic function below the level of the injury. Losses may involve lack of voluntary motor control of the skeletal muscles, loss of sensation, and loss of autonomic function. The extent of these losses depends upon the level of the spinal cord at which the injury occurred and the amount of residual neural damage.

PHYSICAL AND NEUROLOGICAL CONSEQUENCES

Spinal cord injuries that occur at the cervical level of the spine (neck) will result in quadriplegia or quadriparesis (complete or partial paralysis as well as sensory loss of the trunk and all four extremities); higher cervical level injuries also produce loss of control of the muscles involved in respiratory function and thus require respirator assistance. Injuries at the thoracic, lumbar, and sacral levels (upper, middle, and lower back) result in paraplegia and paraparesis (complete or partial paralysis and sensory loss of the lower extremities). In addition, spinal cord damage above the second sacral vertebra often results in loss of bowel and bladder control.

A complete spinal cord lesion is characterized by damage in the spinal cord that leaves no neurofibers in the cord intact and results in a total disruption of neurotransmission below the site of the lesion. In such cases there is no motor, sensory, or autonomic function below the lesion. Since severed or degenerated spinal cord neurons do not regenerate, these losses are permanent; no methods for regaining function are known at present. An incomplete lesion is characterized by damage in the cord that severs or degenerates some neural tracts and leaves others intact. In such cases, some combination of motor, sensory, and/or autonomic function is present at various sites below the injury depending upon the location and number of severed or degenerated neurons. As with complete lesions, losses that are due to incomplete lesions are permanent. In addition, injuries to the spinal cord can result in compression of neural tissue and swelling of the cord that cause functional losses below the site of the injury. Losses from these causes, however, can be followed by a spontaneous recovery over time with restoration of some or all of the function.

The prognosis for return of function after spinal cord injury cannot always be predicted. Although modern diagnostic methods such as X rays, myelograms, and computerized tomography (CT) scans provide valuable information, the exact nature of the neural damage is often difficult to determine accurately. Assessment of functional losses at time of injury is not sufficient for prediction of recovery because both severed or degenerated neurons in the cord that cannot recover and compressed nerve tissue that can recover may contribute to the cause of the initial functional losses. Rapid return of motor and sensory function in the first week after injury is a good prognostic indicator. Losses remaining after 6 months are likely to be permanent.

INCIDENCE

Spinal cord injury represents a significant national problem. Reports from the National Spinal Cord Injury Data Research Center suggest that there are over 250,000 spinal cord injury victims presently living in the United States, with approximately 10,000 new traumatic injuries occurring each year (Young & Northrup, 1979). The majority of injuries involve damage to the cervical spine resulting in quadriplegia. The next most frequent injury involves the thoracic–lumbar spine resulting in functional losses to the lower extremities. The impact of these injuries in catastrophic physical losses, cost in dollars, and dramatic psychological and social consequences is devastating. More than 80% of those people receiving spinal cord injuries are males and over 60% are between 10 and 29 years of age. The life expectancy of the spinal cord injured person is 30.2 years past the injury (DeVivo, Fine, Maetz, & Stover, 1980), leaving most victims to face the majority of their adult lives with significant unrecoverable functional losses.

ETIOLOGY

Injuries to the spinal cord are usually the result of severe trauma to the spine. Vehicular accidents are the greatest cause (48.3%) of spinal cord injuries. The other causes include falls (22.1%), sports activities (14.2%), penetrating wounds such as gunshot and stab wounds (12.5%), and various other events (2.9%) (McCollough, Green, Klose, Goldberg, & Klose, 1981). Although it is apparent that some spinal cord injuries are the result of a coincidental sequence of events not under the control of the person, most appear to be related to the imprudent behavior of the injured person. Some authors have made references to the psychological or behavioral antecedents of this type of injury (Fordyce, 1964; Grzesiak & Zaretsky, 1979; Knorr & Bull, 1970; Kunce & Worley, 1966; Peter, 1975); however, there is very little research on this topic.

Fordyce (1964) investigated the relationship between personality characteristics and the manner of the onset of injury among spinal cord injured males. The circumstances leading to the spinal cord injury of 58 males were scaled by judges on a continuum of imprudent to prudent behavior. Two groups of 12 subjects at either extreme of imprudent–prudent behavior were compared on seven Minnesota Multiphasic Personality Inventory (MMPI) measures. The results suggested that the men whose injuries were judged to be related to imprudent behavior showed significantly more impulse-dominated behavior than did the men judged as relatively prudent. Kunce and Worley (1966) found that spinal cord injured persons who were active agents in their accidents scored higher on the aviator key of the Strong Vocational Interest Blank (i.e., indicating higher levels of adventurousness, boldness, and assertiveness) than did injured persons who were passive in their accidents.

The results of these studies are quite important, as they suggest that certain measurable behavioral factors may increase the risk of spinal cord injury. It is indeed unfortunate that, although it is believed that behavioral factors play an important role in the etiology of spinal cord injury, there have not been more studies that have attempted to identify these factors. Prevention of spinal cord injuries, which is of crucial importance, requires well-designed behavioral research to identify the behavioral risk factors involved in spinal cord injury and to develop the methodology for changing these factors in high-risk groups.

PSYCHOLOGICAL CONSEQUENCES

Spinal cord injuries have dramatic psychological effects. A substantial literature regarding these effects has been published. Some of the literature has been based on personal experience; the remainder has attempted to identify psychological effects either by means of structured interviews or psychometric measurement procedures with patients. The result has been that many different authors generally have identified similar psychological effects such as denial, depression, and anxiety. There has been great disagreement, however, as to whether the occurrence of these psychological factors are related to individual differences among patients' preinjury personalities alone or whether all spinal cord injured persons undergo a systematic series of stages, each with related psychological reactions (Trieschmann, 1980). This disagreement has important implications for treatment. The stage model (Dunn, 1975; Hohmann, 1975; Knorr & Bull, 1970; Peter, 1975; Siller, 1969) posits that a spinal cord injured person must successfully resolve the psychological issues associated with each stage in order to achieve psychological adjustment to the disability. Treatment strategies then should be geared to promote this progression. The individual differences model suggests that it is necessary to identify the psychological effects experienced by each spinal cord injured person and then develop a treatment to diminish those particular psychological reactions (e.g., Berger & Garrett, 1952; Mueller, 1962).

The earliest attempt to use systematic measurement methods to obtain quantifiable data on the psychological consequences of spinal cord injuries was reported by Thom, VonSalzen, and Fromme (1946) who studied 109 males with spinal cord injuries. These investigators employed (a) a $1\frac{1}{2}$-hour psychiatric interview with each patient; (b) conferences with physicians, nurses, attendants, and technicians engaged in the care of the patients; (c) observations of patients during daily activities; and (d) informal chats with the patients. There were no patients with psychiatric syndromes, and there were no characteristic personality trends or patterns found among the patients. However, 45% of the patients showed some manifestation of depression; some patients also showed dependence and frustration. Finally, it was reported that less dramatic reactions to the disability were related to better pretraumatic personalities.

In a subsequent attempt to study the psychological reactions of spinal cord injury patients, Nagler (1950) observed 500 spinal cord injury patients over a 5-year period. Formal interviews were administered to 200 patients. The remaining patients were observed during neurological examination, on ward rounds, at bedside, and in informal conversation. Nagler identified several types of psychological reactions. These reaction types included (a) anxiety and reactive depression, (b) psychosis, (c) indifference, (d) psychopathic reaction, (e) dependency, and (f) acceptance of disability. The validity of these reaction types is difficult to determine because the specific methods of measurement and statistical analysis were not reported.

Wittkower, Gingras, Mergler, Wigdor, and Lepine (1954) examined 50 spinal cord injured persons using a relatively specific method of measurement. Each subject was given a 5-hour psychiatric interview and was administered the Rorschach, Thematic Apperception Test, Level of Aspiration Test, Rosenzweig Picture Frustration Test, Wechsler–Bellevue, Bender–

Gestalt, and the Draw-A-Person Test. Unfortunately, the actual data were not reported. The authors merely concluded that spinal cord injured persons consistently display denial, distortion of body image, anger, and depression.

Weiss and Diamond (1966) employed methodology superior to that of previous research attempts. These investigators compared the scores of 90 spinal cord myelopathy patients on the Bell Adjustment Inventory and the Bernreuter Personality Inventory with the nondisabled normative data from these instruments. The patient sample included 28 persons whose paralysis was due to spinal cord trauma and 62 persons whose paralysis was due to disease resulting in spinal cord lesions. Onset of disability ranged from 18 to 65 years. T-test comparisons between the patients' Bell Adjustment Scale scores and the scale norms revealed a significant difference in the social adjustment parameter; this suggested that the patients were significantly more aggressive in social contacts than a nondisabled population. Comparisons of patients' emotional adjustment and home adjustment scores to normative data revealed no significant differences. The data from the Bernreuter Personality Inventory showed that the patients were significantly less self-sufficient and significantly more socially oriented than a nondisabled population. However, the patients showed no significant neurotic tendencies relative to nondisabled norms.

The results of the Weiss and Diamond (1966) investigation did not show any psychological adjustment problems in the patient sample, with the exception of relatively low feelings of self-sufficiency. The generally negative results may have been due primarily to either of two factors. One factor was the large proportion of subjects whose spinal cord lesions were due to disease. In such cases the onset of disability is usually slow and progressive, which allows for gradual patient adjustment. The other factor was the long time period since onset of the disability in the sample. The patients may have had sufficient time to adjust to their injuries and thus may not have been representative of the spinal cord injured population (see Watson & Kendall, Chapter 3). If this were the case, the findings would suggest that normal psychological adjustment to disabilities may be a realistic expectation for those paralyzed by spinal cord injuries.

Cook (1979) performed a study similar to that of Weiss and Diamond (1966). The Mini–Mult (an abbreviated form of the MMPI) and the State–Trait Anxiety Inventory were administered to 118 spinal cord injury patients less than 1 year after injury. Comparisons to normative data revealed that the spinal cord injury group scores were within normal limits. Thus, unlike some of the early studies (e.g., Nagler, 1950), there was no evidence that spinal cord injury patients show high levels of anxiety or depression. Nevertheless, similar to the Wittkower et al. (1954) results, one-third of the patients showed denial of emotional responses. The finding that only 30% of the sample showed denial was somewhat surprising. However, the denial of emotions measured by the Mini–Mult is not equivalent to denial of the reality of disability, which is theorized to account for decreased emotional response to the functional losses (see Wittkower *et al.*, 1954).

Kerr and Thompson (1972) studied a large number of patients with acute paraplegia over their entire course of rehabilitation. At the initial observation, 129 of the subjects were within 3 months postinjury, 77 were between 3 months and 1 year postinjury, and 5 were between 1 and 2 years postinjury. The methods of observation, measurement, and data analysis were not clearly specified in the article; nevertheless, conclusions and some data were reported. It was suggested that patients underwent a series of adjustment stages. The first stage was characterized by initial mental shock, fear, and anxiety. These reactions were ascribed to patients' lack of information regarding prognosis and/or misunderstanding of provided information. Grief and mourning were identified as attributes of the second stage. Kerr and Thompson suggested that professionals should attempt to support these reactions rather than foster their repression. Aggression or rebellion were labeled as features of the third stage. Aggression was viewed as a means with which the patients reject dominance by others and thus leads to the establishment of maturity and adult relationships with others. It was concluded that passage through the stages noted above was a natural and mandatory progression; only those who successfully completed all stages were credited with acceptance of disability.

Kerr and Thompson (1972) have provided the only longitudinal investigation of a large number of spinal cord injury patients. It is most unfortunate that the investigators did not report sufficient information regarding their measurement techniques. Hence, it is difficult to assess the validity of their conclusions.

In summary, the literature on the psychological consequences of spinal-cord injury does not provide substantial data from well-designed investigations to support the conclusions offered by investigators. However, there appears to be general agreement among the investigators that spinal cord injured patients tend to exhibit definite psychological reactions such as anxiety, depression, and denial. Regardless of the methodological deficiencies of the literature, all rehabilitation specialists accept the importance of psychological factors in the rehabilitation of the spinal cord injured person. Without psychological adjustment and the ability to cope with the spinal cord injury, it is not possible to meet the goals of patient attainment of the greatest independent functioning and highest quality of life possible given the physical limitations of the injury. The following discussion will examine the treatment interventions that have been studied in the literature concerning the rehabilitation of spinal cord injury patients.

Treatment Interventions

Treatment interventions for the spinal cord injured initially begin with emergency medical procedures applied by the ambulance crews at the scene of the accident. These procedures are followed by treatment in a hospital emergency room and subsequent placement either in an intensive-care unit or an acute-medicine unit, depending on the patient's condition. The entire focus during this initial phase of the treatment is to maintain life, treat and prevent secondary medical complications, and prevent further damage to the cord by decompression and stabilization of the spine.

Throughout the initial treatment period, which varies greatly depending on the condition of the patient, little if any attention is given to the patient's psychological reactions. The possible consequences of the spinal cord injury usually are not presented to the patient for two main reasons: (a) an accurate prediction of recovery usually cannot be determined initially, and (b) those treating the patient usually feel that presenting the possible consequences of the injury would elicit severe depression (to which they are not trained to respond) and thus produce a detrimental effect on the acute medical care. The patient is not given access to a psychologist during this period in most institutions. As a result, the patient must confront the uncertainty of life or death and the possibility of permanent disability without psychological intervention. This is most unfortunate because most individuals cannot easily cope with these issues. The possibility that presentation of information during acute care might result in devastating depression has never been demonstrated or even investigated.

Once the patient is medically stable, the process of rehabilitation begins. The patient usually is transferred to a rehabilitation center or unit and, in almost all cases, comes to rehabilitation expecting to regain total function. The patient usually is neither prepared to cope with permanent physical losses nor feels a need to learn to cope given his or her confidence in attaining full functional recovery. When the patient is confronted with the true probabilities of functional return, he or she is likely to refute the information.

The focus of rehabilitation is to help the patient regain as much physical function as the neurological impairment will allow, and to become as functionally independent as possible through (a) the use of substituting and strengthening unaffected muscle, (b) learning new skills, and (c) utilizing adaptive devices to compensate for permanent physical losses. Therefore, the patient's ability to cope with the permanent losses is a key factor in the rehabilitation process. The patient will neither be compliant with nor motivated for any treatment that focuses on learning functional skills to compensate for physical losses if he or she cannot accept or cope with the permanent losses.

The process of rehabilitation involves an interdisciplinary team approach with physicians, physical therapists, occupational therapists, psychologists, social workers, vocational counselors, nurses, and recreation therapists working toward the overall goals of rehabilitation in an integrative manner. The role of the psychologist on the team is of major importance; it is to apply the principles of behavioral science to the spinal-cord injured person for the purpose of helping him or her to cope with the physical and functional losses and attain the goals of the rehabilitation program.

PSYCHOTHERAPEUTIC INTERVENTIONS

Almost every article concerning the rehabilitation of the spinal cord in-jured person refers to the importance of psychotherapeutic interventions. Similarly, almost all of the articles that report the outcome of rehabilitation programs identify a psychotherapeutic component. However, the specific nature of these psychotherapeutic interventions and their respective suc-cesses in resolving the problems that they address are usually never reported.

An example of the lack of specific process and outcome information may be found in Grayson's (1950) discussion of psychotherapeutic intervention with individual spinal cord injury patients. Grayson stressed the importance of psychotherapeutic intervention for the *acceptance* of the disability by spinal cord injury patients. He suggested that psychotherapy should examine the meaning of the disability for a particular patient, and should entail an educa-tional process concerning the patient's emotional reactions to the disability. The process of this therapeutic approach consists of (*a*) exploring the pa-tient's psychological resources, (*b*) determining the obstacles that prevent the patient's use of his or her psychological resources, and (*c*) aiding the patient in the dissolution of these obstacles. Grayson's approach is most positive. However, he failed to describe in detail the techniques that may be used to identify the patient's strengths and to accomplish the dissolution of the perceived obstacles. In addition, Grayson did not indicate the effective-ness of his therapeutic approach. Unfortunately, the deficiencies associated with Grayson's (1950) early report may be found in many contemporary papers regarding the use of psychotherapeutic interventions with individual patients (e.g., Maki, Winograd, & Hinkle, 1976) as well as with patient groups (Mann, Godfrey, & Dowd, 1973; Rohrer, Adelman, Puckett, Toomey, Talbert, & Johnson, 1980; Romano, 1976; Wittkower *et al.*, 1954).

Unlike the investigators noted above, Miller, Wolfe, and Spiegel (1975) performed an investigation of the effectiveness of group therapy with spinal cord injury patients that used experimental and control groups. The subject sample consisted of 31 spinal cord injury patients between the ages of 15 and 30 years, 15 of whom were paraplegics and 16 of whom were quadriplegics. The subjects were divided into two groups, an experimental group consisting of 18 patients who were given group therapy twice a week for 1 month and a control group of 13 patients who were not provided with group therapy. Unfortunately, patients were assigned to groups on the basis of self-selection rather than in a random fashion. Patients who expressed interest in group therapy were included in the experimental group and those who chose not to be group members were included in the control group. All subjects were administered a spinal cord knowledge inventory prior to the beginning of group therapy within the first 2 weeks of their hospitalization. This inventory was developed by the investigators to measure knowledge and attitudes about disability. It also included 7-point rating scales concerning self-concept, perceived family support since injury, and hospital care and services. The inventory was again administered to all subjects at the termination of group therapy. The group therapy consisted of the presentation of factual information regarding the physiological consequences of the spinal-cord injury and a discussion of sexual functioning. The results indicated that both the experimental and control groups showed significant increases in knowledge regarding spinal-cord injury and disability. However, the experimental group showed a much greater pre- to posttherapy increase in knowledge ($p < .0005$) than did the control group ($p < .05$). The experimental group also showed a significant increase in self-concept ratings, whereas the control group showed no change. In addition, the control group's ratings of hospital care and services as well as family support tended to decrease across inventory administrations.

The results of the Miller *et al.* (1975) study must be viewed with caution because the investigators did not employ random subject assignment. Patient self-selection may have introduced some confounding variables that actually were responsible for the positive results shown by the subjects who received group therapy. For example, patients who were highly motivated or eager to obtain accurate information were more likely to have selected the experimental rather than the control condition. Other deficiencies associated with the study included (*a*) the use of an inventory that had not been assessed with regard to reliability, (*b*) failure to directly compare the inventory responses of the two subject groups at posttherapy with adequate control for possible pretherapy group differences, (*c*) lack of an attention–placebo control group, and (*d*) the absence of any follow-up assessment (see Watson & Kendall, Chapter 3).

Roessler, Milligan, and Ohlson (1976) attempted to determine the effectiveness of a personal achievement skills training program for the spinal cord injured. This program used a structured group format that focused on individuals' awareness of values, capacities, and acceptance of others as well as their own needs and skills in communication, problem and goal definition, and constructive action. Each phase of the program was divided into specific behavioral steps; however, a detailed explanation of these steps was not provided. Ten spinal cord injury patients were randomly assigned to a personal achievement skills training group and 10 patients were assigned to a no-treatment control group. Self-report measures of psychological adjustment were administered to patients at pre- and posttherapy. They were not supplemented by more direct measures of the skills taught to training group patients. Regardless of the measurement flaw, the attrition rate in both the experimental and control groups was so great that it was not possible to analyze the data.

Summary

Considering the psychological impact of spinal cord injury and the coping skills required to deal with the severe associated losses, it is most unfortunate that there has not been adequate research on the effectiveness of psychotherapeutic interventions. The deficiencies of the research discussed previously might be due to the limited funding available for rehabilitation research or to the fact that, until recently, few psychologists have been interested in rehabilitation research. Nevertheless, the paucity of adequate research concerning psychotherapeutic interventions has produced two negative consequences. First, although nearly all rehabilitation specialists acknowledge that psychological factors influence patients' recoveries, the crucial psychological variables involved have not been adequately identified. In addition, although most rehabilitation programs include psychotherapeutic interventions for their patients, proper investigation of the efficacy of these interventions have not been performed. The empirical evaluation of specific therapeutic techniques in well-designed experimental paradigms that include adequate measurement procedures is absolutely necessary to establish the validity of those techniques. The development of a sophisticated evaluation literature also is necessary to ensure the introduction of new therapeutic interventions and to promote the use of interventions that are shown to be effective among rehabilitation professionals.

THERAPEUTIC INTERVENTIONS FOR SEXUAL DYSFUNCTION

Spinal cord injuries result in sexual dysfunctions that vary as functions of the completeness of the lesion and of patient gender. In males, fertility usually is lost, and the ability to have erections initially is lost. Depending upon the level and completeness of the lesion, erections may reappear in the form of reflex erections or, in some cases, limited psychogenic erections. The neuromuscular losses also present practical problems in sexual activity for the male (e.g., inability to perform thrusting motions). Females usually retain their fertility and experience fewer practical problems resulting from neuromuscular losses. However, sensory losses tend to limit the pleasure derived from sexual experiences, and orgasm is a rare occurrence. It is important to realize that patients of both genders retain sexual functioning capabilities to some degree and that their dissatisfactions with sexual behavior usually result from psychological factors and insufficient theoretical, technical, and practical information. It is essential that spinal cord injured patients learn to cope with the physical limitations involved with sexual dysfunction and develop meaningful and satisfying sexual relationships if the rehabilitative process is to be considered complete.

Trieschmann (1980) has presented a good review of sexuality and spinal cord injury. She has divided postinjury sexual function into sex drives, sex acts, and sexuality. With respect to sex drives, the literature suggests that there are large individual differences among patients that appear to be related more to preinjury sexual behavior and attitudes rather than to the nature of the injury. In addition, although sex drives may be somewhat diminished by injury, sexual pleasure is not necessarily reduced. The literature indicates that capacity for involvement in sexual acts following spinal cord injury varies greatly according to the extent and location of damage to the cord. However, patients' abilities to perform sexual acts successfully may be dramatically increased by the provision of information regarding the physiology of sexual functioning with specific neurological damage and the use of specially designed (a) adaptive devices and (b) techniques for positioning and stimulation that lead to reflex responses and pleasurable sensations. Trieschmann (1980) has defined sexuality as the degree to which the spinal cord injured person perceives himself or herself as sexually attractive. The literature suggests that patients' perceptions of their sexuality impacts greatly on their relationships with others, as well as on their ability to participate in sexual and social behavior. In summary, the degree of sexual dysfunction induced by spinal cord injury is determined by physiological and, more importantly, psychological factors. If patients may learn to cope with the physical losses related to sexual dysfunction, they may increase their ability to perform sexual acts and to experience sexual satisfaction.

There is a clear need for effective and reliable interventions for teaching spinal cord injured patients to cope with sexual dysfunction. Similar to the literature regarding psychotherapeutic intervention, several articles have been published that have proposed intervention models; few investigators, however, have reported outcome data and even fewer have utilized experimental designs. For example, both Romano and Lassiter (1972) and Isaacson and Delgado (1974) have discussed the components of sexual counseling programs that were developed to meet the needs of discharged spinal cord injury patients as assessed by follow-up surveys. Both programs included educational components and various procedures for facilitating the development of communication skills between the patients and their sexual partners. Unfortunately, neither report included any information concerning the evaluation of program effectiveness. Several other sexual counseling programs have been discussed in the literature that have (a) included flexible training formats to respond to individual differences among patients (Comarr & Vigue, 1978a, 1978b; Evans, Halar, DeFreece, & Larsen, 1976; Hoch, 1977); (b) used a spinal cord injured person and sexual partner as coping models for the patients and their partners (i.e., a couple that had worked adaptively to overcome their sexual difficulties; Eisenberg & Rustad, 1976); and (c) included a sexual desensitization component and a pretraining assessment of patients' sexual knowledge, attitudes, and behavior (Cole, Chilgren, & Rosenberg, 1973). None of the reports cited, however, included program evaluation data.

Unlike the majority of authors who have discussed therapeutic interventions for sexual dysfunction, Halstead, Halstead, Salhoot, Stock, and Sparks (1978) examined the effects of sexual attitude reassessment workshops on the attitudes of both disabled and nondisabled participants regarding various sexual activities. The workshops, designed to help participants become more comfortable with their own sexuality, consisted of a $2\frac{1}{2}$-day program utilizing a multimedia approach that presented a variety of sexual topics. Attitudes and feelings toward these and other topics were then explored and exchanged in a series of small group discussions. The effectiveness of 15 workshops involving 650 disabled and nondisabled participants was evaluated by obtaining pre- and postworkshop attitude ratings from participants concerning sexual activities. Attitudes were assessed by means of nine rating scales. Each scale consisted of a description of a different sexual activity and a 5-point scale ranging from "I feel great about it" (1) to "I am repulsed by it" (5). The results indicated that, relative to the preworkshop assessment, the participants showed more positive attitudes toward each sexual activity described by the rating scales following completion of the workshop. The disabled participants showed significantly more positive attitudes toward four of the nine activities and the nondisabled produced significantly more positive attitudes regarding eight of the nine activities.

The Halstead et al. (1978) study demonstrated that a sexual attitude reassessment workshop can effectively change disabled persons' attitudes toward specific sexual activities. A major deficiency of the study, however, was its lack of data regarding whether or not the changes in the disabled participants' sexual attitudes produced more satisfactory sexual functioning. Measurement of satisfaction with sexual functioning and of actual sexual behavior at pre- and postworkshop as well as at a follow-up period would have produced most valuable data.

Another examination of the effectiveness of sexual attitude reassessment workshops with the spinal cord injured was performed by Held, Cole, Held, Anderson, and Chilgren (1975). The workshop format included (a) selected films on aspects of human sexuality, sexual therapy, and sexuality of the disabled; (b) a multimedia presentation of pornography in saturation amounts for desensitization purposes; (c) didactic and panel discussions that provided information on the sexual feelings of the spinal cord injured and that included disabled persons and their partners as discussants; and (d) small group discussions that allowed the participants to discuss their feelings and integrate the presented material. Fifty-three of the participants completed a sexual attitude questionnaire prior to and 6 weeks after the workshop. Nine sexual activities were rated on 5-point scales similar to those used by Halstead et al. (1978). The results indicated that the participants reported significantly more positive attitudes regarding four of the nine activities from the pre- to postworkshop assessments. A no-treatment control group consisting of 18 first-year medical students showed no significant attitude changes with regard to any of the sexual activities.

The Held et al. (1975) investigation produced results that were quite similar to those of Halstead et al. (1978) despite the fact that Held et al. used a 6-week follow-up assessment of participants' attitudes rather than an immediate postworkshop assessment. Unfortunately, the investigation failed to use scales or behavioral check lists for the assessment of sexual behavior and satisfaction with sexual function that, if administered at pre- and postworkshop as well as at follow-up, would have provided valuable information on the effectiveness of the sexual attitude reassessment workshop in facilitating sexual adjustment. It should be noted that Held et al.'s use of a control group might suggest that the mere administration of the rating scales over time did not change participants' sexual attitudes. However, the use of medical students rather than spinal cord injured persons as control subjects precluded any conclusions regarding the actual cause of the reported attitude changes. It would have been desirable to have randomly assigned spinal cord injured persons undergoing rehabilitation to either a workshop treatment condition or a nonworkshop control group and to have assessed persons' sexual attitudes, functioning, and satisfaction at pre- and postworkshop as well as at long-term follow-up. This approach would have provided a more valid test of the effects of the workshop intervention on the coping abilities and sexual functioning of the spinal cord injured.

Melnyk, Montgomery, and Over (1979) recently performed a controlled study of attitude changes of spinal cord injured persons following participation in a sexual counseling program. Twenty-six spinal cord injured persons (both paraplegics and quadriplegics of both genders) with sexual dysfunction were assigned either to an experimental group or a control group. The experimental group was given six seminars of sexual attitude and identity reassessment seminars that consisted of 3-hour structured meetings concerning various topics (i.e., the development of a list of problem areas, self-guided imagery training for sensuality and communication, communication and sex education, and sexual techniques and sexual problems in spinal-cord injury). The control group was not provided with any counseling or attention from the seminar leaders. Subjects' attitudes regarding 12 sexual activities were measured with 5-point rating scales both prior to the counseling program and at 8 weeks following completion of the program. In addition, the experimental subjects were administered the A-State Anxiety Scale prior to the first seminar and following the first and sixth seminar. The results indicated that the control subjects produced significantly more favorable attitudes toward 2 of the sexual activities during the course of the investigation. The experimental subjects showed a significant and favorable attitude change regarding 3 of the activities, 1 of which was associated with positive change by the control group. The experimental subjects showed no changes in anxiety from pre- to posttreatment periods.

The Melnyk *et al.* (1979) investigation illustrated the importance of the use of control groups in treatment outcome research. The significant and positive attitude change shown by the experimental subjects on three of the scales might lead one to conclude that the counseling program may produce more positive sexual attitudes among spinal cord injured persons. However, the control group data indicate that spinal cord injured persons may undergo some positive attitude changes over time in the absence of any intervention. In light of these findings, it would have been particularly interesting to have assessed the sexual attitudes of the two subject groups at a 6-month follow-up. Several other methodological improvements also would have been useful. First, it would have been desirable to have included an attention–placebo control group in order to control for the effects of therapist attention and subjects' expectations of positive benefits. Second, data collection regarding subjects' actual sexual behavior and feelings of satisfaction would have provided valuable information concerning the effects of the counseling program. The final improvement would have been the use of a between-group analysis in addition to the within-group analysis reported by the investigators.

Summary

The rehabilitation of sexual functioning has been recognized only recently as an important part of the overall treatment of the spinal cord injured.

Nevertheless, a substantial literature has been published that attests to the importance of the treatment of sexual dysfunction and that suggests the need for intervention programs to help spinal cord injured persons to develop the coping skills necessary to deal with their physical losses and increase their sexual behavior and satisfaction. The literature reviewed by Trieschmann (1980) indicates that the crucial factors that interfere with persons' abilities to perform sexual acts and experience sexual pleasure are emotional responses to the physical losses, negative attitudes, and lack of information concerning sexual functioning as well as specific adaptive devices and techniques. The intervention programs that have been developed to help the spinal cord injured cope better with sexual dysfunction generally have addressed each of the crucial factors identified by Trieschmann. Unfortunately, the few programs that have been evaluated have assessed outcome only on the basis of attitudinal, rather than behavioral, change. Furthermore, none of the outcome studies has used adequate experimental designs. It is necessary to perform controlled investigations that include the use of attention–placebo control groups, behavioral outcome measures, and long-term follow-up assessments before it can be determined if current intervention programs may help spinal cord injured persons to learn the coping skills necessary for successful sexual adjustments.

BEHAVIORAL INTERVENTIONS

It was noted earlier in this chapter that the process of spinal cord injury rehabilitation in part requires the learning of new skills and the use of adaptive devices. Thus, it would seem advantageous to apply the principles of operant and classical conditioning to the treatment of some specific problems related to spinal cord injury (Fordyce, 1971; Trieschmann, 1980). The limited amount of research regarding the use of learning theory in spinal-cord rehabilitation efforts has produced some impressive results. The following discussion first examines investigations of the use of operant and classical conditioning to promote increases in desired behaviors. The discussion then reviews the use of biofeedback to help spinal cord injured persons learn to control various physiological responses.

Operant Conditioning

Taylor and Persons (1970) described the application of operant techniques to increase the performance of desired behaviors by two spinal cord injury patients. In one case, a quadriplegic patient wished to increase his educational level in order to cope better with his disability. The staff considered the patient's goal to be unrealistic because he did not have the persistence necessary to perform well in college. The authors attempted to increase the amount of time the patient spent reading in order to help him prepare better for college study. Initial measurement indicated that the patient read less than 30 minutes a day. During the next 10 weeks, the rehabilitation staff provided social attention to the patient contingent on the time he spent reading each day. The patient's average daily reading time increased to 3 hours and 9 minutes during the tenth week. The second case described by the authors was that of a quadriplegic patient whose preinjury tendency to show dependent behavior and to ruminate about psychotic behavior increased after injury. The staff rewarded the patient with social attention only for nonpsychotic conversation. Following the initiation of the regimen, the patient displayed increased self-confidence and self-esteem and showed less dependency, depression, obsessiveness, and preoccupation with physical problems. In addition, comparisons of the patient's admission and discharge MMPI scores revealed significant improvement on 8 of the 10 clinical scales.

Taylor and Persons' (1970) case presentations are dramatic and suggest the power of operant techniques to produce behavioral changes. However, the failure to use the appropriate control procedures for a single-subject investigation (Kazdin, 1978) prevents the attribution of the reported changes solely to the reinforcement contingencies instituted by the rehabilitation staff. A second flaw associated with the case presentations was the failure to reassess the patients at some point following termination of the reinforcement system. Termination of the system might have resulted in a decrease in patients' performance of desired behaviors and thus would have shown the use of operant conditioning techniques to be of little long-term value.

Operant techniques also have been used to help spinal cord injured patients to increase daily fluid intake. A high daily fluid intake often is recommended to patients for prevention of urinary tract infections, which are a leading cause of death among the spinal cord injured. Fowler, Fordyce, and Berni (1969), for example, attempted to increase the fluid intake of a female patient whose actual daily fluid intake was only two-thirds of the prescribed 3000-cc amount. The patient was asked to self-monitor and record her daily fluid intake on a continuous basis. Her fluid intake record was made public in the form of a graph. In addition, the treatment staff responded positively to increases in drinking behavior and did not provide attention to decreases in drinking. The patient's fluid intake increased dramatically in less than a month to a daily average of 3500 cc and was maintained at 3000 cc 2 months later at discharge. These results were replicated by Sand, Fordyce, Trieschmann, and Fowler (1970) with another patient who did not comply with a fluid-intake regimen. Unfortunately, neither Fowler et al. (1969) nor Sand et al. (1970) reported follow-up data regarding fluid intake after the behavioral contingencies were removed.

Sand, Fordyce, and Fowler (1973) studied the relative effects of operant conditioning and verbal explanation upon patients' fluid intakes. Ninety-three spinal cord injury patients were divided into a reinforcement group consisting of 24 patients and a verbal explanation group consisting of 69 patients. The reinforcement subjects received praise from the treatment staff when they achieved a daily intake quota of 3000 cc. The subjects' daily intake records also were displayed in public. The verbal information subjects only received an explanation from the treatment staff regarding the importance of fluid intake and the daily intake quota. The results indicated that the reinforcement group alone produced significant increases in fluid intake. Although one might conclude that operant methods more effectively elicit patient compliance with fluid intake regimens than the traditional practice of giving patients rational explanations of the need for high fluid intake, Sand *et al.* (1973) failed to provide data regarding maintenance of fluid intake after removal of the reinforcement contingencies. Controlled investigations that include follow-up assessments must be performed before any conclusions may be made regarding the relative effectiveness of operant techniques and information provision in facilitating high fluid intake.

Decubitus ulcers, also known as bed sores, are another major problem confronting the spinal cord injured person. Lacking sensation, a spinal cord injured person is likely to remain in the same sitting or lying position without shifting weight or making slight changes in position. These changes are absolutely necessary to prevent the constant pressure of the bone on the skin surface from causing lesions in the soft tissue between the bone and the skin. These lesions can become quite large and are susceptible to infection; in addition, the person must be confined to bed for long periods for healing to occur. In some cases, the lesions require a surgical skin graft. With proper attention to weight shifting, decubitus ulcers can be prevented. However, patient compliance to a routine of continual weight shifting is sometimes difficult to attain. Malament, Dunn, and Davis (1975) applied a negative reinforcement technique to prevent decubiti in five paraplegic patients. In order to help these patients intermittently relieve pressure from their ischium, a training device was developed that would emit a 68–80-dB tone for 30 seconds if the patient remained seated continuously for 10 minutes. The device was triggered by a pressure-sensitive switch placed under a seat cushion. Each sounding of the tone was recorded automatically on a counter. The tone could be prevented or terminated if the patient relieved pressure from the seat cushion by pushing up for at least 4 seconds. Each push-up of 4 or more seconds duration also was recorded automatically on a counter. During the first phase of the experiment, the patients were unobtrusively monitored during their normal daily routines with the tone deactivated to obtain a base-line record of the number of 10-minute periods in which the patients failed to perform a push-up. During the second phase, the alarm was activated and the patients were informed concerning the training device and instructed to keep the tone from sounding. In the third phase, the tone was deactivated without the patients' knowledge in order to assess the effect of the treatment. Two weeks after the completion of the third phase, two of the patients were evaluated to see if their push-up behavior was maintained (two of the other three patients were discharged early while the third did not undergo the second and third phases of training because of the display of adequate push-up behavior during the first phase of the experiment). Results showed that one patient's push-up behavior substantially increased and the number of tone soundings decreased nearly to zero during the second phase; these results were maintained in the third and follow-up phases. The remaining patient's consistency of push-up behavior increased (although the mean number of push-ups actually decreased relative to the first phase levels) and the number of tone soundings substantially decreased during the second phase. Again, these changes were maintained during the third and follow-up periods.

The Malament *et al.* (1975) study demonstrated that operant techniques may be used to help patients learn and perform behavior necessary for the prevention of disabling medical conditions. The data from the third phase and the follow-up period suggested that the use of the training device may produce long-term effects upon patients' push-up behavior. However, a longer interval between the end of the third phase and follow-up would have allowed for more definitive conclusions concerning long-term effects. It also would have been useful to have compared the effectiveness of the training device with that of information provision or other traditional methods with regard to compliance with weight-shifting regimens.

Rottkamp (1976) performed a comparative study of behavior modification and traditional training techniques upon the body positioning of spinal cord injured patients. The patients assigned to the behavior modification condition received instruction in and a demonstration of proper body positioning as well as positive reinforcement for changes in body position; those assigned to the control condition only received instruction in and a demonstration of proper body positioning. The behavior modification subjects showed (a) significantly more frequent body-position changes, (b) fewer requests for assistance during body changes, and (c) significantly decreased intervals of prolonged skin pressure (with an improved status of pressure lesions) as a function of the reinforcement contingencies. Thus, Rottkamp (1976) provided positive evidence for the effectiveness of behavioral techniques relative to that of traditional instruction in helping patients prevent medical complications and reduce unnecessary disability.

The task of increasing muscle strength and endurance, which is a major focus of rehabilitation for the spinal cord injured, also may be facilitated by the application of behavior therapy techniques. Fordyce, Sand, Trieschmann, and Fowler (1971) demonstrated that the exercise work endurance of a paraplegic woman could be increased by making rest periods contingent on the amount of exercise work performed in physical therapy rather than upon the duration of exercise work. This finding is important because the behavioral contingencies in physical and occupational therapy often are coincidentally arranged and thus result in reinforcement of poor performance rather than peak performance. Fordyce *et al.*'s (1971) findings, however, suggest that the identification of the specific patient behaviors in physical or occupational therapy that facilitate attainment of therapeutic goals and the introduction of reinforcement contingencies to shape and increase these behaviors may produce substantial patient improvement.

Trotter and Inman (1968) performed a controlled investigation of the effectiveness of reinforcing desired patient behavior in physical therapy. Twenty-four subjects (12 quadriplegics and 12 paraplegics) were matched according to disability, sex, level of spinal cord lesion, hand dominance, and initial muscle strength, and then were randomly assigned to either an experimental or a control group. All subjects received the same general therapeutic program for biceps or triceps strengthening except that the experimental subjects' program incorporated verbal and visual reinforcement for specific therapeutic gains. The reinforcement consisted of praise for each measurable change in strength and weekly review of the ongoing graph of amount of weight lifting achieved by each subject. It should be noted that the weekly gains in strength were related to each subject in terms of how close he was at that point to attaining specified functional goals (e.g., crutch walking, propelling a wheelchair, self-care). The control subjects received no specific verbal or visual reinforcement. Therapist–patient verbal interactions were allowed to occur as they do in traditional physical therapy. The results showed that the control subjects gained an average of only 2.40-lb lifting capability from pre- to posttreatment whereas the experimental subjects gained an average of 10.29-lb lifting capability. An analysis of variance indicated that these differences in gained muscle strength were highly significant. The dramatic results illustrate the powerful clinical effects that can be achieved by the application of learning principles to extant physical or occupational therapy programs.

The techniques described above also have been used to facilitate patient training in the use of orthotic devices (orthopedic appliances used to improve functioning of moveable parts of the body such as arms or legs). Trombly (1966) used operant conditioning to train two quadriplegic patients to use an upper extremity myoelectric orthosis effectively. These devices are quite complex and often are difficult to master. Most patients become frustrated when their repeated efforts do not result in a functional response, and therefore reject the orthotic device. Trombly's training program included breaking down the behaviors required to operate the orthotic device into easily accomplishable steps and giving verbal praise to the patients when they accomplished each step. Both patients learned to operate the complex device. A follow-up assessment of one patient indicated that use of the orthotic device was maintained at home after discharge. The results of this study suggest that operant conditioning techniques may effectively be used to provide spinal cord injured patients with greater functional control over the environment. The case study nature of the Trombly (1966) report, however, makes it necessary to perform controlled investigations before firm conclusions may be established concerning the effects of positive reinforcement on patients' use of orthotic devices during and following occupational therapy.

Classical Conditioning

Ince, Brucker, and Alba (1976, 1977, 1978a, 1978b) attempted to apply a classical conditioning paradigm to establish neurogenic bladder voiding in response to a neutral stimulus in complete spinal cord injury patients. The patients, who had no control over voiding, initially were administered a neutral stimulus of mild electric current to the leg, which did not produce urination. The patients then were administered more intensive electrical stimulation to the lower abdomen over the bladder, which did produce urination. Reapplication of the neutral stimulus continued to produce no response, indicating that the more intensive stimulus did not sensitize the bladder. The neutral stimulus and bladder stimulation then were paired over a number of trials after which the previously neutral stimulus alone produced voiding.

The results of the experiments described above have important theoretical implications because they establish for the first time that humans are capable of learning to regulate a spinal reflex in the absence of brain control. Further research may develop methods for establishing control of other physiological functions by use of external stimuli below the level of spinal cord injury. The results of the experiments also have practical implications, as they demonstrate that classical conditioning may be applied to produce a reliable voiding with low residual urine in the bladder and thus decrease the chance of urinary tract infections. Unfortunately, however, the results fell short of one of the authors' intended goals of allowing the patients to be free of drainage devices and to use normal toilet facilities by applying the small electrical device to the leg. Spontaneous voiding, which began to occur when stimulus applications were applied at intervals more than 4 hours apart, rendered independence from drainage devices impractical.

Biofeedback

The application of behavioral paradigms to help persons learn specific voluntary control over physiological responses, a process commonly known as biofeedback training, has not been used extensively with spinal cord injury patients. The reason for the lack of biofeedback applications may be attributed to neurological theory. Spinal cord neurons that are severed have a zero probability of return of function, and neurons that suffer reparable damage require time for repair. Given these anatomical limitations, it has long been accepted that any motor neuron firing below the damaged cord at any point in time is considered to represent the total response possible and is not subject to modification by learning paradigms. However, Brudny, Korein, Levidow, Grynbaum, Lieberman, and Friedmann (1974) described the application of electromyographic (EMG) biofeedback to two quadriplegic spinal cord injury patients. Both patients had had only minimal and nonfunctional movement of their arms since injury 3 years prior to the study and previously had received physical therapy. Visual and audio EMG feedback was provided from muscles in one arm incorporating a shaping procedure designed to relax spastic muscle and strengthen weak muscle. It was reported that both patients showed improvement as a result of the EMG feedback application; only one case, however, was described in detail. A 2-year follow-up revealed that the effect of biofeedback training was maintained and that the patient was able to perform useful functions. Nonetheless, it appeared that the patient also showed improved functioning in the arm that was not the target of training.

Nacht, Wolf, and Coogler (1982) reported on the application of EMG biofeedback training to an incomplete spinal cord injury patient during the acute phase of his injury. The EMG training was performed after the patient underwent a surgical procedure that included a laminectomy and insertion of Harrington rods. The feedback consisted of an oscilloscope display of EMG activity from the gluteus medius and gluteus maximus muscles during eight sessions of training. An 8-month follow-up indicated that a large increase in motor neuron recruitment had occurred. Although the increases in EMG activity measured at follow-up in this study are impressive, the use of a single-case noncontrolled design makes it impossible to determine the EMG activity change that may be attributed to the feedback application. Spinal cord injury patients tend to show increased EMG activity several months after surgeries such as laminectomies because of the reduction of pressure on the cord.

The limited applications of EMG biofeedback for enhancing the voluntary control of motor neuron activity below the level of the injury have been associated with large functional gains. The designs of the studies described, however, make it unclear whether EMG biofeedback produced any significant gains that otherwise would not have occurred. Preliminary results from research in the author's laboratory reveal that some patients produce significant gains that would not be attainable without EMG biofeedback training.

However, the parameters and neurological mechanisms associated with these gains are not totally clear.

Biofeedback training has been applied successfully to treat postural hypotension in spinal cord injured persons. Postural hypotension is a particularly distressing phenomenon that occurs in high-thoracic and cervical level spinal cord injury patients. The injuries suffered by these patients produce autonomic disregulation, which in turn causes blood to pool in the lower extremities. As a result, some of the patients may not sit upright and others may not stand. Brucker and Ince (1977) provided blood pressure feedback to a spinal cord injury patient with a complete lesion at the third thoracic vertebra whose postural hypotension was so severe that he could not stand and walk with his crutches and braces after 2 years of rehabilitation. However, after 11 biofeedback training sessions, the patient learned to increase his blood pressure voluntarily 20 mm Hg on command. At 1-month follow-up, he was able to increase his blood pressure as much as 45 mm Hg on command and thus could stand and walk with his braces and crutches for 4-hour periods. The ability to stand clearly was due to the learned control of blood pressure because when the patient was told not to increase his blood pressure the postural hypotensive effect would return.

On the basis of the dramatic result just described, Brucker, Miller, Pickering, and Ince (Brucker, 1980) performed a well-controlled experiment in which they attempted to establish learned voluntary control of blood pressure among 10 complete spinal cord injury patients by providing them with feedback of blood pressure levels on a heartbeat-by-heartbeat basis. The results indicated that the patients were able to produce significant voluntary increases in blood pressure that were not mediated by skeletal muscle or respiratory mechanisms. The learned blood pressure control allowed the patients, who formerly were unable to sit upright because of the hypotension, to use electric wheelchairs and to increase significantly their functional abilities and assimilation into the community.

The results reported by Brucker (1980) and Brucker & Ince (1977) are particularly important for several reasons. First, they demonstrate that a behavioral technique can be effectively used to treat a devastating and dangerous physiological consequence of spinal cord injury for which there is no known successful medical or pharmacological intervention. Second, they indicate that there may be mechanisms by which information can be transmitted past the injured part of the cord that may have wide-ranging implications for treatment paradigms designed to facilitate return of function. Finally, the results show that learned voluntary control of autonomic responses, heretofore considered improbable on the basis of neurological theory, is possible for the spinal cord injured person and may be possible for persons without spinal cord injuries as well.

Summary

The work that has been performed concerning the use of behavioral interventions with the spinal cord injured, although very limited in quantity, has demonstrated some dramatic and significant results. Several operant conditioning investigations have demonstrated that rewarding therapeutically beneficial behaviors and withdrawing reinforcement following the display of negative behaviors may produce increased compliance with therapeutic regimens (e.g., Fowler *et al.*, 1969; Malament *et al.*, 1975; Rottkamp, 1976; Sand *et al.*, 1973). In addition, the application of operant conditioning principles may be used to increase substantially the endurance or functional outcome of various therapeutic procedures (e.g., Fordyce *et al.*, 1971; Trombly, 1966; Trotter & Inman, 1968). Considering the strong evidence described above, it is surprising and unfortunate that operant techniques are not more routinely utilized in physical therapy and medicine. Additional research concerning the effectiveness of these techniques in physical therapy, occupational therapy, rehabilitation nursing, and medicine might lead to further applications of behavioral techniques to the problems and goals of the disciplines noted previously. The work on learned control of physiological responses by means of classical conditioning and biofeedback training is an extremely new and theoretically controversial area in the rehabilitation literature. With the exception of the studies regarding learned control of blood pressure for postural hypotension, this research area is still in an early stage of development. Nonetheless, the literature suggests that behavioral techniques may be applied to restore neurological functions; this application may prove to be a significant and dramatic contribution to medicine. In all, the use of behavioral interventions represents a most pragmatic approach to helping persons cope with spinal cord injury in that it provides a method by which persons may develop greater functional control over their overt behaviors, physiological processes, and the environment.

Conclusions

Spinal cord injuries, which have a substantial frequency of occurrence in the young, result in devastating functional losses that currently are not restorable by medical techniques. Although the neurological and physiological consequences of spinal cord injury are well known, the psychological consequences are assumed by many to be severe—but they are not carefully documented. Numerous authors essentially have reported their personal observations and interpretations of patients' psychological responses to injury. Other authors have employed psychometric devices; however, the measurement studies have used relatively poor methodological procedures. Nonetheless, there is a surprising consensus among authors that patients tend to respond to spinal cord injury with displays of depression, anxiety, and denial. There is also a consensus that psychological factors have great impact on the rehabilitative process and that patients require psychological intervention to cope effectively with their injuries, although there are not sufficient data to warrant these conclusions.

The interventions for the spinal cord injured consist of acute medical care to prevent death and medical complications, followed by rehabilitation training to help patients utilize their personal resources and those of present technology to attain the greatest functional capability possible given the permanent neurological losses. The behavioral sciences play a most important role in the rehabilitation process, for it is often the psychological and behavioral variables that most highly determine patient outcome during rehabilitation. While almost all rehabilitation institutions provide psychological interventions to patients, the majority of the published reports concerning psychotherapeutic interventions and therapeutic interventions for sexual dysfunction lack adequate measurement and methodological procedures. However, the literature concerning the use of behavioral techniques with problems resulting from spinal cord injuries (e.g., noncompliance, postural hypotension) generally has incorporated appropriate measurement techniques and adequate experimental designs. This literature also has produced some highly significant and dramatic therapeutic results.

It is clear that the psychological and the associated behavioral consequences of spinal cord injury are highly significant and important not only because of their severity, but because they represent the limiting factors in patients' responses to the rehabilitation process. Thus, interventions directed toward the psychological and behavioral consequences of injury are crucial to individuals' attempts to cope effectively with their functional losses. The research described in this chapter suggests that the application of the principles of learning may prove to be a powerful technique with which to address some of the currently unresolvable problems of spinal cord injured patients. Through careful and innovative research, behavioral scientists may provide the next major advances in the treatment and functional recovery of the spinal cord injured.

References

Berger, S., & Garrett, J. Psychological problems of the paraplegic patient. *Journal of Rehabilitation*, 1952, *18*, 15–17.
Brucker, B. S. Biofeedback and rehabilitation. In L. P. Ince (Ed.), *Behavioral psychology in rehabilitation medicine: Clinical applications*. Baltimore: Williams & Wilkins, 1980.

Brucker, B. S., & Ince, L. P. Biofeedback as an experimental treatment for postural hypotension in a patient with a spinal cord lesion. *Archives of Physical Medicine and Rehabilitation*, 1977, *58*, 49–53.

Brudny, J., Korein, J., Levidow, L., Grynbaum, B., Lieberman, A., & Friedmann, L. Sensory feedback therapy as a modality of treatment in central nervous system disorders of voluntary movement. *Neurology*, 1974, *24*, 925–932.

Cole, T. M., Chilgren, R., & Rosenberg, P. A new programme of sex education and counseling for spinal cord injured adults and health care professionals. *Paraplegia*, 1973, *11*, 111–124.

Comarr, A. E., & Vigue, M. Sexual counseling among male and female patients with spinal cord and/or cauda equina injury, Part I. *American Journal of Physical Medicine*, 1978, *57*, 107–122. (a)

Comarr, A. E., & Vigue, M. Sexual counseling among male and female patients with spinal cord and/or cauda equina injury, Part II. *American Journal of Physical Medicine*, 1978, *57*, 215–227. (b)

Cook, D. W. Psychological adjustment to spinal cord injury: Incidence of denial, depression, and anxiety. *Rehabilitation Psychology*, 1979, *26*, 97–104.

DeVivo, M. J., Fine, P. R., Maetz, H. M., & Stover, S. L. Prevalence of spinal cord injury: A reestimation employing life table techniques. *Archives of Neurology*, 1980, *37*, 707–708.

Dunn, M. E. Psychological intervention in a spinal cord injury center: An introduction. *Rehabilitation Psychology*, 1975, *22*, 165–178.

Eisenberg, M. G.,.& Rustad, L. C. Sex education and counseling program on a spinal cord injury service. *Archives of Physical Medicine and Rehabilitation*, 1976, *57*, 135–140.

Evans, R. L., Halar, E. M., DeFreece, A. B., & Larsen, G. L. Multidisciplinary approach to sex education of spinal cord-injured patients. *Physical Therapy*, 1976, *56*, 541–545.

Fordyce, W. E. Personality characteristics in men with spinal cord injury as related to manner of onset of disability. *Archives of Physical Medicine and Rehabilitation*, 1964, *45*, 321–325.

Fordyce, W. E. Behavioral methods in rehabilitation. In W. S. Neff (Ed.), *Rehabilitation psychology*. Washington, D.C.: American Psychological Association, 1971.

Fordyce, W. E., Sand, P. L., Trieschmann, R. B., & Fowler, R. S. Behavioral systems analyzed. *Journal of Rehabilitation*, 1971, *37*, 29–34.

Fowler, R. S., Fordyce, W. E., & Berni, R. Operant conditioning in chronic illness. *American Journal of Nursing*, 1969, *69*, 1226–1228.

Grayson, M. The concept of "acceptance" in physical rehabilitation. *Military Surgeon*, 1950, *107*, 221–226.

Grzesiak, R. C., & Zaretsky, H. H. Psychology in rehabilitation: Professional and clinical aspects. In R. Murray & J. C. Kijek (Eds.), *Current perspectives in rehabilitation nursing*. St. Louis, Mo.: C. V. Mosby, 1979.

Halstead, L. S., Halstead, M. G., Salhoot, J. T., Stock, D. D., & Sparks, R. W. Sexual attitudes, behavior and satisfaction for able-bodied and disabled participants attending workshops in human sexuality. *Archives of Physical Medicine and Rehabilitation*, 1978, *59*, 497–501.

Held, J. P., Cole, T. M., Held, C. A., Anderson, C., & Chilgren, R. A. Sexual attitude reassessment workshops: Effect on spinal cord injured adults, their partners and rehabilitation professionals. *Archives of Physical Medicine and Rehabilitation*, 1975, *56*, 14–18.

Hoch, Z. Sex therapy and marital counseling for the disabled. *Archives of Physical Medicine and Rehabilitation*, 1977, *58*, 413–415.

Hohmann, G. Psychological aspects of treatment and rehabilitation of the spinal cord injured person. *Clinical Orthopaedics and Related Research*, 1975, *112*, 81–88.

Ince, L. P., Brucker, B. S., & Alba, A. Behavior techniques applied to the care of patietns with spinal cord injuries with an annotated reference list. *Behavioral Engineering*, 1976, *3*, 87–95.

Ince, L. P., Brucker, B. S., & Alba, A. Conditioning bladder responses in patients with spinal
    cord lesions. *Archives of Physical Medicine and Rehabilitation*, 1977, *58*, 59–65.
Ince, L. P., Brucker, B. S., & Alba, A. Conditioning responding of the neurogenic bladder.
    Psychosomatic Medicine, 1978, *40*, 14–24. (a)
Ince, L. P., Brucker, B. S., & Alba, A. Reflex conditioning in a spinal man. *Journal of
    Comparative and Physiological Psychology*, 1978, *92*, 796–802. (b)
Isaacson, J., & Delgado, H. E. Sex counseling for those with spinal cord injuries. *Social
    Casework*, 1974, *55*, 622–627.
Kazdin, A. E. Methodological and interpretive problems of single-case experimental designs.
    Journal of Consulting and Clinical Psychology, 1978, *46*, 629–642.
Kerr, W. G., & Thompson, M. A. Acceptance of disability of sudden onset in paraplegia.
    Paraplegia, 1972, *10*, 94–102.
Knorr, N. J., & Bull, J. C. Spinal cord injury: Psychiatric considerations. *Maryland State
    Medical Journal*, 1970, *19*, 105–108.
Kunce, J., & Worley, B. Interest patterns, accidents, and disability. *Journal of Clinical Psy-
    chology*, 1966, *22*, 105–107.
Maki, R. J., Winograd, M., & Hinkle, E. Counseling/psychotherapy approach in rehabilitation
    of a spinal cord injury population. *Archives of Physical Medicine and Rehabilitation*, 1976,
    57, 548. (Abstract)
Malament, I. B., Dunn, M. E., & Davis, R. Pressure sores: An operant conditioning approach
    to prevention. *Archives of Physical Medicine and Rehabilitation*, 1975, *56*, 161–165.
Mann, W., Godfrey, M. E., & Dowd, E. T. The use of group counseling procedures in the
    rehabilitation of spinal cord injured patients. *The American Journal of Occupational Ther-
    apy*, 1973, *27*, 73–77.
McCollough, N. C., Green, B. A., Klose, K. J., Goldberg, M. L., & Klose, C. Spinal cord
    injury in South Florida. *The Journal of the Florida Medical Association*, 1981, *68*,
    968–973.
Melnyk, R., Montgomery, R., & Over, R. Attitude changes following a sexual counseling
    program for spinal cord injured persons. *Archives of Physical Medicine and Rehabilitation*,
    1979, *60*, 601–604.
Miller, D. K., Wolfe, M., & Spiegel, M. Therapeutic groups for patients with spinal cord
    injuries. *Archives of Physical Medicine and Rehabilitation*, 1975, *56*, 130–135.
Mueller, A. D. Psychologic factors in rehabilitation of paraplegic patients. *Archives of Physical
    Medicine and Rehabilitation*, 1962, *43*, 151–159.
Nacht, M. B., Wolf, S. L., & Coogler, C. E. Use of electromyographic biofeedback during the
    acute phase of spinal cord injury. *Physical Therapy*, 1982, *62*, 290–294.
Nagler, B. Psychiatric aspects of cord injury. *American Journal of Psychiatry*, 1950, *107*, 49–56.
Peter, A. R. Psychosocial aspects of spinal cord injury. *Maryland State Medical Journal*, 1975,
    24, 65–69.
Roessler, R., Milligan, T., & Ohlson, A. Personal adjustment training for the spinal cord
    injured. *Rehabilitation Counseling Bulletin*, 1976, *19*, 544–550.
Rohrer, K., Adelman, B., Puckett, J., Toomey, B., Talbert, D., & Johnson, S. W. Rehabilita-
    tion in spinal cord injury: Use of a patient-family group. *Archives of Physical Medicine and
    Rehabilitation*, 1980, *61*, 225–229.
Romano, M. D. Social skills training with the newly handicapped. *Archives of Physical Medi-
    cine and Rehabilitation*, 1976, *57*, 302–303.
Romano, M. D., & Lassiter, R. E. Sexual counseling with the spinal-cord injured. *Archives of
    Physical Medicine and Rehabilitation*, 1972, *53*, 568–572.
Rottkamp, B. C. An experimental nursing study: A behavior modification approach to nursing
    therapeutics in body positioning of spinal cord-injured patients. *Nursing Research*, 1976,
    25, 181–186.

Sand, P. L., Fordyce, W. E., & Fowler, R. S. Fluid intake behavior in patients with spinal-cord injury: Prediction and modification. *Archives of Physical Medicine and Rehabilitation*, 1973, *54*, 254–262.

Sand, P. L., Fordyce, W. E., Trieschmann, R. B., & Fowler, R. S. Behavior modification in the medical rehabilitation setting: Rationale and some applications. *Rehabilitation Research and Practice Review*, 1970, *1*, 11–24.

Siller, J. Psychological situation of the disabled with spinal cord injuries. *Rehabilitation Literature*, 1969, *30*, 290–296.

Taylor, G. P., Jr., & Persons, R. W. Behavior modification techniques in a physical medicine and rehabilitation center. *Journal of Psychology*, 1970, *74*, 117–124.

Thom, D. A., VonSalzen, C. F., & Fromme, A. Psychological aspects of the paraplegic patient. *Medical Clinics of North America*, 1946, *30*, 473–480.

Trieschmann, R. B. *Spinal cord injuries*. New York: Pergamon Press, 1980.

Trombly, C. A. Principles of operant conditioning related to orthotic training of quadriplegic patients. *American Journal of Occupational Therapy*, 1966, *20*, 217–220.

Trotter, A. B., & Inman, D. A. The use of positive reinforcement in physical therapy. *Physical Therapy*, 1968, *48*, 347–352.

Weiss, A. J., & Diamond, M. D. Psychologic adjustment of patients with myelopathy. *Archives of Physical Medicine and Rehabilitation*, 1966, *47*, 72–76.

Wittkower, E. D., Gingras, G., Mergler, L., Wigdor, B., & Lepine, A. A combined psychosocial study of spinal cord lesions. *Canadian Medical Association Journal*, 1954, *71*, 109–115.

Young, J. S., & Northrup, N. E. *Statistical information pertaining to some of the most commonly asked questions about SCI*. Phoenix: National Spinal Cord Injury Data Research Center, 1979.

12

Respiratory Disorders*

THOMAS L. CREER

Introduction

At one time or another, we all experience various types of respiratory disorders. If we are fortunate, the distress will be restricted to occasional heavy breathing or wheezing when climbing up a flight of stairs, or to the cold we seem to catch at least once a year. With better physical conditioning, we might discover that we have less respiratory distress when climbing stairs; unfortunately, we may still have that annual cold, no matter the amount of vitamin C we ingest.

We know that, in most instances, there are steps we can take to alleviate the occasional periods of acute respiratory distress we experience. We can always exercise or reduce our weight; this, in turn, should help us in situations requiring physical exertion. With the common cold, we can take two aspirin and go to bed. Time is our ally; we know that a common cold eventually will disappear. These expectations are not held by individuals with chronic respiratory conditions, however. People afflicted with such disorders anticipate that they will suffer from their affliction, either on an intermittent or a regular basis. In most cases, people can learn to cope with their disorder and live full, productive lives. For some individuals, on the other hand, the respiratory condition eventually will result in death.

This chapter describes the three chronic respiratory conditions grouped together under the label chronic obstructive pulmonary disease (COPD): asthma, chronic bronchitis, and emphysema. In particular, the discussion

*The writing of this chapter was supported in part, by Grant HL 22021 and Grant HL 27402 from the Division of Lung Diseases, National Institute of Heart, Lung, and Blood.

COPING WITH
CHRONIC DISEASE
313

focuses on asthma. The decision to emphasize asthma is not meant to negate the importance of either chronic bronchitis or emphysema. Rather, it reflects the fact that considerably more attention has been directed by behavioral scientists to asthma than to the other two conditions.

Asthma

From what I have heard from others, and as is known to your highness, I conclude that this disorder starts with a common cold, especially in the rainy season, and the patient is forced to gasp for breath day and night, depending upon the duration of the onset, until the phlegm is expelled, and flow completed and the lung wall cleared

Moses Maimonides

Moses Maimonides (Sampter, 1969, p. 5) was a physician who lived between the years of 1135 and 1204. His treatise is considered a classic in the area of asthma and allergy; although his description of asthma would not serve in diagnosing the disorder, it is an accurate description.

The difficulties associated with the study of asthma do not begin in describing patients during attacks; rather, they begin in attempting to define the disorder. A medical definition of asthma must outline the causes of the affliction and the way these causes induce the disorder. Because asthma is largely an enigma, attempts to define the affliction have always sparked contention and arguments. The problem was highlighted in the early 1970s when a panel of experts was assembled and charged with the task of arriving at a uniform definition of asthma. After considerable debate, the group concluded that asthma could not be adequately defined (Porter & Birch, 1971). They did provide yet another description of asthma but, as pointed out by Young (1980), it brought us no closer to a precise definition of the ailment, nor to an explanation of the ancient but accurate saying, "All that wheezes is not asthma."

CHARACTERISTICS OF ASTHMA

It will become apparent that the assessment of asthma and asthma-related behaviors is at the core of this chapter. Problems in assessment are inherent in any phenomenon as complex as asthma, especially when there is no consensual agreement regarding a definition of the disorder. It is necessary, however, to use some sort of definition as a guide to the present discussion of asthma. The definition most appropriate for this purpose was offered by Chai (1975). He defined asthma as an intermittent, variable, and reversible airway obstruction. Characteristics of Chai's definition are depicted in Figure 12.1, which portrays characteristics of the asthma suffered by a hypothetical patient. Each characteristic merits a brief discussion.

Frequency

The number of attacks occurs on an intermittent or an aperiodic basis. A patient may suffer a series or burst of attacks over a brief period and then not suffer an asthmatic episode for a long duration of time. The hypothetical patient presented in Figure 12.1 suffered three attacks, with two attacks occurring within a brief time period and the final occurring after a relatively long passage of time. The continuum of time varies from patient to patient; it could be that our hypothetical patient suffered three attacks during a single week, or that the episodes were experienced over the course of a year. A peculiarity of asthma is that it can occur at any time over the course of a patient's life. Thus, a patient who has suffered a number of attacks in a short span of time may go a number of years without experiencing an asthmatic episode. Creer (1979) recounted the story of an elderly patient who complained that he recently had experienced his first attack "since Roosevelt was President." Further conversation with the man revealed that the patient was not referring to Franklin Delano, but to his cousin Theodore!

A number of factors are involved in determining the frequency of attacks experienced by any given patient. Patients classified as suffering extrinsic or allergic asthma may experience attacks only during a particular season of the year. If they are allergic to a certain pollen, for example, their attacks may coincide with the season when that pollen is most prevalent. For the remainder of the year, the patient may not experience any more respiratory discomfort than that experienced by the nonasthmatic individual. In fact,

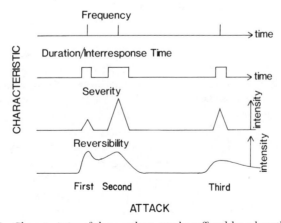

FIGURE 12.1   Characteristics of three asthma attacks suffered by a hypothetical patient.

unless the patient reveals that he or she has a history of asthma, the physician would find it difficult to confirm the diagnosis of asthma (Williams, 1980).

Another group of patients have what is referred to as intrinsic or idiopathic asthma. This form of asthma is not associated with allergens, but may result from infections or other physiological factors. Unlike patients with extrinsic or allergic asthma who experience attacks on a seasonal basis, patients with intrinsic or idiopathic asthma may suffer attacks year-round or on what is referred to as a perennial basis. The problem with the categorization scheme used in the preceding is that the broad separation of asthma into two groupings neglects the large overlap between the two categories (e.g., Reed & Townley, 1978; Williams, 1980). In other words, there are a number of patients who are described as suffering a mixed type of asthma, that is, they experience attacks triggered by both intrinsic and extrinsic factors. As a consequence of this flaw in classifying asthmatic patients, Reed and Townley (1978) have proposed that asthma be conceived as a disorder with three components: "(1) the stimuli that provoke airway obstruction; (2) the person on whom the stimuli act, with the physiologic and biochemical steps that link the stimulus to the response; and (3) the physiologic and pathologic response that constitutes obstruction [p. 660]." This particular method of categorizing phenomena, familiar to behavioral scientists, seems to be a more propitious way to classify asthmatic patients than does a system based solely upon stimuli provoking attacks.

The intermittent nature of asthma presents problems to the behavioral scientist who wishes to work with an asthmatic population. One major problem is that there is no standardized way of defining what is or what is not an attack. In most instances, the decision as to what constitutes an asthmatic episode is left to the patient. Needless to say, this introduces a problem to assessment in that patients vary in their perceptions of an attack. The difficulties are twofold (Creer & Kotses, in press):

1. Not all patients are *aware* of the physical changes that herald the onset of an attack. Rubinfeld and Pain (1976) found patients who claimed they were asthma-free when, in actuality, objective pulmonary physiology indices showed they were exhaling less than 50% of their predicted expiratory rates. With some patients, this may be due to a lack of sensory input, for example, lack of hypoxic drive to the effect that an attack has started.

2. In most cases patients are aware they are experiencing physical changes, but they may have difficulty in correctly *interpreting* sensory input. A number of possibilities can occur with the onset of an attack (Creer, 1980; Creer & Kotses, in press): (a) the patient may misinterpret sensory signals and decide he or she is not suffering an attack, thus delaying treat-

ment of the episode; (b) the context in which the attack occurs may influence the decision-making process of the patient (more on this topic in the following); (c) the patient may interpret physical changes as portending the onset of an attack when, in actuality, the changes serve as signals for other phenomena (e.g., the patient who, having formerly experienced a high-anxiety-arousing attack, associates further episodes of anxiety as signals for attacks); and (d) the patient correctly determines that certain changes do signal an attack and initiates treatment.

There are methods by which patients may be taught to make the latter decision. The most widely used method to improve the correlation between subjective feelings of asthma and objective indices of bronchial obstruction was described in a classic study by Chai, Purcell, Brady, and Falliers (1968). They suggested that the Wright Peak Flow Meter, an instrument that assesses the maximum airflow a person can produce and maintain for 10 msec, can be used to provide information on a person's pulmonary functions. The instrument is portable and can be used in almost any environment, including the home. With the meter, information can be gathered about the pulmonary obstruction experienced by an asthmatic patient.

More recently, Renne, Nau, Dietiker, and Lyon (1976) took a different tack: children were provided with peak flow meters and asked to record the values they thought they could produce at different times during the day. The study employed a reinforcement paradigm in which the youngsters were informed they would be given scrip exchangeable either for gifts or for the opportunity to chart estimates of their pulmonary functioning as they approximated pulmonary data obtained by the experimenters. Renne and his colleagues reported success in teaching asthmatic children to correlate their subjective feelings of asthma with objective measurements of pulmonary obstruction.

Flow rates, as obtained with the Mini-Wright Peak Flow Meter—a smaller and less expensive version of the original instrument—were employed by Taplin and Creer (1978) to teach patients to predict more precisely the probable occurrence of an asthma attack. Based upon a calculation of base rates of attacks and flow rates obtained in the morning and evening, two conditional probabilities were calculated for each asthmatic youngster. These probabilities estimated first the likelihood of an attack in a 12-hour period following a flow rate score equal to or less than the critical value, and second the likelihood of an attack within a 12-hour period following a peak flow score greater than the critical value. Results of the study suggested that peak flow data collected from a patient increased the predictability of asthma attacks suffered by that individual. It should be noted that other, less expensive instruments—the Pulmonary Monitor and the Peak Flow Whistle—also can be used to teach patients to monitor their pulmonary physiology better (Burns, 1979; Chiaramonte & Prabhu, 1981).

A second major problem posed by the intermittent nature of asthma occurs when the investigator plans to assess the effect of an independent variable on the disorder. The difficulty can develop in gathering either baseline or follow-up data. In collecting base-line information, the investigator may discover that attacks occur too infrequently to permit him or her to meet the criteria required of a base line (e.g., Gelfand & Hartmann, 1975). Possible solutions to this problem include obtaining base-line data over an extended period of time, a tack that may not be feasible in many investigations, or attempting to recruit as subjects only those patients with perennial asthma. Recruiting patients who suffer asthma on a year-round basis would resolve the difficulty if it were not for the fact that many of these patients suffer both perennial *and* seasonal asthma. In other words, they suffer attacks throughout the year and there also is a seasonal component to their attacks in that the frequency of asthmatic episodes can increase during particular times of the year. This presents a paradox that repeatedly occurs in working with an asthmatic population. To illustrate this paradox, consider an investigator who, having gathered appropriate base-line data, introduces an independent variable of some type, for example, an intervention procedure such as relaxation. The results of this variable may, according to the data, show an effect, for example, a decrease in the rate of asthmatic episodes. Before rejoicing at these results, the investigator must be certain that the changes that occurred were, indeed, due to the intervention procedure he or she applied. It could well be that the decrease in attacks was the result of introduction of the independent variable, but it also is possible that the changes occurred because of a second independent variable *not* under the control of the experimenter. To continue with the illustration, it is highly possible that the changes were not the result of teaching the patients to relax, but instead were a reflection of another, uncontrolled independent variable, such as the changing of seasons. What may be even more likely to have occurred is that, unknown to the investigator, a physician may have altered a number of patients' medications in some manner so that the result is a reduction in the frequency of their attacks. Medications, if taken as prescribed, can be the most powerful independent variable used to change the rate of asthma attacks. The task of the behavioral scientist is somehow to control, through cooperation with the patient's physician, when medications are to be altered. As was demonstrated in a study by Miklich, Renne, Creer, Alexander, Chai, Davis, Hoffman, and Danker-Brown (1977), this is not always an easy matter to resolve. What does the behavioral scientist do if, as in the situation faced by Miklich and his colleagues, a better and more effective medication becomes available? Should an asthmatic patient be denied the drug even though it could be potentially beneficial to his or her health? Or, on the other hand, should the behavioral scientist complete his or her study? These are the kinds of questions that are apt to be raised when an attempt is made to hold medications stable for the sake of studying the efficacy of a behavioral technique.

The question of how long follow-up data should be obtained following application of an independent variable also has no simple answer. Several years ago, Leigh (1953) advocated the initiation of long-term projects, lasting 5, 10, and 15 years, to assess the effect of various intervention strategies on asthma. The idea is laudable, particularly in light of the intermittent nature of the disorder. However, there are two major problems that prevent adoption of Leigh's suggestion:

1. It would be difficult to follow any patient for a prolonged period of time. Asthmatic patients are not only mobile in the sense that they are apt to move around the country seeking a climate more beneficial to their disorder, but they also tend to switch physicians in their search for the elusive "cure" for asthma.

2. More importantly, a patient's asthma is apt to change over a period of time. Although it remains difficult to forecast the course of any patient's asthma, there is evidence that some children do improve, or outgrow the disorder, as they age. However, the exact number of youngsters who outgrow their asthma remains unknown. The Task Force on Asthma assembled by the National Institute of Allergic and Infectious Diseases points out that there is considerable discrepancy in findings on this topic: the range of estimates of those who become free of asthma as adults range from 26% to 78% (Young, 1980).

Duration and Interresponse Time

While the terms *duration* and *interresponse time* are not part of the definition of asthma, they are important characteristics of the disorder. Duration simply means how long an attack or asthmatic episode lasts; interresponse time refers to the time that elapses between attacks (i.e., frequency of attacks). These complementary measures are useful in the assessment of the asthmatic patient, although they are not free from problems. At what point, for example, does one begin measuring the onset of an attack? Does an attack begin from the moment the patient claims to be experiencing respiratory distress or does one start when pulmonary obstruction is indicated on an index such as peak flow rate? These are questions that must be answered before using duration as a dependent measure.

It may be that, as has been done in hospital settings (Creer, 1970; Creer,

Weinberg, & Molk, 1974; Hochstadt, Shepard, & Lulla, 1980), the investigator may wish to use the duration and frequency of the patient's hospitalizations as dependent variables. There are three advantages to using such data as dependent measures (Creer, 1979): (a) the number and duration of hospitalizations experienced by the patient over a period of time may be an excellent guide to the severity of the disease; for example, the higher the frequency of attacks requiring hospitalization, the greater is the severity (Chai *et al.*, 1968); (b) the data are considered as reliable and valid when the experimenter has access to a patient's medical record; and (c) an analysis can be made, over a period of time, of the pattern of asthma suffered by the individual. This information, in turn, has implications for the diagnosis and treatment of the disorder.

There is a major disadvantage to using duration and frequency of hospitalizations as dependent measures for asthma: the variables can be manipulated by factors in the hospital setting that are unrelated to the disease process per se. For example, three studies (Creer, 1970; Creer *et al.*, 1974; Hochstadt *et al.*, 1980) have demonstrated that the reduction of reinforcement for illness behavior in the hospital—through the systematic application of a time-out procedure—resulted in a decrease in both the number and duration of hospitalizations for asthma. Thus, unless monitored carefully, the validity of the use of the frequency and duration of hospitalizations as indices of chronic respiratory disease, particularly asthma, may be questioned.

Maimonides was the first to suggest that, with proper treatment, the interval between two asthma attacks might be lengthened. However, the index was not used as a dependent measure with asthmatic patients until it was employed by Hochstadt *et al.* (1980). They analyzed the hospital records of seven asthmatic youngsters described as "overusers" of the hospital in that they: (a) verbalized the intent to develop asthma symptoms in order to be admitted when a friend was hospitalized or a special event was planned; (b) stated a preference to remain in the hospital rather than to return home; (c) predicted a quick return to the hospital following their discharge; and (d) prolonged their hospitalizations by developing symptoms of asthma when told of their impending discharge. The analysis revealed that the mean interval between hospitalizations was 48.9 days for these children. The time-out procedure suggested by Creer (1970), consisting of the removal of comic books, TV, and the opportunity to interact socially with other patients, then was applied each time one of the children was admitted to the hospital over the course of a year. The results by Hochstadt and his coworkers (1980) indicated that the mean interval between hospitalizations increased from 48.9 days to 85.3 days with application of the time-out procedure. Again, the reader must be cautioned that this change does not reflect an underlying change in the patient's asthma; rather, it demonstrates how a particular dependent measure of the disorder can be manipulated by environmental factors extraneous to the process of the disorder.

Variability

Attacks vary in severity from mild episodes, characterized by a feeling of tightness in the chest or a slight wheeze, to status asthmaticus or steadily worsening asthma (Creer, 1979). The latter can result in death, primarily through the formation of mucus plugs that literally stop breathing. Williams (1980) suggested that the variability of asthma has been the principal reason the disorder has eluded precise definition. He explained that whereas the conventional definition of asthma as a variable airway obstruction is sufficiently broad to embrace all patients afflicted with the condition, it necessarily overlaps with other forms of COPD.

The severity of asthma varies both from patient to patient and from episode to episode within the same patient. Both the interindividual and intraindividual variations in severity have implications for the behavioral scientist. In the first place, patients can be categorized along a continuum from those who suffer occasional mild wheezing to those in whom obstruction is more or less a permanent feature. For the patients in the former category, asthma may be little more than a nuisance; they may suffer some discomfort during their infrequent and mild attacks, but the condition may not interfere to any extent with their daily lives. The situation is just the opposite for those on the other end of the spectrum, however. Jones (1976) has noted that for these persons, asthma is characterized by persistent respiratory debilitation rather than by definitive attacks of asthma. As might be expected, the disorder becomes a prepotent factor in dictating the life-style of these individuals. Behavioral scientists are apt to become involved with such patients in attempting to help them cope with a debilitating physical condition. In this respect, the patients present behavioral problems similar to those afflicted with more severe forms of COPD, particularly emphysema (Dudley, Glaser, Jorgenson, & Logan, 1980a).

As depicted in Figure 12.1, attacks also can vary in severity from episode to episode within the same person. Thus, the patient may suffer a mild attack, followed by a more severe attack the next time he or she experiences the disorder. More than likely, however, the patient will suffer several mild attacks in succession, followed by a severe episode. The behavioral problem that is apt to result from such a schedule can be briefly summarized as follows: a patient, having experienced several mild attacks of asthma, will alter his or her behavior. Compliance with medications may begin to deteriorate or the patient may unnecessarily expose himself or herself to known precipitants of attacks. As a consequence, the patient may acquire expectations that only mild attacks are apt to occur and, therefore, be unprepared to manage a severe attack. The solution to this problem is to teach the patient how to appropriately respond to any attack, no matter the intensity of the episode. Such self-instruction by patients can become a key ingredient in the self-management of the disorder (Creer, 1980; Creer, Renne & Chai, 1982).

A final, but very important, point should be noted about assessing the severity of asthma attacks: there is no standardized way to classify an attack as mild, moderate, or severe. A number of different gauges have been suggested across the years, ranging from the amount of medications taken by the patient during an episode to the length of time he or she was hospitalized with the attack. None of the methods is widely used, however. One potentially valuable method of classifying an attack as mild, moderate, or severe was suggested by the parents of children enrolled in a large self-management project for asthma (Creer, 1980). These parents used the decrease in peak expiratory flow rates, as obtained with a peak flow meter, to determine if an attack was mild, moderate, or severe. If the decrease was a certain number of liters per minute, but not enough to reach the lowest value on the meter (60 l/min), the attack was described as mild; if, on the other hand, the decrease was such that it could no longer be recorded with the meter, that is, the child could no longer produce a reading that topped 60 l/min, the attack was regarded as moderate. Parents considered attacks as severe when they fulfilled two criteria. The first criterion, as with attacks referred to as moderate, was that the youngster's peak flow values decreased so that they could no longer be recorded with a peak flow meter. In addition, the parents described how the decrease in peak flow values was observed over a relatively brief period of time—in a matter of a few minutes or hours. In other words, the second criterion for a severe attack was that the youngster's peak expiratory flow rates show a sudden and large decrement. This method of operationalizing the severity of asthma attacks requires refinement, but it does offer possibilities.

Reversibility

The airway obstruction that constitutes an asthma attack results from a narrowing of the large and/or small airways; it is caused by smooth-muscle spasm, swelling of tissue, excessive mucus secretion, dried mucus plugs, or a combination of these factors (Creer, 1979). Reversibility denotes that the airway obstruction can be reversed either spontaneously or with adequate treatment. The reversibility component of the disorder is a hallmark of asthma (McFadden, 1980b); it differentiates the condition from other respiratory conditions such as emphysema.

Two aspects of reversibility should be noted. First, it is a relative condition. As was noted earlier, there are patients who always seem to have some airway obstruction. However, there must be some reversal of the airway obstruction, either spontaneous or resulting from proper treatment, for a patient to be diagnosed as suffering asthma. Second, the fact that attacks can spontaneously remit provides a major obstacle in the assessment of the condition, particularly when the aim is to determine the effect of a particular intervention strategy on asthma. The literature is replete with reports of success in treating asthma, particularly individual cases of the disorder, in which spontaneous remission cannot be ruled out as the significant component in the production of such results (Creer, 1979). Behavioral scientists, in particular, show a proclivity for making this error.

A discussion of spontaneous remission would be incomplete without mention of how this characteristic has contributed to an abundant array of techniques for treating asthma. Standing on one's head, applying mustard plasters, balancing a penny on one's forehead, and smelling the aroma of certain woods all have been advocated as remedies for attacks. What seems to occur is a chance pairing between a particular stimulus and the spontaneous remission of asthma. This results in the superstitious belief that these procedures actually aborted the episode. There is one procedure that is used in various parts of the United States, although it lacks any demonstrated value in the treatment of asthma. The procedure is to have a patient carry around a small dog, usually a chihuahua. Apparently, the dog emits a wheezing-like sound that some have likened to the wheezing that occurs during attacks. By carrying around these dogs, the rationale is that there will be a transference of symptoms in that the child will wheeze less and the dog will wheeze more. Although the procedure may seem logical to some who favor psychoanalysis, the procedure actually can induce or intensify attacks in asthmatic youngsters allergic to animal dander (*Asthma and the other allergic diseases*, 1979).

CHARACTERISTICS OF ASTHMATIC PATIENTS

A number of patient characteristics could be described in this section. However, four topics—compliance, emotions, treatment, and context— have been selected for discussion. These topics are depicted for a hypothetical patient in Figure 12.2. Two variables, treatment and context, normally might not be conceived of as patient characteristics; they are included in this discussion, however, because of the large behavioral component involved in both variables.

Compliance

Compliance can be defined as how well a patient adheres to instructions provided by his or her physician. With asthmatic patients, the topic includes

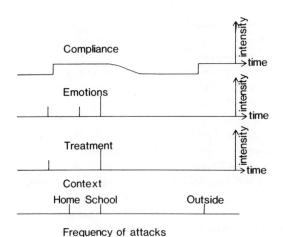

FIGURE 12.2   Characteristics of a hypothetical asthma patient.

behaviors extending from the avoidance of known precipitants of attacks to adherence to medication regimens. Since a description of all of the behaviors that constitute compliance is beyond the scope of the present discussion, the focus will be on medication compliance.

There are a number of reasons asthmatic patients fail to comply with medication instructions (Creer, 1979). These range from the expense of the drugs to the side effects they induce. Perhaps the problem of compliance can best be illustrated by returning to Figure 12.2. This shows that the patient began complying with medication instructions shortly before the first attack. He continued to adhere to these instructions until after the second episode. Thereafter, there was a decline in compliance until, for a period, he did not take his medications at all. In fact, he resumed taking the drugs only with the onset of his third attack.

If we asked our hypothetical patient why he became noncompliant, he might offer any number of explanations. Some might be nothing more than weak excuses ("I forgot"), but other reasons might be compelling arguments for noncompliance. The following represent three such arguments.

First, there are the expenses entailed in purchasing the medications. Drugs taken on a continuing basis for the treatment of chronic respiratory disorders, including asthma, easily can exceed $100 a month. Unless there is assistance available to many patients and their families, these patients simply will fail to take asthma medications as prescribed.

Second a number of side effects regularly occur as a result of taking asthma medications. Many of these side effects are physical, ranging from cataracts, which can result from the prolonged use of corticosteroids (Dunand, Chai,

Weltman, Spauling, & Meltzer, 1975), to the insomnia, lightheadedness, tremors, and even seizures that may be seen with patients who take pre-scribed theophylline or theophylline-based products to control their asthma (Brandon, 1977). It could well be that many patients view such physical changes as more disruptive than the asthma they occasionally suffer.

Other patients experience side effects from their asthma medications that might be considered relatively psychological in nature. These patients com-plain that it is difficult for them to concentrate on a task for any period of time. Observations of some asthmatic children in the classroom did confirm this complaint: the youngsters seemingly did lack attending skills and, there-fore, were off-task much of the time (Creer & Yoches, 1971). Recently, the problem has been more closely investigated by Bill Suess and his colleagues (Suess & Chai, 1981; Suess, Chai, Kalisker, & Stump, 1982). In the latter study, tests of visual retention and paired associate learning were admin-istered to three groups of children: (a) asthmatic children receiving the-ophylline therapy; (b) asthmatic youngsters receiving a theophylline–steroid combination therapy; and (c) nonasthmatic children not receiving any known medications. Data gathered by Suess and his coworkers indicated that 6 to 8 hours after the administration of medication, the performance of the youngsters receiving the theophylline–steroid combination treatment was significantly poorer relative to that of the other two groups. No signifi-cant differences were found between the three groups, however, approx-imately 24 and 48 hours after the theophylline–steroid therapy group re-ceived the preparation. These results suggest that the youngsters who received steroids for the control of asthma experienced interference with their cognitive processes for at least up to 6 to 8 hours after ingestion of the medicine.

Finally, an analysis of Figure 12.2 shows a pattern of compliance displayed by many asthmatic patients: they take their medicine only when suffering attacks. The remainder of the time, the patients tend to be noncompliant. There are two points that should be emphasized about the response pattern of our hypothetical patient; these points represent the third compelling argument for medication noncompliance. First, the hypothetical patient is behaving in a manner consistent with his, and our, reinforcement history. From childhood on, we are taught to take medicine only when ill, a practice strengthened by medication containers that are difficult to open even when we are well. Many asthmatic patients, on the other hand, are suddenly told to forget this lifelong practice and to take medicine on a regular basis, even when they feel well. Needless to say, there are asthmatic patients who do not forget what they were originally taught and thus are noncompliant. The second point that should be emphasized concerning the response pattern shown in Figure 12.2 is that the hypothetical patient, like many other patients, frequently is reinforced for not complying with medication instructions. The figure shows that the hypothetical patient went for a period of time without experiencing an attack. Under these circumstances, the patient was not punished for being noncompliant, but was reinforced by good health for noncompliant behavior. In summary, patients' premorbid reinforcement histories and long interresponse times may be causally related to their noncompliance with medication regimens.

A splendid conclusion to this discussion of compliance would be to offer a strategy guaranteed to alter noncompliance in asthmatic patients. This, however, is not possible: the reasons for failure to comply with medical instructions are too numerous and complex to warrant the use of a global strategy. And, as with other diseases or physical disorders (Dunbar & Agras, 1981), patterns of noncompliance are hard to change. The general tack that has been suggested by Creer (1979) for improving compliance in COPD patients includes steps that can be taken by physicians, such as prescribing less expensive medications with fewer side effects, and by behavioral scientists, such as establishing a system for monitoring and recording compliant behaviors. This strategy has yielded promising results, but there is, as yet, no thorough and systematic investigation of how medication compliance can be improved in COPD patients, including those with asthma.

Emotions

There are so many meanings for the term *emotion* that another only would add to the confusion. What is meant as emotional responding should become clearer as the discussion continues. Figure 12.2 depicts that our hypothetical patient experienced three emotional episodes. Two of the emotional episodes are unrelated to the patient's attacks; the third occurred concurrently with an asthmatic episode. This pattern of emotional and asthma episodes points out several factors: first, not every emotional reaction experienced by a person with asthma will lead to an attack. In the present case, none of the patient's emotional reactions is related to the onset of an attack. Second, emotional factors and their role in either the precipitation or exacerbation of an attack varies from person to person. There are many patients whose emotions are totally unrelated to their asthma; with others, including our hypothetical patient, emotional reactions may be more involved with the exacerbation of ongoing attacks rather than the precipitation of asthmatic episodes. Finally, as will be noted later, the context in which emotions are aroused is a significant variable in determining whether or not an attack will occur.

Any discussion of emotions and asthma is apt to become, in the words of Chai (1974), "very emotional! [p. 410]." The contention regarding the relationship between emotions and asthma does not center on whether or not emotions can affect asthma; those who suffer attacks or attempt to treat the distress of an asthma episode are well aware of the role emotions can play in either triggering or exacerbating an attack. The argument instead concerns the possible mechanism or mechanisms by which emotions interact with asthma. Here is a mystery, despite the fact that the link between emotions and asthma was made by Aretaeus in the second century A.D. (Rosenblatt, 1976).

Elsewhere (Creer, 1979) I have argued that "behavioral components of emotional responding trigger asthma either through mechanical means, probably through stimulation of the vagus nerve, or through exercise [p. 158]." There is evidence to support these views. On one hand, it has long been known that such behaviors as coughing, crying, laughing, and shouting can precipitate attacks in some patients. A number of investigators (e.g., McFadden, 1980a) have attributed the occurrence of such behaviors to stimulation of the vagus nerve, which in turn prompts the bronchial constriction that characterizes asthma.

Another possible link between emotions and asthma is exercise. It has been estimated by some observers that perhaps 90% of asthmatic children suffer exercise-induced attacks (Ghory, 1975). The exact mechanism for exercise-induced asthma is as yet unknown (e.g., Cropp, 1978), although airway cooling has been suggested as a probable culprit (McFadden, 1980a, 1980b). What is important for this discussion is that many patients have observed that the same behaviors they perform when exercising are the same as those they would exhibit if emotionally aroused (Creer, 1979). In other words, the patients describe how they shout, laugh, or jump around if excited; they might exhibit the same behavioral pattern, however, if they were playing basketball or on a playground.

It must be emphasized that the position that the overt manifestions of emotional responding can elicit asthma episodes is strongly behavioral and is dependent upon *what* the person does when emotional. It can explain most attacks of asthma suffered by patients, but not all emotionally related asthma episodes. The induction of asthma through suggestion, a number of demonstrations of which were made by Luparello and his colleagues (e.g., Luparello, Lyons, Bleecker, & McFadden, 1968), attest to the involvement of cognitive processes in some forms of emotionally aroused asthma. Hence, it is likely that cognitive and other physical processes, such as hyperventilation, hypocapnea, and changes in adrenal medullary or cortical functions, as well as vagus nerve activity, are involved in various forms of emotionally aroused asthma (Reed & Townley, 1978).

A sine qua non of attempts to alter inappropriate emotional behavior is to teach the patients responses that are incompatible with such behavior. This

approach—entailing the use of systematic desensitization—has proven useful with asthmatic patients (Creer, 1979); it seems particularly appropriate in
changing the panic that, occurring concurrently with an attack, can exacerbate the episode (Creer, 1974, 1978; Creer et al., 1982).

Treatment

Here, the term *treatment* refers to what the patient does to treat his or her
attacks. Figure 12.2 shows that our hypothetical patient appropriately treated himself during only one attack (the second asthmatic episode). He did not
treat himself during either the first or third attacks, a fact suggesting that any
treatment he did receive was provided by someone else or that the attacks
remitted spontaneously. At the same time, the patient did treat himself
when he did not actually suffer an asthmatic episode. This is commonly seen
when asthmatic individuals use a nebulizer when it is not really necessary to
do so.

The performance of our hypothetical patient in treating his asthma is not
atypical. On the one hand, many patients do not know the steps they should
take to alleviate the distress of an incipient attack. They wait for the episode
to subside or, in the event that it intensifies, they seek treatment in the
emergency room of a hospital. It is difficult to break this treatment-seeking
pattern with many patients, particularly adults. They stoically adopt the
philosophy of waiting out the episode or, if required, going to an emergency
room. As with the case of medication noncompliance, the patients normally
are reinforced for their treatment-seeking behavior. If the attack spontaneously remits, the patients not only are freed of respiratory distress, but
they are saved the expense of medical treatment. If, however, treatment is
required, the patients also are reinforced by going to an emergency room. As
Aelony (1980) pointed out, the emergency room treatment consists of the
administration of drugs and techniques that rapidly begin reversing the
asthmatic condition. This therapy, Aelony emphasized, is available only in
an emergency room. Under such circumstances the patients are reinforced
both by an alleviation of their distress and by what is, in many situations, a
less expensive way to treat the attack—an occasional visit to an emergency
room versus regular visits to a physician.

Many adult asthmatics, on the other hand, treat themselves with medications when they really are not suffering an attack. They particularly tend to
overuse nebulized drugs, consuming small canisters of medication in a frac-
tion of time recommended. There are a number of reasons for such behavior.
Some patients actually may believe they are experiencing the symptoms of
an attack and initiate treatment; others may want the supposed high they
claim to experience with ingestion of the medicine. In both cases, the medi-

cation is used inappropriately. Prolonged usage of nebulized medications in such a manner can have serious consequences for the asthmatic patient, including death.

The best way to teach a patient how to treat his or her asthma is to instruct the individual in self-management procedures. Such self-management instruction programs have proliferated in recent years, particularly those designed to teach children how to manage their asthma. The results generally have been excellent. In a study described by Creer and Leung (1981), for example, significant changes in costs of the disease and school attendance were noted as a result of the implementation of a self-management program for asthmatic children. The data showed a 66% reduction in health care costs for families involved with the program and an improvement in children's school attendance from an average absentee rate of 17.5 days during a year's base-line period to 6.4 days in the year following participation in the program. Self-management of asthma, as well as of other forms of COPD, does indeed offer a ray of hope for the future.

Context

Context refers to the circumstances under which an attack occurs. The context includes not only the setting, but the behavior of the individual as well. (In fact, it probably entails some sort of interaction between the setting and the behavior of the individual.) Figure 12.2 shows that our hypothetical patient suffered his attacks while at home, school, and outside. The individual probably did not suffer an attack each time he was in one of these settings; yet, on at least three occasions, there was an interaction of some sort between the person and the environment such that an asthmatic episode occurred. Perhaps the interaction was purely physical in that a high level of dust in the home or grass pollen outdoors triggered the attacks. It certainly would be impossible to rule out such stimuli as interacting with the person to produce asthma.

There are times, however, when even if known precipitants of a patient's attacks are present, he or she does not suffer an attack. For example, almost any asthmatic person, or members of his or her family, can relate how the patient could have suffered what might have been a serious attack under circumstances in which medical assistance was unavailable. Perhaps the person began to wheeze on a camping trip and discovered that he or she had forgotten to bring medication. One would think that the patient would have suffered a very severe asthmatic episode in such a situation (and in some instances, this indeed may have been the case). However, many informants are apt to say that despite these circumstances the patient managed himself or herself such that a full-blown episode did not occur, or was controlled until assistance was obtained. A better example of context has been described by Groen (1976). He noted that survivors reported the rarity of asthma attacks among inmates of Nazi concentration camps. Many of these people undoubtedly suffered from asthma; they managed, however, to avoid attacks in a setting in which such episodes could have had tragic consequences.

There are other times, nonetheless, when a patient will complain of asthma, even when there is no observable evidence that he or she actually is suffering an episode. Creer (1977) described such a case—a youngster who repeatedly claimed he was having an attack in the absence of any measurable symptoms. It was only after repeated experiences of this nature that it was possible to piece together why the youngster made such claims: the context for his reports of asthma appeared to be linked to events occurring at school, the most notable of which were examinations.

Despite its role in setting the stage for the occurrence or nonoccurrence of attacks, the context within which asthmatic episodes occur virtually has been ignored by researchers investigating the disorder. It is a potent independent variable and, as such, worthy of systematic investigation. Certainly, it must be considered in designing a behavioral study on the relationship of behavioral factors to asthma.

Chronic Bronchitis and Emphysema

Chronic bronchitis is defined as persistent coughing on most days for at least 3 months of the year for 2 or more consecutive years (Ruth, 1975). The cough is usually loose and rattling; it generally is worse in the morning and evening than during the rest of the day. Snider (1976) has pointed out that chronic bronchitis may be associated with airway obstruction, ranging from a mild abnormality detectable only with sophisticated physiological instruments, to severe chronic airway obstruction with a profound disruption of lung function. In the latter case, chronic bronchitis can be a threat to life itself.

Unlike asthma and chronic bronchitis, which are defined in terms of the observable manifestations of the disorders, emphysema is defined in terms of pathology. That is, emphysema is defined as an abnormal and permanent enlargement of respiratory air spaces (the structures beyond the terminal bronchiole or small branches of the bronchial tree) that is accompanied by disruptive changes in breathing (American Thoracic Society, 1962). Functionally, the disorder is characterized by a shortness of breath, called *dyspnea*, that results both from the difficulty in expelling air from the lungs and from the poor distribution of the inhaled air throughout these organs (American Lung Association, 1975). In advanced states, death is the final outcome of emphysema.

Compared to asthma, there have been few attempts by behavioral scientists to work with patients afflicted by chronic bronchitis or emphysema. There is a twofold reason for this: first, neither chronic bronchitis nor emphysema is considered to have a psychosomatic component in the sense that psychological factors are thought to be causally related to the afflictions. As noted throughout this discussion, the same cannot be said for asthma. Second, the behavioral aspects of both chronic bronchitis and emphysema always have been overshadowed by the physical and medical problems presented by these disorders that pose a threat to life. Despite the fact that behavioral scientists have shown relatively little interest in designing interventions for patients with chronic bronchitis or emphysema, studies linking behavioral and psychological variables to COPD have been performed and may be conceptualized as representing four levels of investigation: description, demonstration, correlation, and behavioral intervention.

DESCRIPTION

An initial step in investigation is to describe the phenomenon in question, in this case the behaviors or psychological processes displayed by patients with chronic bronchitis, asthma, or emphysema. A number of researchers have provided such a description, with the result that a set of behaviors or behavioral patterns, common to COPD patients, has been identified by Agle and Baum (1977), Creer (1979), and Dudley, Glaser, Jorgenson, and Logan (1980a, 1980b, 1980c). Behaviors associated with COPD include anxiety, depression, alcoholism, body preoccupation, paranoid states, and a decrease in sexual functioning. Strategies that can be taken to resolve such problems also have been identified by Creer (1979), Dudley and his coworkers (1980b), and Windsor, Green, and Roseman (1980).

DEMONSTRATION

This level of investigation provides an empirical statement of the "if . . then" variety about the phenomenon in question. Demonstration studies are important because they often reveal the operation of a process or procedure that has not yet been fully defined and quantified (Johnston & Pennypacker, 1980). The best example of a demonstration project is the work by Thomas Petty (1978) and his colleagues on the rehabilitation of patients with COPD. A study reported by Sahn and Petty (1978), for example, reported that the longevity of COPD patients was extended by virtue of their participation in a rehabilitation program. There are no behavioral outcome data from the studies performed by Petty's (1978) research group; however, their work illustrates the medical sophistication required to work with a COPD population.

CORRELATION

According to Johnston and Pennypacker (1980), correlational inquiry requires the identification and measurement of multiple values of the variables in question. From such information, statements such as "when x_1 occurs, y_1 occurs," can be made.

A number of investigations have attempted to correlate psychological variables to COPD by administering a variety of psychometric instruments to patients afflicted with the condition. An example of such a study is that reported by McSweeney, Heaton, Grant, Cugell, Solliday, Petty, and Timms (1980). A number of instruments, including the Minnesota Multiphasic Personality Inventory (MMPI), the Katz Adjustment Scale, and the Sickness Impact Profile (SIP) were administered to 166 COPD patients involved in a study comparing nocturnal versus continuous oxygen therapy. The results showed that the patients were depressed, preoccupied with their physical condition, and, in general, dissatisfied with life. In addition, significant and positive correlations were found between patients' scores on the SIP and their scores on the Halstead Neuropsychological Impairment Index and two other measures of brain dysfunction. Significant and negative correlations were found between patients' SIP scores and three measures of pulmonary and cardiac functioning (e.g., maximum workload achieved during exercise). It was suggested that some of the negative emotional sequelae of COPD might result from an inadequate supply of oxygen to the portions of the brain that mediate emotional behavior.

BEHAVIORAL INTERVENTION

There have been few attempts to develop behavioral interventions for patients with COPD. Nevertheless, a promising beginning has been made, primarily through efforts to teach these patients how better to care for themselves and cope with their disorder. Atkins, Kaplan, and Timms (1982) have performed what is probably the best study concerning an attempt to change the behavior of patients with COPD. The aim of the study was to improve the low rates of compliance to exercise programs chronically exhibited by the COPD population. Fifty-six patients were randomly assigned to one of five experimental groups: behavior modification, cognitive behavior modification, cognitive modification, social support control, and no treatment control. Persons assigned to the experimental groups participated in various six-session programs designed to increase their adherence to an exercise program; individuals assigned to the no treatment control group, however, were given an exercise prescription but no training with regard to the implementation of the regimen.

A wealth of data were gathered by Atkins and her colleagues. First, the three treatment groups showed significant increases in exercise, in comparison to the two control groups, over the initial 9 weeks of the program. In addition, individuals in the cognitive behavior modification group performed significantly greater walking than did people in the other two treatment groups. Second, patients in the three treatment groups showed significant increases in exercise tolerance, in comparison to individuals in the two control groups, at a 3-month follow-up. In addition, significant differences between the treatment and control groups were observed with respect to scores on a general health status index and changes in patients' self-efficacy judgments. Finally, Atkins and her coworkers demonstrated, through an imaginative cost-effectiveness analysis, that the behavioral program for exercise compliance in COPD patients resulted in increments in health status at a cost comparable to other widely advocated programs.

The study by Atkins and her colleagues is unique in another sense: there was a sufficient COPD population to warrant use of a group design. The use of group designs in behavioral intervention studies with COPD patients is, unfortunately, quite unusual. A number of problems preclude the use of group designs with COPD, extending from an insufficient number of available subjects to problems that arise in attempting to match one patient with another. As a result, single-subject designs appear to have a prominent role in the future study of COPD, including asthma. This role has been emphasized both by physicians (Clark, 1977) and behavioral scientists (Creer, 1979; Creer, Renne, & Christian, 1976). In fact, Clark (1977) emphatically stated, at a meeting of the Research Committee of the British Thoracic and Tuberculosis Association, that in asthma research "patients should wherever possible be used as their own controls and comparisons between subjects should be kept to a minimum [p. 226]." Clark had a number of reasons for making such a suggestion, including the problems noted above as well as difficulties in defining asthma.

Conclusions

The remarks by Clark (1977) bring the present discussion full circle. A number of problems in COPD have been highlighted; few solutions have been offered. Perhaps this situation is as it should be. We are just at the beginning of an epoch in which behavioral methodology holds promise for COPD patients. We can take comfort, however, in the fact that we are pioneers, and that our future will be "limited only by our horizons of human concern and imagination [Creer, 1979, p. 288]."

Acknowledgments

The author is indebted to Harry Kotses for his comments regarding an earlier version of the manuscript, and to James R. Hall for his assistance in the preparation of the figures.

References

Aelony, Y. Why patients with asthma go to the emergency room. *Journal of the American Medical Association, 1980, 243,* 732.

Agle, D. P., & Baum, G. L. Psychological aspects of chronic obstructive pulmonary disease. *Medical Clinics of North America, 1977, 61,* 749–758.

American Lung Association. *Introduction to lung diseases* (6th ed.). New York: American Lung Association, 1975.

American Thoracic Society Committee on Diagnostic Standards for Nontuberculous Diseases. Definitions and classifications of chronic bronchitis, asthma, and pulmonary emphysema. *American Review of Respiratory Disease, 1962, 85,* 762–768.

Asthma and the other allergic diseases: NIAID Task Force Report. (NIH Publication No. 79-387). Washington, D.C.: National Institutes of Health, May 1979.

Atkins, C. J., Kaplan, R. M., & Timms, R. M. *Behavioral programs for exercise compliance in chronic obstructive pulmonary disease.* Manuscript submitted for publication, 1982.

Brandon, M. L. Newer medications to aid treatment of asthma. *Annals of Allergy, 1977, 39,* 117–129.

Burns, K. L. An evaluation of two inexpensive instruments for assessing airway flow. *Annals of Allergy, 1979, 43,* 246–249.

Chai, H. Intermediary mechanisms in asthma: Some informal comments on the pathogenesis of the breathing disturbances. *Clinical Pediatrics, 1974, 13,* 409–412.

Chai, H. Management of severe chronic perennial asthma in children. *Advances in Asthma and Allergy, 1975, 2,* 1–12.

Chai, H., Purcell, K., Brady, K., & Falliers, C. J. Therapeutic and investigational evaluation of asthmatic children. *Journal of Allergy, 1968, 41,* 23–36.

Chiaramonte, L. T., & Prabhu, S. L. Peak flow whistle: Preliminary report. *Annals of Allergy, 1981, 47,* 95–98.

Clark, T. J. H. Definition of asthma for clinical trials. *British Journal of Diseases of the Chest, 1977, 71,* 225–227.

Creer, T. L. The use of a time-out from positive reinforcement procedure with asthmatic children. *Journal of Psychosomatic Research, 1970, 14,* 117–120.

Creer, T. L. Biofeedback and asthma. *Advances in Asthma and Allergy, 1974, 1,* 6–11.

Creer, T. L. Psychologic aspects of asthma. *Respiratory Therapy*, 1977, 7, 15–18; 86; 88.

Creer, T. L. Asthma: Psychologic aspects and management. In E. Middleton, Jr., C. E. Reed, & E. F. Ellis (Eds.), *Allergy: Principles and practice*. St. Louis, Mo.: C. V. Mosby, 1978.

Creer, T. L. *Asthma therapy: A behavioral health care system for respiratory disorders*. New York: Springer, 1979.

Creer, T. L, Self-management behavioral strategies for asthmatics. *Behavioral Medicine*, 1980, 7, 14–24.

Creer, T. L., & Kotses, H. Asthma: Psychologic aspects and management. In E. Middleton, Jr., C. E. Reed, & E. F. Ellis (Eds.), *Allergy: Principles and practice* (2nd ed.). St. Louis, Mo.: C. V. Mosby, in press.

Creer, T. L., & Leung, P. *The development and evaluation of a self-management system for children with asthma*. Paper presented at Self-management Educational Programs for Childhood Asthma, University of California at Los Angeles, Los Angeles, June 1981.

Creer, T. L., Renne, C. M., & Chai, H. The application of behavioral techniques to childhood asthma. In D. C. Russo & J. W. Varni (Eds.), *Behavioral pediatrics: Research and practice*. New York: Plenum, 1982.

Creer, T. L., Renne, C. M., & Christian, W. P. Behavioral contributions to rehabilitation and childhood asthma. *Rehabilitation Literature*, 1976, 37, 226–232; 247.

Creer, T. L., Weinberg, E., & Molk, L. Managing a problem hospital behavior: Malingering. *Journal of Behavior Therapy and Experimental Psychiatry*, 1974, 5, 259–262.

Creer, T. L., & Yoches, C. The modification of an inappropriate behavioral pattern in asthmatic children. *Journal of Chronic Diseases*, 1971, 24, 507–513.

Cropp, G. J. A. Exercise-induced asthma. In E. Middleton, Jr., C. E. Reed, & E. F. Ellis (Eds.), *Allergy: Principles and practice*. St. Louis, Mo.: C. V. Mosby, 1978.

Dudley, D. L., Glaser, E. M., Jorgenson, B. N., and Logan, D. L. Psychosocial concomitants to rehabilitation in chronic obstructive pulmonary disease. Part 1. Psychosocial and psychological considerations. *Chest*, 1980, 77, 413–420. (a)

Dudley, D. L., Glaser, E. M., Jorgenson, B. N., & Logan, D. L. Psychosocial concomitants to rehabilitation in chronic obstructive pulmonary disease. Part 2. Psychosocial treatment. *Chest*, 1980, 77, 544–551. (b)

Dudley, D. L., Glaser, E. M., Jorgenson, B. N., & Logan, D. L. Psychosocial concomitants to rehabilitation in chronic obstructive pulmonary disease. Part 3. Dealing with psychiatric disease (as distinguished from psychosocial or psychophysiologic problems). *Chest*, 1980, 77, 677–684. (c)

Dunand, P., Chai, H., Weltman, D., Spaulding, H., & Meltzer, G. Posterior polar cataracts and steroid therapy in children. *Journal of Allergy and Clinical Immunology*, 1975, 55, 123. (Abstract)

Dunbar, J. M., & Agras, W. S. Compliance with medical instructions. In J. M. Ferguson & C. B. Taylor (Eds.), *Comprehensive handbook of behavioral medicine* (Vol. 3). New York: Spectrum, 1981.

Gelfand, D. M., & Hartmann, D. P. *Child behavior: Analysis and therapy*. New York: Pergamon, 1975.

Ghory, J. E. Exercise and asthma: Overview and clinical impact. *Pediatrics*, 1975, 56, 844–860.

Groen, J. J. Present status of psychosomatic approach to bronchial asthma. In O. Hill (Ed.), *Modern trends in psychosomatic medicine: 3*. Boston: Butterworths, 1976.

Hochstadt, N., Shepard, J., & Lulla, S. H. Reducing hospitalizations of children with asthma. *The Journal of Pediatrics*, 1980, 97, 1012–1015.

Johnston, J. M., & Pennypacker, H. S. *Strategies and tactics of human behavioral research*. Hillsdale, N.J.: Erlbaum, 1980.

Jones, R. S. *Asthma in children*. Acton, Mass.: Publishing Sciences Group, 1976.

Leigh, D. Asthma and the psychiatrist: A critical review. *International Archives of Allergy and Applied Immunology,* 1953, *4,* 227–246.

Luparello, T., Lyons, H. A., Bleecker, E. R., & McFadden, E. R., Jr. Influences of suggestion on airway reactivity in asthmatic subjects. *Psychosomatic Medicine,* 1968, *30,* 819–825.

McFadden, E. R., Jr. Asthma: Airway reactivity and pathogenesis. *Seminars in Respiratory Medicine,* 1980, *1,* 287–296. (a)

McFadden, E. R., Jr. Asthma: Pathophysiology. *Seminars in Respiratory Medicine,* 1980, *1,* 297–303. (b)

McSweeney, A. J., Heaton, R. K., Grant, I., Cugell, D., Solliday, N., Petty, T., & Timms, R. Chronic obstructive pulmonary disease: Socioemotional adjustment and life quality. *Chest,* 1980, *77,* 309–311. (Supplement)

Miklich, D. R., Renne, C. M., Creer, T. L., Alexander, A. B., Chai, H., Davis, M. H., Hoffman, A., & Danker-Brown, P. The clinical utility of behavior therapy as an adjunctive treatment for asthma. *The Journal of Allergy and Clinical Immunology,* 1977, *60,* 285–294.

Petty, T. L. (Ed.). *Chronic obstructive pulmonary disease.* New York: Marcel Dekker, 1978.

Porter, R., & Birch, J. (Eds.). *Identification of asthma.* London: Churchill Livingston, 1971.

Reed, C. E., & Townley, R. G. Asthma: Classification and pathogenesis. In E. Middleton, Jr., C. E. Reed, & E. F. Ellis (Eds.), *Allergy: Principles and practice.* St. Louis, Mo.: C. V. Mosby, 1978.

Renne, C. M., Nau, E., Dietiker, K. E., & Lyon R. *Latency in seeking asthma treatment as a function of achieving successively higher flow rate criteria.* Paper presented at the meeting of the Association for the Advancement of Behavior Therapy, New York, December 1976.

Rosenblatt, M. B. History of bronchial asthma. In E. B. Weiss & M. S. Segal (Eds.), *Bronchial asthma: Mechanisms and therapeutics.* Boston: Little, Brown, 1976.

Rubinfeld, A. R., & Pain, M. C. F. Perception of asthma. *Lancet,* 1976, *1,* 882–884.

Ruth, W. E. Examination of the chest, lungs, and pulmonary system. In M. H. Delp & R. T. Manning (Eds.), *Major's physical diagnosis* (8th ed.). Philadelphia: W. B. Saunders, 1975.

Sahn, S. A., & Petty, T. L. Results of a comprehensive rehabilitation program for severe COPD. In T. L. Petty (Ed.), *Chronic obstructive pulmonary disease.* New York: Marcel Dekker, 1978.

Sampter, M. (Ed.). Moses Maimonides. In *Excerpts from classics in allergy.* Columbus, Ohio: Ross Laboratories, 1969.

Snider, G. L. The interrelationships of asthma, chronic bronchitis, and emphysema. In E. B. Weiss & M. S. Segal (Eds.), *Bronchial asthma: Mechanisms and therapeutics.* Boston: Little, Brown, 1976.

Suess, W. H., & Chai, H. Neuropsychological correlates of asthma: Brain damage or drug effects? *Journal of Consulting and Clinical Psychology,* 1981, *49,* 135–136.

Suess, W. M., Chai, H., Kalisker, A., & Stump, N. *Mnemonic effects of asthma medications in children.* Manuscript submitted for publication, 1982.

Taplin, P. S., & Creer, T. L. A procedure for using peak expiratory flow rate data to increase the predictability of asthma episodes. *The Journal of Asthma Research,* 1978, *16,* 15–19.

Williams, M. H., Jr. Clinical features. *Seminars in Respiratory Medicine,* 1980, *1,* 304–314.

Windsor, R. A., Green, L. W., & Roseman, J. M. Health promotion and maintenance for patients with chronic obstructive pulmonary disease: A review. *Journal of Chronic Diseases,* 1980, *33,* 5–12.

Young, P. *Asthma and allergies: An optimistic future (DHEW Publication No. [NIH] 80-388).* Washington, D.C.: U.S. Government Printing Office, 1980.

PART III

General Issues in Coping with Chronic Disease

13

Coping with Chronic Pain

LAURENCE A. BRADLEY

Introduction

The experience of pain is associated with a large number of chronic diseases. With respect to cancer, for example, "moderate to severe pain is experienced by about a third of patients during the intermediate stage of their disease and by two-thirds or more during the terminal stage [Noyes, 1981, p. 57]." Persons also may suffer chronic pain due to (*a*) peripheral neuropathies produced by diabetes mellitus, (*b*) cardiovascular disease (angina pectoris), and (*c*) spinal cord or head injuries. In addition, some chronic pain syndromes may be iatrogenic in nature (e.g., pain due to aseptic necrosis or reflex sympathetic dystrophy following irradiation treatments for cancer), whereas others may be due to chronic diseases about which little is known (e.g., rheumatoid arthritis).

The purpose of the present chapter is to summarize the behaviorally oriented pain control literature that has implications for helping patients with chronic disease better cope with their pain experiences. Thus, the chapter first provides a review of the literature regarding behavioral approaches to the control of chronic benign pain. Particular emphasis is given to the efficacy of self-control treatment approaches that might have implications for the process of coping with pain due to chronic disease. The few studies that have appeared in the literature to date with regard to the use of self-management techniques for the control of pain associated with chronic disease are then reviewed; a detailed examination of the literature concerning arthritic pain that is secondary to hemophilia and pain resulting from rheumatoid arthritis is included. Finally, the chapter provides a summary of the findings that are relevant to clinical practice as well as suggestions for future research.

Behavioral Approaches to the Control of Chronic Benign Pain

Chronic benign pain may be defined as pain that persists for a period of 6 or more months and is not the result of a malignant disease process (Bradley, Prokop, Gentry, Van der Heide, & Prieto, 1981; Ziesat, 1981). It should be noted, however, that chronic benign pain is not equivalent to pain associated with a conversion reaction. Many patients with chronic benign pain suffer varying degrees of organic pathology (White, Bradley, & Prokop, in press; Ziesat, 1981). Indeed, many investigators consider chronic benign pain to be an independent disorder rather than a symptom (Brena, 1978; Ziesat, 1981).

The chronic benign pain patient who is referred for behaviorally oriented treatment typically is an individual who has undergone one or more medical or surgical treatments that have failed to produce long-term positive results. The three major techniques used to treat chronic benign pain, if medical or surgical interventions have failed, are inpatient contingency management, electromyographic (EMG) and electroencephalographic (EEG) biofeedback, and cognitive–behavioral therapy (Genest & Turk, 1979; Ziesat, 1981). Nearly all of the treatment outcome studies available in the literature, however, have examined treatment programs that have included one or more of the behaviorally oriented therapeutic approaches already noted as well as other interventions such as chemotherapy, vocational rehabilitation, sexual or marital counseling, and physical therapy (Keefe, 1982). Thus, it has not been possible to determine the components of these multimodal treatment programs that may be responsible for producing patient change (Bradley & Prokop, 1982).

The following discussion first briefly reviews the literature regarding the multimodal behavioral treatment of chronic benign pain (excluding various forms of headaches and temporomandibular joint syndrome) that features the use of contingency management (operant conditioning) procedures in combination with biofeedback training or other interventions. It then examines the relatively small literature regarding the outcomes produced by multimodal self-management programs that emphasize patient use of various coping strategies to control or cope better with chronic benign pain.

MULTIMODAL INPATIENT CONTINGENCY MANAGEMENT PROGRAMS

Fordyce and his colleagues were the first persons to apply the principles of operant conditioning to chronic benign pain sufferers in an inpatient contingency management program (Fordyce, 1976; Fordyce, Fowler, De-

Lateur, Sand, & Trieschmann, 1973; Fordyce, Fowler, Lehmann, & De-
Lateur, 1968; Fordyce, McMahon, Rainwater, Jackins, Questal, Murphy, &
DeLateur, 1981). The precepts underlying the inpatient contingency man-
agement programs developed by Fordyce and others are:

1. Nociception and the actual pain experience are unobservable. The only
observable manifestations of pain are pain behaviors defined as "all forms of
behavior generated by the individual commonly understood to reflect the
presence of nociception, including speech, facial expression, posture, seeking health care attention, taking medications, and refusing to work [Fordyce,
1978, p. 54]."

2. Acute pain behaviors function as respondents that "occur as direct and
automatic responses to specific antecedent stimuli [Fordyce & Steger, 1979,
p. 133]." However, these pain behaviors also may serve as operants that are
followed by direct (e.g., social attention) and indirect (e.g., escape from an
aversive work situation) consequences that reward and maintain the display
of pain behaviors in the absence of antecedent stimuli.

3. Pain behavior in the absence of antecedent stimuli also may be displayed as a function of observational learning and nonreinforcement of well
behavior.

4. The goals of inpatient contingency management of chronic benign
pain, then, are to achieve sufficient control over the patient's environment
such that (a) reinforcement is withdrawn from pain behaviors (particularly
medication usage and excessive health care utilization; (b) reinforcement
is made contingent upon well behaviors (e.g., increases in activity level,
decreases in medication intake and verbal expressions of pain); and (c)
persons in the home environment are trained to reinforce the display of
well behavior and to withdraw reinforcement upon the display of pain behavior.

Fordyce and his colleagues (Fordyce et al., 1973) presented outcome data
regarding 36 patients who received between 4 and 12 weeks of inpatient
contingency management treatment and an average of 3 weeks of outpatient
treatment. The patients showed a significant increase from pretreatment to
the end of outpatient treatment in uptime (i.e., time spent standing, walking, or engaged in similar behavior), and exercise performance. The patients
also showed a significant decrease in intake of narcotic analgesics, nonnarco-
tic analgesics, and hypnosedative medication from pretreatment to the end
of inpatient treatment. Thirty-one of the patients completed a follow-up
questionnaire at an average period of 22 months posttreatment. The patients' self-reports suggested that they had maintained their increased activity levels and decreased medication intake.

The Fordyce et al. (1973) investigation suffered from several methodological flaws. First, the investigation failed to include a no-treatment and an attention–placebo control group (see Watson & Kendall, Chapter 3). In addition, a self-report questionnaire was used to assess patient behavior at follow-up. Reliance on patient self-report precludes acceptance of the follow-up data as accurate; indeed, several recent studies have shown that there often is great disagreement between patients' self-reports of their behavior and direct unobtrusive measures of the same behavior (Kremer, Block, & Gaylor, 1981; Ready, Sarkis, & Turner, 1982; Taylor, Zlutnick, Corley, & Flora, 1980). Finally, it should be noted that 50% of the patients failed to respond to the follow-up questionnaire item regarding medication usage. Thus, even if the patients' self-reports were accurate, a substantial number of patients may have increased their medication intake following treatment.

Despite the limitations of the Fordyce *et al.* study described in the preceding, the investigation has served as a model for nearly all the studies published since 1973 that have examined the outcomes produced by inpatient contingency management programs. Table 13.1 presents a summary of these outcome studies.

Table 13.1 shows that inpatient contingency management programs appear to produce positive changes in the medication intake and activity levels of *some* patients. However, none of the investigations summarized in the table included adequate control procedures. In addition, the majority of the investigations produced data consisting of patient self-reports or observations of patient behavior that had not been assessed with regard to reliability or accuracy. The absence of reliable and accurate behavioral outcome data is particularly distressing because the purpose of inpatient contingency management is to alter environmental stimuli systematically in order to produce reliable and desirable changes in patient behavior.

Another methodological deficiency associated with the contingency management literature involves the follow-up assessments of patients' outcomes. Although the majority of the investigations included at least a 6-month posttreatment follow-up evaluation, only one investigation (Seres & Newman, 1976) used direct observation measures of patient behavior both at posttreatment and at follow-up (Newman, Seres, Yospe, & Garlington, 1978). The lack of consistency between the assessment measures used during treatment and at follow-up is important because it is not possible to make a valid determination of the maintenance of treatment outcome unless the follow-up measures are identical to those assessed at the completion of treatment (Prokop & Bradley, 1981). It also should be noted that several of the investigations that included follow-up assessments were characterized by a high rate of subject attrition (i.e., Ignelzi, Sternbach, & Timmermans, 1977; Newman *et al.*, 1978; Roberts & Reinhardt, 1980). The highly positive follow-up data reported in these investigations may have been inflated due to attrition among patients who showed relatively little improvement or who were unable to maintain the gains they had achieved during treatment.

Finally, none of the contingency management investigations included assessments of patients' covert experiences (e.g., belief in their ability to control pain or increase activity levels; see Bradley & Prokop, 1982) that might have been related to patients' outcomes It is necessary for investigators to examine the relationships between patients' covert experiences and their treatment outcomes in a consistent manner across investigations in order to determine if any pretreatment or posttreatment covert experiences might serve as predictors of outcome. If some predictive relationships are found, it might be useful to add to contingency management programs a treatment component designed to change patients' cognitions in a positive fashion and thus possibly enhance the long-term effects of treatment.

In summary, the literature suggests that one or more of the treatments that typically are included in inpatient contingency management programs appear to produce positive behavioral changes among chronic benign pain patients. This conclusion must be regarded as tentative, however, in that (a) all of the studies failed to adequately control for placebo factors; (b) it is impossible to determine what specific treatments included in the contingency management programs may have been responsible for producing the reported outcomes; and (c) the stability of the reported outcomes was never adequately established. Several recent reviews have provided criticisms of the literature that are similar to those noted in the preceding (Block, 1982; Grzesiak, in press; Keefe, 1982; Sanders, 1979; Turk & Genest, 1979; Turner & Chapman, 1982; Ziesat, 1981).

MULTIMODAL SELF-MANAGEMENT PROGRAMS

It is clear that inpatient contingency management is not an appropriate choice of treatment for individuals who suffer pain resulting from chronic diseases such as those described in the present volume. Nonetheless, several investigators have relied in part on treatments described in the contingency management literature in order to develop self-management training programs for chronic benign pain that have relevance for patients with pain due to chronic disease.

The self-management training programs that have been developed to date, unlike the inpatient contingency management programs, have no single underlying set of principles. However, Genest and Turk (1979) have noted that both the contingency management and self-management approaches to pain treatment involve: (a) the assessment and alteration of patients' cognitions regarding their pain problems; (b) the development, acquisition, and rehearsal of new cognitive and behavioral skills for coping

TABLE 13.1

Capsule Summary of the Major Outcome Studies Produced by Multimodal Inpatient Contingency Management Programs

Authors	Sample	N	Additional interventions	Design	Posttreatment results	Follow-up period	Follow-up results	Methodological weaknesses
Anderson, Cole, Gullickson, Hudgens, & Roberts (1977)	Diverse syndromes	34	Family therapy; occupational therapy; vocational evaluation and counseling; outpatient supportive therapy	Single-sample outcome	Not reported	6 mo–7 yr	25 patients were free of analgesics	No control group; no description of outcome data or of the manner in which analgesic use at follow-up was verified
Cairns, Thomas, Mooney, & Pace (1976)	Low-back pain	90	Occupational therapy	Single-sample outcome	70% indicated decreased pain or increased activity level	$M = 10$ mo	Changes in pain and activity levels maintained; 58% reported less analgesic medication intake than at pretreatment; 75% of patients selected for vocational training were either work-	No control group; all data consisted of self-reports given at follow-up

(continued)

ing or in a training program

Study	Syndrome	N	Treatment	Design	Results	Follow-up	Comments
Chapman, Brena, & Bradford (1981)	Diverse syndromes	100 completed program; 19 dropped out	Sympathetic nerve blocks; coping skills training	Single-sample outcome	Significant decreases from pretreatment in self-reports of pain; significant increases in self-reports of activities of daily living; no changes on McGill Pain Questionnaire	$M = 21$ mo	Posttreatment results maintained; 47% of patients were not using any narcotic analgesics, sedatives, anxiolytics, phenothiazines, or pentazocine	No control group; all data consisted of self-reports; follow-up conducted both by mail ($N = 48$) and by telephone ($N = 40$)
Fordyce, Fowler, De-Lateur, Sand, & Trieschmann (1973)	Diverse syndromes	36	Vocational rehabilitation; occupational therapy; outpatient treatment ($M = 3$ wk)	Single-sample outcome	Significant increases from pretreatment in uptime, walking, sit-ups, and weaving; significant decreases in narcotic analgesic, analgesic, and hyposedative intake	$M = 22$ mo	Present self-reports of pain significantly lower than retrospective estimates of pain at admission; changes in activity level and medication intake maintained	No control group; all follow-up data consisted of self-reports; 50% nonresponse rate to follow-up questionnaire item regarding medication intake

TABLE 13.1 (Continued)

Authors	Sample	N	Additional interventions	Design	Posttreatment results	Follow-up period	Follow-up results	Methodological weaknesses
Greenhoot & Sternbach (1974)	Diverse syndromes	54	Group therapy; relaxation training; biofeedback; vocational rehabilitation; some patients received surgery	Single-sample outcome	Decreases from pretreatment in self-reports of pain, and Hs, D, Hy, and Pt scales of MMPI; increases in self-reports of walking time and distance as well as number of exercises	See Ignelzi, Sternbach, & Timmermans (1977)	Not reported	No control group; all data consisted of self-reports
Ignelzi, Sternbach, & Timmermans (1977)	Diverse syndromes	32–36	Not reported	Single-sample outcome; follow-up to Greenhoot & Sternbach (1974)	Not reported	3 yr	Significant decreases from pretreatment in self-reports of pain estimates and medication intake; significant increases in physical activity	No control group; all data consisted of self-reports; 33–41% of original sample failed to complete follow-up measures

346

Newman, Seres, Yospe, & Garlington (1978)	Low-back pain	36	Not reported	Single-sample outcome; follow-up to Seres & Newman (1976)	Not reported	18 mo	Significant increases from pretreatment in exercise performance; significant decreases in self-reports of medication intake; 40% of patients free of medication usage; majority of patients reported pain unchanged or worse relative to pretreatment but claimed they were able to cope with pain better	No control group; medication data consisted of self-reports
Roberts & Reinhardt (1980)	Diverse syndromes	26; 8 did not comply	Occupational therapy	Controlled multisample outcome	Not reported	1–8 yr	Significantly greater number of treated than no-treatment-control subjects met	All data consisted of self-reports; the two control groups were not adequate

(continued)

TABLE 13.1 (Continued)

Authors	Sample	N	Additional interventions	Design	Posttreatment results	Follow-up period	Follow-up results	Methodological weaknesses
							criteria for success (e.g., employed, no financial compensation); treated subjects reported significant decreases from pre-treatment in medication use, number of reclining hours, and scales Hs, D, and Hy of MMPI, as well as significant increases in number of standing and working hours	as one consisted of patients who had been rejected for treatment and the other consisted of patients who had been accepted for treatment but had refused to enter program

Study	Syndrome	N	Treatment	Design	Outcome	Follow-up	Follow-up results	Comments
Seres & Newman (1976)	Low-back pain	100	Education, biofeedback, body mechanics, and relaxation training	Single-sample outcome	Only 5% of patients took prescription medication compared to 87% at pretreatment; substantial increases in straight leg raising and other exercises from pre- to posttreatment	3 mo	22% of patients took prescription medication; all increases in exercise maintained; 80% of patients reported they no longer sought medical care for back pain; 75% agreed to disability claim closure	No control group
Sternbach & Timmermans (1975)	Diverse syndromes	113	See Greenhoot & Sternbach (1974)	Multisample outcome	Patients who received surgery showed significantly greater reductions from pre- to posttreatment on scales Hy and Ma of MMPI, pain estimates, and a chronic	Not reported	Not reported	No control group; all data consisted of self-reports; posttreatment activity levels of surgery patients assessed during second postoperative week; no fol-

(continued)

TABLE 13.1 *(Continued)*

Authors	Sample	N	Additional interventions	Design	Posttreatment results	Follow-up period	Follow-up results	Methodological weaknesses
					invalidism scale than did nonsurgery patients; non-surgery patients reported greater increases in activity levels than surgery patients			low-up assessment
Swanson, Floreen, & Swenson (1976)	Diverse syndromes	31	Not reported	Single-sample outcome; follow-up to Swanson, Swenson, Maruta, & McPhee (1976)	Not reported	3–6 mo	The majority of 21 of the "successful" (as measured by nurses' ratings) patients who were followed maintained or increased their improvements with respect to pain estimates and medication usage; 17	All data consisted of self-reports; 13 patients were interviewed and completed questionnaire—there was close correspondence between their interview and questionnaire responses but this may have been due to a

350

| Swanson, Maruta, & Swenson (1979) | Diverse syndromes | 200 | See Swanson, Swenson, Maruta, & McPhee (1976) | Single-sample outcome | Significant decreases from pretreatment in self-reports of pain; significant increases in self-reports of uptime; 117 patients showed moderate to marked improvement on nurses' ratings of their attitudes, medication | 1 yr; included 75 patients who had been rated as improved | worked full-time or showed increase in work activity; 18 had maintained or improved sleep; 17 had not sought further medical treatment since end of treatment | self-selection artifact |
| | | | | | | 65% of patients (25% of original sample) maintained improvement | | No control group; all follow-up data consisted of self-reports |

(continued)

TABLE 13.1 (Continued)

Authors	Sample	N	Additional interventions	Design	Posttreatment results	Follow-up period	Follow-up results	Methodological weaknesses
					reduction, and physical function			
Swanson, Swenson, Maruta, & McPhee (1976)	Diverse syndromes	34; 16 failed to complete program	Vocational rehabilitation, biofeedback, relaxation training, and other psychological treatments	Single-sample outcome	Significant reductions from pretreatment in patients' pain estimates as well as nurses' measures of patient uptime and ratings of patient pain and manipulative behavior; 27 of 34 patients showed moderate to marked improvement on nurses' ratings of their attitudes, medication reduction, and physical function	Not reported	Not reported	No control group; only data that did not consist of self-reports were those based on nurses' ratings; nurses' ratings were not assessed for reliability

with pain that will enhance patients' expectations of personal efficacy with regard to pain control; and (c) techniques for the maintenance and generalization of positive therapeutic change. The major differences between the contingency management and self-management approaches to pain treatment appear to be that the latter place the responsibility for improvement on the patient rather than on the treatment staff and family members (Keefe, 1982) and emphasize that it is necessary to change patients' perceptions of pain as an uncontrollable event in order to effect behavioral change (Genest, 1978).

Table 13.2 presents a summary of the studies that have been published within the past 6 years concerning the outcomes produced by multimodal self-management programs. The table shows that, similar to the results of the inpatient contingency management investigations, the multimodal self-management programs appear to produce positive changes in the subjective pain estimates and psychosocial functioning of *some* chronic benign pain patients. Only one of the investigations (Rybstein-Blinchik, 1979), however, used an adequate attention–placebo treatment to control for the nonspecific effects of treatment and patients' expectancies of change. Indeed, the Rybstein-Blinchik (1979) investigation demonstrated that patients' expectancies of change did not vary across the four treatment conditions; thus, the treatment effects associated with the "relevant" cognitive strategy (i.e., redefining pain sensations as less somatically oriented feelings such as "numbness" or "aroused" and providing self-rewards for successful redefinition efforts) were not artifacts of different beliefs among patients regarding the potential efficacy of their respective treatments.

The multimodal self-management investigations suffered from several methodological weaknesses in addition to the lack of control procedures cited above. For example, Table 13.2 reveals that only two studies (Rybstein-Blinchik, 1979; Rybstein-Blinchik & Grzesiak, 1979) used reliable and direct observations of patients' pain behaviors as well as patients' self-reports of pain as outcome measures. Both of these investigations demonstrated that a cognitively oriented treatment strategy may produce decreases in patients' pain behaviors and their subjective self-reports of pain.

It should be noted that the Rybstein-Blinchik investigations did suffer from a methodological flaw that was common to nearly all of the self-management studies. That is, neither the Rybstein-Blinchik (1979) nor the Rybstein-Blinchik and Grzesiak (1979) report included an adequate follow-up assessment. It is impossible to determine, then, whether the reported results were maintained over long periods of time following the completion of treatment. It is particularly important to assess the long-term maintenance of treatment gains in outcome studies involving chronic pain patients because there is strong evidence that some family members tend to reinforce the pain behaviors displayed by patients (Block, Kremer, & Gaylor, 1980a; For-

TABLE 13.2

Capsule Summary of the Major Outcome Studies Produced by Multimodal Self-Management Programs

Authors	Sample	N	Interventions	Design	Posttreatment results	Follow-up period	Follow-up results	Methodological weaknesses
Gottlieb, Koller, & Alperson (1982)	Low-back pain	78	Biofeedback training; counseling in self-control techniques for management of stress and anxiety; self-paced medication reduction; patient-involved case conferences; physical therapy; vocational rehabilitation; education	Single-sample outcome	Not reported	1 year	Employment at pretreatment and follow-up increased from 8 to 45%; 86% of unemployed and 53% of employed patients reported pain to be a major psychologically disabling factor at follow-up; 37% of unemployed and 3% of employed patients reported taking medications for pain relief at follow-up; 70% of un-	No control group; all data consisted of self-reports obtained in telephone interviews

Study	Pain type	N	Treatment	Design	Outcome	Follow-up	Results		Comments
Gottlieb, Strite, Koller, Madorsky, Hockersmith, Kleeman, & Wagner (1977)	Low-back pain	72	Biofeedback training; individual, group, and family psychotherapy; self-paced medication reduction; physical therapy; vocational counseling; education	Single-sample outcome	Significant increases from pretreatment on ratings of functional improvement and clinical objectives by nurses, physical therapists, and psychologists; only 50 patients met criteria for success	1 mo	33 of 40 successful patients maintained gains in all areas; 38 maintained successful levels of vocational restoration: 19 of 23 patients contacted at 6 mo posttreatment were employed or in training	employed and 34% of employed patients reported being treated for back pain	No control group; all data consisted of ratings for which there were no reliability checks or self-reports of vocational activity; length of follow-up period was inadequate
Hartman & Ainsworth (1980)	Diverse syndromes	10	Autogenic exercises; alpha biofeedback; stress inoculation training	Uncontrolled, two-sample outcome	Patients who received stress inoculation training after	4–6 wk	Posttreatment differences were maintained		No control group; all data consisted of self-reports; base-

(continued)

355

TABLE 13.2 (Continued)

Authors	Sample	N	Interventions	Design	Posttreatment results	Follow-up period	Follow-up results	Methodological weaknesses
					alpha biofeedback showed significantly greater reductions in self-reports of pain than did patients who received stress inoculation training followed by alpha biofeedback			line period was inadequate because patients received autogenic exercises; length of follow-up period was inadequate
Herman & Baptiste (1981)	Diverse syndromes	75	Education; group discussion; relaxation training assisted by autogenic training and systematic desensitization	Single-sample outcome	Significant decreases from pretreatment in self-reports of pain and depression; 79% of patients were rated by their case managers as more than 39% im-	6 mo	41 of 50 patients contacted at follow-up had been judged as "successful" at posttreatment—35 reported they had maintained gains or	No control group; case managers' ratings were not assessed for reliability; use of telephone interviews at follow-up lacked reliability; high

				proved in various categories of functioning (i.e., were "successful")		made further improvements in functioning; 28% of all patients who were unemployed at pretreatment had returned to work by follow-up	attrition rate during follow-up, especially among "failures"
Keefe, Block, Williams, & Surwit (1981)	Low-back pain	111	EMG-assisted relaxation training; psychotropic medication; self-paced medication reduction	Single-sample outcome	Significant reductions from pretreatment in frontal EMG levels and self-reports of pain and tension; chart review showed 49% of patients reduced analgesic and narcotic analgesic medication intake and 63% showed increased activity levels	Not reported	No control group; activity level data based on an examination of interview notes; no follow-up assessment

(continued)

357

TABLE 13.2 (*Continued*)

Authors	Sample	N	Interventions	Design	Posttreatment results	Follow-up period	Follow-up results	Methodological weaknesses
Khatami & Rush (1978)	Diverse syndromes	5; 1 failed to complete program	EMG biofeedback and relaxation training; cognitive therapy; family therapy	Single-sample outcome	Significant decreases relative to pretreatment in self-reports of pain, analgesic intake, hopelessness, and depression	6 and 12 mo	All gains were maintained at both follow-up periods	No control group; all data consisted of self-reports
Malec, Cayner, Harvey, & Timming (1981)	Diverse syndromes	40	Occupational and physical therapy; education; medication tapering; vocational rehabilitation; coping-skills training	Single-sample outcome	Not reported	6 mo–3 yr	10 of 27 patients met criteria for success (drug-free; employed full or part-time or continuing 50%–100% of prescribed exercise program as well as reporting an increase in recreational activities; no increase in	No control group; all data consisted of self-reports; follow-up conducted both by mail and by telephone; success criteria were developed without an underlying rationale

(continued)

Study	Syndrome	N	Treatment	Design	Outcome	Follow-up	(pain at follow-up)	Comments
Rybstein-Blinchik (1979)[a]	Diverse syndromes	44	Attention–placebo control; cognitive therapy with a "somatization," "irrelevant," or "relevant" relabeling-training strategy; other treatments unspecified	Multisample outcome	Patients who received cognitive therapy with "relevant" relabeling strategy used significantly fewer and milder verbal pain descriptors than did patients in other conditions; "relevant" condition patients also showed significantly fewer pain behaviors than patients in other conditions	Not reported	Not reported	No follow-up assessment
Rybstein-Blinchik & Grzesiak (1979)[a]	Diverse syndromes	5	Stress inoculation training; cognitive relabeling of	Single-sample outcome	Not reported	1 mo	Substantial decreases from pretreatment in self-reports	No control group; length of follow-up period was inadequate

359

TABLE 13.2 (Continued)

Authors	Sample	N	Interventions	Design	Posttreatment results	Follow-up period	Follow-up results	Methodological weaknesses
			pain; other treatments unspecified				of pain and observers' recordings of pain behavior	
Turner, Heinrich, McCreary, & Dawson (1979)[b]	Low-back pain	43	Cognitive–behavioral therapy; progressive relaxation training; waiting list attention–placebo control	Multisample outcome	Patients who received either cognitive–behavioral therapy or progressive relaxation training showed pre- to posttreatment decreases in self-reports of physical and psychosocial	1 mo	Gains in physical and psychosocial dysfunction maintained; cognitive–behavioral patients produced significantly lower self-reports of pain than did progressive-relaxation patients	All data consisted of self-reports; length of follow-up period was inadequate; the attention–placebo consisted of a weekly telephone conversation with a therapist, which may have

been an inadequate control for the attention provided to cognitive–behavioral and progressive-relaxation patients

dysfunction as well as pain; cognitive–behavioral patients rated themselves as significantly more improved than progressive relaxation patients with regard to pain tolerance and participation in normal activities

[a] The patients used in the Rybstein-Blinchik investigations were drawn from physical therapy wards and thus received additional treatments that were not specified in the published reports.

[b] Turner (1982) recently published a 1½–2 year follow-up of 70% of the patients who received either cognitive-behavioral therapy or progressive relaxation training. The follow-up, conducted by mail, revealed that patients in both treatment groups greatly decreased their use of the health care system and back pain treatments since pretreatment. Patients in both groups also showed significant decreases in self-reports of pain from pretreatment to follow-up. However, only the cognitive-behavioral patients showed pretreatment to follow-up increases in the number of hours spent working at a job each week.

dyce, 1976; Mohamed, Weisz, & Waring, 1978; Shanfield, Heiman, Cope, & Jones, 1979; Swanson & Maruta, 1980). Table 13.2 shows only two investigations that included follow-up assessments at 6 months posttreatment (Herman & Baptiste, 1981; Khatami & Rush, 1978). Unfortunately, Herman and Baptiste (1981) lost one-third of the original patient sample to attrition at the 6-month follow-up assessment. Khatami and Rush (1978) successfully followed five patients for 12 months after the completion of treatment. It was stated that all five patients maintained their gains at the follow-up assessment; this report must be viewed with great caution, however, since the data consisted entirely of self-reports.

Finally, the self-management training literature may be criticized for the dearth of efforts to measure patients' covert experiences. Despite the fact that one important goal of self-management training is to change patients' behaviors by altering patients' belief in their abilities to control their pain experiences, none of the studies summarized in Table 13.2 included an assessment of relevant patient cognitions prior to, during, or following treatment. The failure to examine patients' covert experiences makes it impossible to determine whether the effects of the various treatment programs may have been mediated by changes in patients' expectations of personal efficacy concerning their pain-control skills (see Bradley & Prokop, 1982; Kendall & Korgeski, 1979). For example, it is not possible to attribute the efficacy of Rybstein-Blinchik's (1979) "relevant" cognitive training strategy to changes in patients' cognitions because Rybstein-Blinchik neglected to include measures of covert experiences in her investigation.

In summary, the literature consistently indicates that training patients to use various combinations of self-management skills appears to elicit self-reports of decreased pain and functional improvement. However, the literature suffers from several methodological deficiencies that render this conclusion tentative. The deficiencies include the lack of: (a) adequate placebo control procedures; (b) reliable and accurate measures of actual patient behavior; and (c) long-term follow-up assessments of patient functioning. In addition, none of the multimodal self-management investigations included assessments of patients' covert experiences that might make it possible to determine if the effects of the training programs were mediated by positive changes in patients' cognitions regarding their pain control skills.

SUMMARY AND IMPLICATIONS FOR CHRONIC DISEASE RESEARCH

A great number of investigations have been conducted since 1973 regarding the efficacy of behaviorally oriented treatments for chronic benign pain. Despite the many methodological weaknesses associated with the literature, there is agreement among medical or health psychologists as well as among some physicians that both inpatient contingency management and self-management training programs are effective treatment modalities for some patients (Keefe, 1982; Urban, 1982).

Unfortunately it is not possible at present to determine which patients are likely to show optimal responses either to a contingency management or a self-management training program. It also is impossible to determine what particular treatment components actually effect patient change, as only two investigations (Rybstein-Blinchik, 1979; Turner, Heinrich, McCreary, & Dawson, 1979) have employed factorial designs that allow comparisons of efficacy among various treatments. Finally, it should be noted that the majority of the studies described previously examined the effects of various multimodal treatment packages on the pain reports or behaviors of patients with heterogeneous chronic benign pain syndromes. The heterogeneity among patients might have been responsible in part for the inconsistency of treatment effects found within the patient samples.

Patient heterogeneity also might be responsible for the great disagreement that currently exists among investigators with respect to which demographic, behavioral, or psychological factors may serve as predictors of patient response to treatment. That is, there is a general consensus among investigators that the chronicity of pain and disability is negatively associated with treatment outcome (Block, Kremer, & Gaylor, 1980b; Keefe, Block, Williams, & Surwit, 1981; Maruta, Swanson, & Swenson, 1979; Painter, Seres, & Newman, 1980; Swanson, Swenson, Maruta, & Floreen, 1978). Disagreement exists among investigators, however, regarding the predictive value of other factors such as patient sex (Painter *et al.*, 1980; Swanson *et al.*, 1978), compensation payments (Block *et al.*, 1980b; Swanson *et al.*, 1978), and Minnesota Multiphasic Personality Inventory (MMPI) scores (Keefe *et al.*, 1981; Maruta *et al.*, 1979). It already has been found that the use of homogeneous patient samples and specific treatment interventions across patients results in more powerful outcome prediction with the MMPI than does the use of heterogeneous patient samples and treatments (Bradley *et al.*, 1981). Thus, the application of specific treatment interventions (e.g., contingency management with EMG biofeedback and occupational therapy) to homogeneous patient samples (e.g., patients with low back pain associated with narrowing of intervertebral space) might allow investigators to delineate relatively powerful predictors of patient outcome as well as produce positive outcomes more consistently across patients. If this were to occur, it then would be possible to perform factorial investigations to determine which specific components of a successful treatment package serve to produce patient change.

Several investigators have begun to apply specific treatment interventions or intervention packages associated with the self-management literature to patients with pain due to various chronic diseases. Chronic diseases, such as diabetes, cancer, and rheumatoid arthritis, tend to produce pain syndromes that appear to be particularly amenable to self-management training interventions. That is, the time-lines (Nerenz & Leventhal, Chapter 2) of these diseases are unpredictable as well as cyclic or chronic. Patients therefore may experience spontaneous exacerbations and dimunitions of their pain experiences as well as their other symptoms. The unpredictable quality of the chronic diseases also may cause patients to experience anxiety and depression that, in turn, may produce increased perceptions of pain and displays of severe pain behaviors. It appears reasonable to assume, then, that treatment interventions that are composed of one or more self-management components may help patients to cope with their pain in an effective and adaptive fashion because these interventions may provide patients with (a) realistic information concerning their conditions; (b) strategies for anticipating and coping with pain and related emotional distress; and (c) increased perceptions of self-efficacy in coping with pain.

The following discussion examines the literature on the behavioral treatments for pain associated with chronic disease that use self-management training strategies. Particular attention is devoted to the literature concerning arthritic pain, in which the most sophisticated outcome studies are found.

Self-Management Approaches to the Control of Pain Due to Chronic Disease

A small number of investigations have been published since 1977 regarding the efficacy of self-management training strategies among chronic disease patients who suffer pain. These include four investigations that have been performed with spinal cord injured patients and amputees as well as six investigations that have been performed with persons suffering from various forms of arthritis. The following discussions first briefly examines the spinal cord injury and phantom limb (postamputation) pain literature. It then provides a detailed review of the investigations that have been performed to date regarding the control of arthritic pain.

SPINAL CORD INJURY AND PHANTOM LIMB PAIN

It has been noted that there are currently over 250,000 spinal cord injury patients in the United States and that approximately 10,000 new spinal cord injuries occur each year (Brucker, Chapter 11; Richards, Meredith, Nepomuceno, Fine, & Bennett, 1980). Various investigators have estimated the incidence of persistent pain after spinal cord injury to vary from 30% to 100%; thus it is clear that intractable spinal cord injury represents a significant clinical problem.

Grzesiak (1977) has reported the only attempt to assess the effectiveness of a self-management intervention on the pain experiences of spinal cord injury patients. Four patients were taught a relaxation–meditation procedure; three of the patients reported the procedure to be effective. Two of the three successful patients continued to report effective use of relaxation–meditation at a 2-year follow-up assessment (the third successful patient could not be located at follow-up). Grzesiak (1982) recently has noted that the successful patients have maintained pain control for more than 5 years following treatment. However, Grzesiak also has suggested that a premorbid history of substance abuse (1982) and causalgialike pain (i.e., characterized by burning sensations) (in press) may predict poor response to relaxation procedures. Richards et al. (1980) also have reported that psychological and family–social environment variables account for a large proportion of the variance in spinal cord injured patients' reports of (a) pain severity and (b) the degree to which pain interferes with performing activities of daily living. The results reported by Grzesiak and the relationship between psychological variables and patients' self-reports of pain intensity indicate further investigation of the use of self-management interventions with spinal cord injury patients is warranted.

Two factors primarily are responsible for the interest in providing self-management treatments to patients with phantom limb pain. First, invasive neurosurgical procedures generally have been shown to be ineffective or impractical (Melzack, 1971). In addition, noninvasive medical procedures, particularly transcutaneous electrical nerve stimulation (TENS), appear to be effective short-term treatments (e.g., Fox & Melzack, 1976; Jeans, 1979; Schuster & Infante, 1980), but they do not consistently produce positive long-term results (e.g., Erikson, Sjölund, & Nielzén, 1979; Melzack, Jeans, Stratford, & Monks, 1980; Richardson, Arbit, & Zagar, 1980; Sternbach, Ignelzi, Deems, & Timmermans, 1976; Taylor, Hallet, & Flaherty, 1981; Wolf, Gersh, & Rao, 1981).

Three reports on the efficacy of EMG biofeedback and relaxation procedures for phantom limb pain have appeared. Dougherty (1980) reported that EMG biofeedback-assisted relaxation of the stump muscles allowed a patient with an above-the-knee amputation of the left leg to control his phantom pain for nearly 4 weeks. Unfortunately, the patient's pain control skills diminished after he reported that his prosthesis caused stump irritation and a return of phantom pain episodes.

Sherman, Gall, and Gormly (1979) described the results produced by several treatment packages consisting of various combinations of progressive muscle relaxation, EMG feedback of stump and frontal muscle tension levels, as well as reassurance and education concerning normal phantom sensations and the relationship between anxiety and pain. These treatment packages were administered to a total of 16 patients with phantom limb pain that was due to single or double amputations of lower or upper extremities. Follow-up assessments ranging from 6 months to 3 years ($M = 1.2$ years) showed that 10 patients reported that they were virtually pain-free and 4 patients stated that their pain had decreased to the extent that they no longer required treatment. In addition, a review of patients' charts suggested that use of analgesic drugs was "eliminated" among the completely successful patients and "sharply reduced" by the patients who reported partial pain relief (p. 52). It should be noted that each of 4 patients whose amputations were due to diabetes reported complete (3) or partial (1) pain relief; 2 of the 4 patients with amputations due to vascular disorders reported complete relief and 1 reported partial relief of pain. McKechnie (1975) reported results similar to those of Sherman et al. (1979) in a case study of the efficacy of relaxation exercises for phantom limb pain; this study, however, did not include a follow-up procedure.

In summary, the multiple case studies produced by Grzesiak (1977) and Sherman et al. (1979) suggest that relaxation-based self-management training interventions may help some persons with spinal cord injuries or phantom limb pain to eliminate or substantially control their pain experiences. It is necessary, however, for investigators to perform controlled outcome studies with long-term follow-up assessments in order to determine the feasibility of providing self-management training interventions to large numbers of patients with pain that is due to spinal cord injury or amputation. These outcome studies should include assessments of treatment efficacy using behavioral and physiological measures as well as patients' self-reports of pain (Bradley et al., 1981; Keefe, 1982; White et al., in press).

Finally, it should be noted that chronic pain induced by spinal cord injury and phantom limb pain are similar to one another in that both result from a disruption of the integrity of the nervous system (Grzesiak, in press) and possible subsequent disruption of endogenous, descending pain control mechanisms (Melzack & Dennis, 1978). It would be useful, then, to determine whether the length of the time interval between injury and initiation of treatment is related to treatment efficacy. The results reported by Sherman et al. (1979) and Richards et al. (1980) suggest that the degree to which self-management interventions are tailored to meet patients' individual needs and the nature of patients' family and social environments also may be related to treatment outcome.[1]

---

[1] My unpublished observations of the use of relaxation-based self-management procedures with a patient following hemicorporectomy (i.e., above-the-hips amputation of the lower extremities and body trunk; see DeLateur, Lehmann, Winterscheid, Wolf, Fordyce, & Simons,

ARTHRITIC PAIN

Investigators who have examined the effectiveness of self-management training interventions for chronic pain associated with arthritis have focused on two types of arthritic disease. Varni and his associates have conducted a programmatic series of investigations with hemophiliacs who have suffered degenerative conditions similar to osteoarthritis resulting from repeated hemorrhages into multiple joint areas (Varni, 1981a, 1981b; Varni, Gilbert, & Dietrich, 1981). Three different investigators, however, have examined the efficacy of various self-management techniques with rheumatoid arthritis patients (Achterberg, McGraw, & Lawlis, 1981; Denver, Laveault, Girard, Lacourciere, Latulippe, Grove, Preve, & Doiron, 1979; Randich, 1982).

Hemophilia

Varni (1981a) has noted that "chronic, severe degenerative arthritis represents the most frequent problem confronting the physician who manages the care of adult hemophiliacs, with an estimated 75 percent of adult hemophiliacs demonstrating one or more affected joints [p. 183]." On the basis of a review of the medical literature regarding arthritis pain management and the results of a survey of hemophilic patients with severe arthritic pain, Varni developed a treatment protocol consisting of three components: (a) progressive muscle relaxation training; (b) meditative breathing exercises; and (c) imagery training (vivid imagination of scenes that patients previously experienced as warm and pain-free). The protocol also entailed home practice of warming imagery at least twice each day for 15 minutes and verbal feedback regarding patients' abilities to increase peripheral skin temperature at the sites of their most severe pain (as measured by a thermal biofeedback unit). Varni's (1981a) first investigation involved two male patients; only one patient, however, underwent the thermal biofeedback assessment. Using a multiple baseline reversal design, it was found that the patients reduced the number of days each week that they experienced arthritic pain at the most affected site from pretreatment means of 6 and 4, respectively, to posttreatment means of 1.0 and .4 and to means of .5 and .2 at an 8-month follow-up assessment. In addition, the patient who underwent the thermal biofeedback assessment increased peripheral skin temperature at the most affected site from a mean of 84.8° F at base line to means of 88.6° F at posttreatment and 90.1° F at the 8-month follow-up assessment. The

---

1969; Leichentritt, 1972) suggest that the changing nature of phantom pain perceptions in the first weeks after injury requires the use of flexible, individualized treatments. The patient's pain experiences also appeared to be influenced by his marital relationship and by the social rewards provided by the treatment staff and others for pain and well behavior.

use of a reversal design demonstrated that the increase in peripheral skin temperature was due to the imagery training. A review of pharamacy records during treatment and at follow-up indicated that both patients produced long-term reductions in their use of analgesic medications. Furthermore, one patient reported cessation of morning stiffness (morning stiffness is commonly associated with osteoarthritis).[2]

Varni (1981b) used a multiple base-line design to examine the efficacy of his treatment intervention with three adult hemophiliacs. Follow-up assessments ranging from 7 to 14 months posttreatment indicated that the patients reported (a) substantial reductions (M = 5.33) in the number of days each week during which they experienced pain; (b) substantial decreases (M = 2.93 on a 10-point scale) in subjective pain intensity ratings; and (c) large, positive changes (Ms = 2.3–2.7 on 6-point scales) with regard to mobility, sleep, and overall general functioning. The thermal biofeedback assessment revealed an average increase in peripheral skin temperature at the most affected site of 4.1° F. An analysis of patients' pharmacy records and medical charts showed a large reduction (M = 4.97) in the number of analgesic tablets ordered by the physicians for the patients despite the fact that plasma protein factor replacement requirements as well as patients' reports of bleeding frequency and acute bleeding-pain intensity did not vary during the course of the study.

Varni et al. (1981) extended the use of the treatment intervention described above to a 9-year-old child with arthritis of one knee secondary to severe hemophilia. It was reported that the patient reduced his mean pain intensity ratings from 7.0 at pretreatment to 2.0 at a 1-year follow-up assessment. During this period of time, the patient also (a) eliminated his use of meperidine (a narcotic analgesic), (b) substantially reduced his use of an acetaminophen–codeine elixir, (c) eliminated the need for hospitalizations for pain and nearly eliminated school absences, (d) increased the range of motion in his arthritic knee and increased quadricep strength, and (e) eliminated all limitation of ambulation on stairs. No assessment of the patient's peripheral skin temperature at the arthritic knee was performed.

In summary, Varni and his associates have produced an excellent series of investigations regarding the efficacy of their relaxation-based self-management procedure. These investigations are particularly noteworthy in that

[2]Varni and Gilbert (1982) recently published a case study in which an adult male hemophiliac was administered the treatment protocol previously described and was instructed to restrict his intake of propoxyphene to a time interval schedule rather than a pain contingent schedule. A 1-year follow-up showed that the patient (a) substantially reduced his ratings of arthritic pain intensity and stress–tension (reductions of 3.2 and 2.7, respectively, on 10-point scales); (b) greatly reduced monthly propoxyphene intake from 17550 mg to 7670 mg (assessed by monitoring pharmacy records); and (c) increased arthritic joint skin temperature by 3.2°F.

they all used multiple measures of outcome (i.e., self-reports of pain intensity and reviews of pharmacy records) and featured long-term follow-up assessments. Indeed, the studies performed with adult patients (Varni, 1981a, 1981b) also included physiological outcome data (i.e., peripheral skin temperature levels) although only the Varni 1981a investigation included a reversal design to assess the specific effects of the imagery training on peripheral skin temperature. The Varni 1981b study also is significant in that it demonstrated that the patients' control of their arthritic pain was not merely an artifact of decreased acute bleeding episodes or altered perceptions of the intensity of acute bleeding pain. Nonetheless, it is necessary to perform additional investigations using larger numbers of patients and appropriate control procedures. It may be that the small group of patients treated by Varni and his associates were particularly highly motivated to reduce reliance upon analgesic medications and adopt self-management procedures. Future research, therefore, may have to be directed toward delineation of hemophilic patients with arthritic pain who may best benefit from provision of a self-management pain control intervention. Finally, because increases in skin temperature at the sites of most severe pain were related to positive patient outcomes, it would be desirable to determine whether (a) thermal biofeedback training alone might be more effective than the imagery component in helping patients to produce increased peripheral skin temperatures, or (b) thermal biofeedback training in combination with imagery training might produce greater increases in skin temperature than would the sole use of either of the two interventions.

Rheumatoid Arthritis

Two investigations have been performed regarding the efficacy of providing rheumatoid arthritis (RA) patients with thermal biofeedback training. Denver et al. (1979) assigned 12 RA patients to one of three conditions: (a) hand-temperature biofeedback and relaxation training; (b) relaxation training only; or (c) a no-treatment control condition. It was found that patients who received hand-temperature biofeedback and relaxation training significantly reduced the variability of their peripheral skin temperature and EMG levels during the course of treatment; they were unable to increase peripheral skin temperature levels consistently across treatment sessions. Nevertheless, it was reported that patients in the biofeedback–relaxation condition significantly increased their tolerance of pain and showed reductions in the time necessary to complete a 50-ft. walk. Unfortunately, it is impossible to determine what factors were responsible for the reported changes in pain tolerance and walking time. It might appear at first that because the biofeedback–relaxation treatment was superior to the relaxation-only treatment, the reported results were due to the effects of the biofeedback training. However, inasmuch as the patients who received biofeedback training were unable to produce reliable increases in hand temperature, it may be that some nonspecific factors associated with the hand-temperature biofeedback and relaxation training condition actually produced the reported outcomes. In addition, the lack of a follow-up assessment makes it impossible to determine whether the changes in walking time and pain tolerance were maintained after treatment.

Achterberg *et al.* (1981) provided 15 RA patients with 12 30-minute sessions of relaxation and finger-temperature biofeedback training as well as a home exercise program and education regarding proper body mechanics and posture. A control group of 8 RA patients received 12 30–40-minute sessions of physiotherapy in addition to the educational intervention and the home exercise program. Both the relaxation–biofeedback and the physiotherapy treatments were conducted over a 6-week period. It was found that patients in both treatment groups showed significant and positive pre- to posttreatment changes in 50-ft. walking time, in self-reports of performance of activities of daily living, and in erythrocyte sedimentation rate. However, only the relaxation–biofeedback patients showed significant and positive pre- to posttreatment changes with respect to (a) the number of nighttime awakenings caused by pain; (b) disability-related work changes; (c) number of involved joints; (d) self-reports of involvement in physical activity; and (e) self-reports of pain severity.

The results of the Achterberg *et al.* study must be viewed with caution for two reasons. First, some of the patients who received biofeedback training were instructed to increase skin temperature levels whereas others were instructed to produce decreases in skin temperature. Assessment of skin temperature levels revealed that the relaxation training allowed patients to produce increases in skin temperature relative to base-line levels during all training sessions and that these temperature increases were relatively unaffected by specific biofeedback instructions. In addition, although the Achterberg *et al.* study is noteworthy for its use of multiple (self-report, behavioral, and physiological) outcome measures, its lack of a long-term follow-up assessment raises concerns regarding the stability of the positive changes achieved by patients in the relaxation–biofeedback condition.

The most recent study regarding the use of self-management training procedures with RA patients was conducted by Randich (1982). Forty-four patients were randomly assigned to one of three groups: (a) an active treatment group that received six group sessions of deep-muscle relaxation training as well as imagery and cognitive strategy training; (b) an attention–placebo control group that received six group-support sessions regarding coping with pain; or (c) a no-treatment control group. It was reported that the active treatment group, relative to the control groups, showed significant and positive changes from pretreatment to an 8-week follow-up assessment in self-reports of daily work, leisure, social, and functional (e.g., walking, reach, grip, self-help, hygiene) activities. No between-group differences were found with regard to self-reports of pain intensity.

Randich's (1982) investigation is the only self-management study in the RA literature that includes an adequately controlled experimental design. It is unfortunate, then, that the investigation did not include any outcome measures based on direct observations of patient behavior. That is, although the reported changes in patients' self-reports of activities of daily living may be atrributed to the active treatment intervention, it is impossible to assume that the patients' self-reports of their behavior were completely accurate (see "Multimodal Inpatient Contingency Management Programs.") Furthermore, the follow-up assessment period was not sufficiently long to determine the stability of the reported results. It also should be noted that, although the active treatment intervention was designed in part to produce changes in patients' perceptions of self-efficacy of pain control, no measures of the patients' covert experiences were used during the course of the study.

In summary, the investigations described previously suggest that providing RA patients with training in deep muscle relaxation and other adjunct procedures may allow them to control their pain experiences better and to increase their physical activity levels. All the investigations, however, suffered from various methodological flaws such as (a) failure to demonstrate that instructions to increase or decrease skin temperature using thermal biofeedback produced reliable changes in peripheral skin temperature levels (Achterberg et al., 1981; Denver et al., 1979); (b) use of weak experimental designs with inadequate control procedures (Achterberg et al., 1981; Denver et al., 1979); (c) failure to use multiple measures of treatment outcome (Denver et al., 1979; Randich, 1982); (d) inadequate follow-up assessment procedures (Achterberg et al., 1981; Denver et al., 1979; Randich, 1982); and (e) failure to assess patients' covert experiences that may be related to treatment outcome (Randich, 1982).

Nevertheless, the results that have been reported suggest that it might be highly productive to perform well-controlled investigations of the long-term effects of providing self-management training to RA patients. Because heat applications are widely prescribed for RA patients and reduced muscle blood flow may lead to the muscle atrophy associated with RA, it would be desirable to perform internally valid tests of the efficacy of training patients to increase peripheral skin temperature at affected joint sites with thermal biofeedback.[3] It also would be desirable to determine (a) whether deep

[3]King and Montgomery (1980, 1981) recently have provided evidence that it is more difficult

muscle relaxation and thermal biofeedback training procedures are differentially effective in helping patients to produce increases in peripheral skin temperature at affected joint sites and (b) if the use of both relaxation and biofeedback training procedures is more effective than the use of either procedure alone. It is essential that all future investigations with RA patients include follow-up periods of at least 6 months. Indeed, in order to assess fluctuations in perceived pain, physical mobility, and peripheral skin temperature control resulting from seasonal changes, it is necessary to use follow-up periods of at least 1 year. Finally, as was noted with regard to the studies of self-management techniques with chronic benign pain patients, it is important to attempt to assess patients' covert experiences during the course of treatment and follow-up.

SUMMARY

The majority of the investigations regarding the use of self-management training procedures for pain that is due to chronic disease produced positive results. Nonetheless, as with the contingency management and self-management approaches to chronic benign pain, the majority of the chronic disease sutides failed to (a) use adequate control procedures; (b) employ multiple measures of treatment outcome, (c) conduct follow-up assessments of sufficient length to determine the stability of the reported outcomes, and (d) assess patients' covert experiences that might be related to treatment outcome.

There also were several attributes unique to the chronic disease studies. First, the patient samples used in these studies were quite small. Thus, it is possible that the selection of a small number of highly motivated patients produced positive results in some investigations (e.g., Varni, 1981a, 1981b; Varni et al., 1981). However, the small sample sizes found in the literature were related to a second unique and positive characteristic of the chronic disease studies. That is, unlike the chronic benign pain investigations, nearly all of the chronic disease studies used homogeneous patient samples; this may have been responsible in part for some of the positive results reported. For example, Grzesiak's (1977) work indicates that a relaxation–meditation training procedure should not be administered to spinal cord injury patients with pain perceptions similar to those of causalgia. The exclusion of patients with causalgialike pain may have contributed to the positive results Grzesiak achieved. Indeed, the additional removal from treatment protocols of pa-

---

for persons to achieve increases in peripheral skin temperature than decreases and that persons may have to rely upon muscular maneuvers in addition to response contingent feedback in order to produce skin temperature increases voluntarily.

tients with premorbid histories of substance abuse may allow Grzesiak or other investigators to produce more powerful outcomes than would be reported without the use of multiple screening procedures. The third unique attribute associated with the chronic disease literature is that the treatment interventions generally consisted of a small number of components such as relaxation training (Grzesiak, 1977), relaxation training, meditative breathing, and imagery training (Varni, 1981a, 1981b; Varni et al., 1981), or relaxation training, EMG biofeedback, education, and reassurance (Sherman et al., 1979). In addition, treatment components in several interventions were designed to produce specific effects upon patients' physiological functioning and pain experiences (e.g., Sherman et al. assumed that feedback of EMG stump levels would reduce stump muscle contractions associated with pain). Thus, the opportunity existed for some investigators to determine if various treatment components actually produced physiological changes and decreased reports of pain. Only Varni (1981a), however, fully demonstrated the relationship between the application of a treatment component and changes in physiological functioning and pain measures.

There are two areas of investigation that have been neglected in the chronic disease literature. First, no investigations have been undertaken of specific interventions with spouses or other family members that may have an impact on patients' outcomes. It may be that if family members receive education concerning chronic disease and pain as well as self-management strategies or undergo treatment designed to enhance their own skills for coping with the effects of chronic disease, it might be possible for the family members to increase patients' compliance with the practice of self-management strategies and thus enhance patients' outcomes. The second area that has been neglected is the use of self-management strategies with patients who suffer from various forms of cancer. As noted at the beginning of this chapter, many cancer patients must endure pain resulting from (a) tumor infiltration of bones, nerves, or hollow viscous areas or (b) cancer therapies (Noyes, 1981). Because the course of cancer is chronic and unpredictable, it seems likely that the use of self-management procedures might prove to be quite beneficial to many patients. The literature concerning self-management of cancer pain currently consists of a small number of uncontrolled trials and case studies of the positive effects produced by hypnotherapy (Barber & Gitelson, 1980; Butler, 1954; Cangello, 1962; Finer, 1979; Lea, Ware, & Monroe, 1960) and EMG and EEG biofeedback (Fotopoulous, Graham, & Cook, 1979). Future investigators should consider that the effects of self-management training with cancer patients might be influenced by individual differences in cancer site and type of medical treatment administered (cf. Freidenbergs, Gordon, Hibbard, Levine, Wolf, & Diller, 1981–1982).

In summary, the literature regarding the use of self-management procedures for the control of pain produced by chronic disease suffers from the
same methodological flaws that are found throughout the chronic benign
pain literature. It is necessary, then, for future investigators to conduct well-
controlled outcome studies that include (a) multiple measures of treatment
outcome; (b) long-term follow-up assessments; (c) assessments of patients'
covert experiences; and (d) larger patient samples than have been utilized to
date. If future investigators continue to use relatively homogeneous patient
samples as well as treatment components that are designed to affect specific
physiological functions related to pain, it may be possible to produce quite
powerful outcome studies with great relevance for clinical practice.

General Suggestions for Clinical Practice

The investigations reviewed in this chapter suggest that it is possible to teach
self-management methods to *some* patients with pain that is due to chronic
disease and thereby reduce patients' self-reports of or behavioral displays of
pain. There is some evidence (e.g., Varni, 1981a) suggesting that patients'
increased control of pain is mediated in part by learned control of physiological functions. Although the results of the chronic disease investigations must
be regarded with caution, practitioners may wish to attempt to assess the
effectiveness of various self-management procedures with their own patients. For this reason a list of recommendations for implementing self-
management training in clinical practice follows:

1. It is necessary to review the medical literature regarding a specific
chronic disease thoroughly before one may legitimately devise a potentially
helpful self-management treatment intervention. It is especially desirable to
include a treatment component designed to produce a specific physiological
effect that may be related to patients' perceptions of pain.

2. It is necessary to assess patients with regard to motivation as well as
psychosocial factors that might influence their abilities to utilize self-management procedures successfully. Education about the treatment intervention and the specific chronic disease for which it has been designed also
should be provided to the patients. Patients who understand the underlying
rationale for an intervention may be more likely to comply with the demands
of the intervention (e.g., home practice of relaxation exercises) than will
patients who do not perceive that the intervention is appropriate for their
specific pain problems. In addition, it seems likely that education also should
be provided to patients' family members; however, no evidence currently
exists to support this assumption.

3. It is desirable to attempt to develop some means for monitoring patients' compliance with the treatment intervention. Assessment of physiological changes that are hypothesized to occur as a function of treatment may be useful. For example, if thermal biofeedback training is used with RA patients, an examination of patients' peripheral skin temperature levels without feedback may provide information concerning patients' compliance with home practice instructions. The use of reversal designs may be of particular value in determining the specific physiological effects of treatment intervention (Varni, 1981a).

4. Detailed records of patients' assessments should be maintained. If possible, these assessments should include multiple measures of treatment outcome.

5. Patient assessments should be performed prior to, throughout, and following treatment. These assessments should be maintained for at least 6 months following treatment; for some chronic diseases, such as rheumatoid arthritis, it is desirable to maintain follow-up assessments for at least 12 months in order to assess seasonal fluctuations in patients' physiological functioning as well as their pain behaviors and experiences.

6. Periodic discussions with the patients and their family members may provide information that will be useful in modifying the treatment intervention to achieve optimal results. These discussions also may lead to the discovery and resolution of patients' or family members' concerns that, in turn, may potentiate the effects of treatment.

7. It would be useful for clinicians to attempt to publish the descriptions of and results produced by their treatment interventions in order to help others design self-management interventions for persons who suffer pain that is due to chronic disease.

References

Achterberg, J., McGraw, P., & Lawlis, G. F. Rheumatoid arthritis: A study of relaxation and temperature biofeedback training as an adjunctive therapy. *Biofeedback and Self-Regulation*, 1981, *6*, 207–223.

Anderson, T. P., Cole, T. M., Gullickson, G., Hudgens, A., & Roberts, A. H. Behavior modification of chronic pain: A treatment program by a multidisciplinary team. *Clinical Orthopedics and Related Research*, 1977, *129*, 96–100.

Barber, J., & Gitelson, J. Cancer pain: Psychological management using hypnosis. *Cancer*, 1980, *30*, 130–136.

Block, A. R. Multidisciplinary treatment of chronic low back pain: A review. *Rehabilitation Psychology*, 1982, *27*, 51–63.

Block, A. R., Kremer, E. F., & Gaylor, M. Behavioral treatment of chronic pain: The spouse as a discriminative cue for pain behavior. *Pain*, 1980, *9*, 243–252. (a)

Block, A. R., Kremer, E. F., & Gaylor, M. Behavioral treatment of chronic pain: Variables affecting treatment efficacy. *Pain*, 1980, *8*, 367–375. (b)

Bradley, L. A., & Prokop, C. K. Research methods in contemporary medical psychology. In P. C. Kendall & J. N. Butcher (Eds.), *Handbook of research methods in clinical psychology.* New York: Wiley, 1982.

Bradley, L. A., Prokop, C. K., Gentry, W. D., Van der Heide, L. H., & Prieto, E. J. Assessment of chronic pain. In C. K. Prokop & L. A. Bradley (Eds.), *Medical psychology: Contributions to behavioral medicine.* New York: Academic Press, 1981.

Brena, S. F. (Ed.). *Chronic pain: America's hidden epidemic: Behavior modification as an alternative to drugs and surgery.* New York: Atheneum, 1978.

Butler, B. The use of hypnosis in the care of the cancer patient. *Cancer*, 1954, *7*, 1–14.

Cairns, D., Thomas, L., Mooney, V., & Pace, J. B. A comprehensive treatment approach to chronic low back pain. *Pain*, 1976, *2*, 301–308.

Cangello, V. W. Hypnosis for the patient with cancer. *American Journal of Clinical Hypnosis*, 1962, *4*, 215–226.

Chapman, S. L, Brena, S. F., & Bradford, L. A. Treatment outcome in a chronic pain rehabilitation program. *Pain*, 1981, *11*, 255–268.

DeLateur, B. J., Lehmann, J. F., Winterscheid, L. C., Wolf, J. A., Fordyce, W. E., & Simons, B. C. Rehabilitation of the patient after hemicorporectomy. *Archives of Physical Medicine and Rehabilitation*, 1969, *50*, 11–16.

Denver, D. R., Laveault, D., Girard, F., Lacourciere, Y., Latulippe, L., Grove, R. N., Preve, M., & Doiron, N. Behavioral medicine: Biobehavioral effects of short-term thermal biofeedback and relaxation in rheumatoid arthritic patients. *Biofeedback and Self-Regulation*, 1979, *4*, 245–246. (Abstract)

Dougherty, J. Relief of phantom limb pain after EMG biofeedback-assisted relaxation: A case report. *Behaviour Research and Therapy*, 1980, *18*, 355–357.

Erikson, M. B. E., Sjölund, B. H., & Nielzén, S. Long-term results of peripheral conditioning stimulation as an analgesic measure in chronic pain. *Pain*, 1979, *6*, 335–347.

Finer, B. Hypnotherapy in pain of advanced cancer. In J. J. Bonica & V. Ventafridda (Eds.), *Advances in pain research and therapy* (Vol. 2). New York: Raven Press, 1979.

Fordyce, W. E. *Behavioral methods for chronic pain and illness.* St. Louis, Mo.: C. V. Mosby, 1976.

Fordyce, W. E. Learning processes in pain. In R. A. Sternbach (Ed.), *The psychology of pain.* New York: Raven Press, 1978.

Fordyce, W. E., Fowler, R. S., DeLateur, B. J., Sand, P. L., & Trieschmann, R. B. Operant conditioning in the treatment of chronic pain. *Archives of Physical Medicine and Rehabilitation*, 1973, *54*, 399–408.

Fordyce, W. E., Fowler, R. S., Lehmann, J. F., & DeLateur, B. J. Some implications of learning in problems of chronic pain. *Journal of Chronic Diseases*, 1968, *21*, 179–190.

Fordyce, W. E., McMahon, R., Rainwater, G., Jackins, S., Questal, K., Murphy, T., & DeLateur, B. J. Pain complaint: Exercise performance relationship in chronic pain. *Pain*, 1981, *10*, 311–321.

Fordyce, W. E., & Steger, J. C. Chronic pain. In O. F. Pomerleau & J. P. Brady (Eds.), *Behavioral medicine: Theory and practice.* Baltimore: Williams & Wilkins, 1979.

Fotopoulos, S. S., Graham, C., & Cook, M. R. Psychophysiologic control of cancer pain. In J. J. Bonica & V. Ventafridda (Eds.), *Advances in pain research and therapy* (Vol. 2). New York: Raven Press, 1979.

Fox, E. J., & Melzack, R. Transcutaneous electrical stimulation and acupuncture: Comparison of treatment for low-back pain. *Pain*, 1976, *2*, 141–148.

Freidensbergs, I., Gordon, W., Hibbard, M., Levine, L., Wolf, C., & Diller, L. Psychosocial aspects of living with cancer: A review of the literature. *International Journal of Psychiatry in Medicine*, 1981–1982, *11*, 303–329.

Genest, M. *A cognitive–behavioral bibliotherapy to ameliorate pain.* Paper presented at the meeting of the American Psychological Association, Toronto, August 1978.

Genest, M., & Turk, D. C. A proposed model for behavioral group therapy with pain patients. In D. Upper & S. M. Ross (Eds.), *Behavioral group therapy: An annual review.* Champaign, Ill.: Research Press, 1979.

Gottlieb, H. J., Koller, R., & Alperson, B. L. Low back pain comprehensive rehabilitation program: A follow-up study. *Archives of Physical Medicine and Rehabilitation*, 1982, *63*, 458–461.

Gottlieb, H., Strite, L. C., Koller, R., Madorsky, A., Hockersmith, V., Kleeman, M., & Wagner, J. Comprehensive rehabilitation of patients having chronic low back pain. *Archives of Physical Medicine and Rehabilitation*, 1977, *58*, 101–108.

Greenhoot, J. H., & Sternbach, R. A. Conjoint treatment of chronic pain. In J. J. Bonica (Ed.), *Advances in neurology* (Vol. 4). New York: Raven Press, 1974.

Grzesiak, R. C. Relaxation techniques in treatment of chronic pain. *Archives of Physical Medicine and Rehabilitation*, 1977, *58*, 270–272.

Grzesiak, R. C. Cognitive and behavioral approaches to management of chronic pain. *New York State Journal of Medicine*, 1982, *82*, 30–38.

Grzesiak, R. C. Rehabilitation of chronic pain syndromes. In C. J. Golden (Ed.), *Annual review of rehabilitation psychology* (Vol. 1). New York: Grune & Stratton, in press.

Hartman, L. M., & Ainsworth, K. D. Self-regulation of chronic pain. *Canadian Journal of Psychiatry*, 1980, *25*, 38–43.

Herman, E., & Baptiste, S. Pain control: Mastery through group experience. *Pain*, 1981, *10*, 79–86.

Ignelzi, R. J., Sternbach, R. A., & Timmermans, G. The pain ward follow-up analyses. *Pain*, 1977, *3*, 277–280.

Jeans, M. E. Relief of chronic pain by brief, intense transcutaneous electrical stimulation: A double-blind study. In J. J. Bonica & D. Albe-Fessard (Eds.), *Advances in pain research and therapy* (Vol. 3). New York: Raven Press, 1979.

Keefe, F. J. Behavioral assessment and treatment of chronic pain: Current status and future directions. *Journal of Consulting and Clinical Psychology*, 1982, *50*, 896–911.

Keefe, F. J., Block, A. R., Williams, R. B., & Surwit, R. S. Behavioral treatment of chronic low back pain: Clinical outcome and individual differences in pain relief. *Pain*, 1981, *11*, 221–231.

Kendall, P. C., & Korgeski, G. P. Assessment and cognitive-behavioral interventions. *Cognitive Therapy and Research*, 1979, *3*, 1–21.

Khatami, M., & Rush, A. J. A pilot study of the treatment of outpatients with chronic pain: Symptom control, stimulus control, and social system intervention. *Pain*, 1978, *5*, 163–172.

King, N. J., & Montgomery, R. B. Biofeedback induced control of human peripheral temperature: A critical review of the literature. *Psychological Bulletin*, 1980, *88*, 738–752.

King, N. J., & Montgomery, R. B. The self-control of human peripheral (finger) temperature: An exploration of somatic maneuvers as aids to biofeedback training. *Behavior Therapy*, 1981, *12*, 263–273.

Kremer, E. F., Block, A., & Gaylor, M. S. Behavioral approaches to treatment of chronic pain: The inaccuracy of patient self-report measures. *Archives of Physical Medicine and Rehabilitation*, 1981, *62*, 188–191.

Lea, P., Ware, P., & Monroe, R. The hypnotic control of intractable pain. *American Journal of Clinical Hypnosis*, 1960, *3*, 3–8.

Leichentritt, K. G. Rehabilitation after hemicorporectomy. *The American Journal of Proctology*, 1972, *23*, 408–413.

Malec, J., Cayner, J. J., Harvey, R. F., & Timming, R. C. Pain management: Long-term follow-up of an inpatient program. *Archives of Physical Medicine and Rehabilitation*, 1981, *62*, 369–372.

Maruta, T., Swanson, D. W., & Swenson, W. M. Chronic pain: Which patients may a pain-management program help? *Pain*, 1979, *7*, 321–329.

McKechnie, R. Relief from phantom pain by relaxation exercises. *Journal of Behavior Therapy and Experimental Psychiatry*, 1975, *6*, 262–263.

Melzack, R. Phantom limb pain: Implications for treatment of pathologic pain. *Anesthesiology*, 1971, *35*, 409–419.

Melzack, R., & Dennis, S. G. Neurophysiological foundations of pain. In R. A. Sternbach (Ed.), *The psychology of pain*. New York: Raven Press, 1978.

Melzack, R., Jeans, M. E., Stratford, J. G., & Monks, R. C. Ice massage and transcutaneous electrical stimulation: Comparison of treatment for low-back pain. *Pain*, 1980, *9*, 209–217.

Mohamed, S. N., Weisz, G. M., & Waring, E. M. The relationship of chronic pain to depression, marital adjustment, and family dynamics. *Pain*, 1978, *5*, 285–292.

Newman, R. I., Seres, J. L., Yospe, L. P., & Garlington, B. Multidisciplinary treatment of chronic pain: Long-term follow-up of low back pain patients. *Pain*, 1978, *4*, 283–292.

Noyes, R. Treatment of cancer pain. *Psychosomatic Medicine*, 1981, *43*, 57–70.

Painter, J. R., Seres, J. L., & Newman, R. I. Assessing benefits of the pain center: Why some patients regress. *Pain*, 1980, *8*, 101–113.

Prokop, C. K., & Bradley, L. A. Methodological issues in medical psychology research. In C. K. Prokop & L. A. Bradley (Eds.), *Medical Psychology: Contributions to behavioral medicine*. New York: Academic Press, 1981.

Randich, S. R. Evaluation of a pain management program for rheumatoid arthritis patients. *Arthritis and Rheumatism*, 1982, *25*, 511. (Abstract)

Ready, L. B., Sarkis, E., & Turner, J. A. Self-reported vs. actual use of medications in chronic pain patients. *Pain*, 1982, *12*, 285–294.

Richards, J. S., Meredith, R. L., Nepomuceno, C., Fine, P. R., & Bennett, G. Psychosocial aspects of chronic pain in spinal cord injury. *Pain*, 1980, *8*, 355–366.

Richardson, R. R., Arbit, J., & Zagar, R. Evaluation of transcutaneous electrical neurostimulation. *Journal of Psychosomatic Research*, 1980, *24*, 79–83.

Roberts, A. H., & Reinhardt, L. The behavioral management of chronic pain: Long-term follow-up with comparison groups. *Pain*, 1980, *8*, 151–162.

Rybstein-Blinchik, E. Effects of different cognitive strategies on chronic pain experience. *Journal of Behavioral Medicine*, 1979, *2*, 93–101.

Rybstein-Blinchik, E., & Grzesiak, R. C. Reinterpretative cognitive strategies in chronic pain management. *Archives of Physical Medicine and Rehabilitation*, 1979, *60*, 609–612.

Sanders, S. H. Behavioral assessment and treatment of clinical pain: Appraisal of current status. In M. Hersen, R. M. Eisler, & P. M. Miller (Eds.), *Progress in behavior modification* (Vol. 8). New York: Academic Press, 1979.

Schuster, G. D., & Infante, M. C. Pain relief after low back surgery: The efficacy of transcutaneous electrical nerve stimulation. *Pain*, 1980, *8*, 299–302.

Seres, J. L., & Newman, R. I. Results of treatment of chronic low-back pain at the Portland Pain Center. *Journal of Neurosurgery*, 1976, *45*, 32–36.

Shanfield, S. B., Heiman, E. M., Cope, D. N., & Jones, J. R. Pain and the marital relationship: Psychiatric distress. *Pain*, 1979, *7*, 343–351.

Sherman, R. A., Gall, N., & Gormly, J. Treatment of phantom limb pain with muscular relaxation training to disrupt the pain-anxiety-tension cycle. *Pain*, 1979, *6*, 47–55.

Sternbach, R. A., Ignelzi, R. J., Deems, L. M., & Timmermans, G. Transcutaneous electrical analgesia: A follow-up analysis. *Pain,* 1976, *2,* 35–41.

Sternbach, R. A., & Timmermans, G. Personality changes associated with reduction of pain. *Pain,* 1975, *1,* 177–181.

Swanson, D W,, Floreen, A. C., & Swenson, W. M. Programs for managing chronic pain. II. Short-term results. *Mayo Clinic Proceedings,* 1976, *51,* 409–411.

Swanson, D. W., & Maruta, T. The family's viewpoint of chronic pain. *Pain,* 1980, *8,* 163–166.

Swanson, D. W., Maruta, T., & Swenson, W. M. Results of behavior modification in the treatment of chronic pain. *Psychosomatic Medicine,* 1979, *41,* 55–61.

Swanson, D. W., Swenson, W. M., Maruta, T., & Floreen, A. C. The dissatisfied patient with chronic pain. *Pain,* 1978, *4,* 367–378.

Swanson, D. W., Swenson, W. M., Maruta, T., & McPhee, M. C. Programs for managing chronic pain. I. Program description and characteristics of patients. *Mayo Clinic Proceedings,* 1976, *51,* 401–408.

Taylor, P., Hallett, M., & Flaherty, L. Treatment of osteoarthritis of the knee with transcutaneous electrical nerve stimulation. *Pain,* 1981, *11,* 233–240.

Taylor, C. B., Zlutnick, S. I., Corley, M. J., & Flora, J. The effects of detoxification, relaxation, and brief supportive therapy on chronic pain. *Pain,* 1980, *8,* 319–329.

Turk, D. C., & Genest, M. Regulation of pain: The application of cognitive and behavioral techniques for prevention and remediation. In P. C. Kendall & J. D. Hollon (Eds.), *Cognitive-behavioral interventions: Theory, research, and procedures.* New York: Academic Press, 1979.

Turner, J. A. Comparison of group progressive-relaxation training and cognitive-behavioral group therapy for chronic low back pain. *Journal of Consulting and Clinical Psychology,* 1982, *50,* 757–765.

Turner, J. A., & Chapman, C. R. Psychological interventions for chronic pain: A critical review. II. Operant conditioning, hypnosis, and cognitive–behavioral therapy. *Pain,* 1982, *12,* 23–46.

Turner, J., Heinrich, R., McCreary, C., & Dawson, E. *Evaluation of two behavioral interventions for chronic low back pain.* Paper presented at the meeting of the American Pain Society, San Diego, September 1979.

Urban, B. J. Therapeutic aspects in chronic pain: Modulation of nociception, alleviation of suffering, and behavioral analysis. *Behavior Therapy,* 1982, *13,* 430–437.

Varni, J. W. Behavioral medicine in hemophilia arthritic pain management: Two case studies. *Archives of Physical Medicine and Rehabilitation,* 1981, *62,* 183–187. (a)

Varni, J. W. Self-regulation techniques in the management of chronic arthritic pain in hemophilia. *Behavior Therapy,* 1981, *12,* 185–194. (b)

Varni, J. W., & Gilbert, A. Self-regulation of chronic arthritic pain and long-term analgesic dependence in a haemophiliac. *Rheumatology and Rehabilitation,* 1982, *21,* 171–174.

Varni, J. W., Gilbert, A., & Dietrich, S. L. Behavioral medicine in pain and analgesia management for the hemophilic child with Factor VIII inhibition. *Pain,* 1981, *11,* 121–126.

White, M. C., Bradley, L. A., & Prokop, C. K. Behavioral assessment of chronic pain. In W. W. Tryon (Ed.), *Behavioral assessment in behavioral medicine.* New York: Springer, in press.

Wolf, S. L., Gersh, M. R., & Rao, V. R. Examination of electrode placements and stimulating parameters in treating chronic pain with conventional transcutaneous electrical nerve stimulation (TENS). *Pain,* 1981, *11,* 37–47.

Ziesat, H. A., Jr. Behavioral approaches to the treatment of chronic pain. In C. K. Prokop & L. A. Bradley (Eds.), *Medical psychology: Contributions to behavioral medicine.* New York: Academic Press, 1981.

14

The Role of the Family in Coping with Childhood Chronic Illness*

JOHN C. MASTERS
MARY C. CERRETO
DEBRA R. MENDLOWITZ

Introduction

Whether we are children or adults, well or ill, family relationships form an important dimension of the social context in which we are born, develop, and die. Our families are influenced by our behavior and circumstances, and they are influential in our growth, development, and functioning. In short there is an ongoing reciprocal relationship between each of us and those whom we call family. Our purpose is to examine this ongoing reciprocal relationship when one family member is chronically ill.

The questions this chapter examines are the role of the family in coping with chronic illness, the ways that families are influenced by the presence of chronic illness in a family member, and, in turn, how families influence the coping and adaptation processes of the ill family member. In the general body of family literature, the reciprocal relationship between an individual and the family unit has been scrutinized most closely from the perspective of family influences on child development; the same is true within the more specific situation of life circumstances surrounding chronic illness. There-

*Preparation of this chapter was partially supported by Training Grant MCT 000 240-17, Bureau of Community Health Services to Mary C. Cerreto and a grant from The Henry R. Luce Foundation to John C. Masters.

381

fore, although it is recognized that the family both influences and is influenced by chronic disease in an adult member, this chapter focuses almost entirely upon the role of the family in relation to childhood chronic illness.

Historically, the examination of the role of the family in coping with and adapting to chronic disease has been beset with the problems inherent in the search for cause-and-effect relationships. Within this linear approach, two questions have been commonly asked: How is family functioning affected by the presence of chronic illness in a child? How is the child's ability to cope with a chronic illness affected by family factors? The literature indicates that answers to each question have been sought separately.

In this chapter we examine the role of the family as both the recipient of stresses attendant to the presence of chronic illness in a child and as the force that ameliorates or exacerbates such stresses. Our premise is that the impact of the illness on family functioning will in turn affect the child's ability to cope and thus have an impact on the illness.

We discuss some of the research that has examined how the family affects and is affected by childhood chronic illness. Despite the vast number of anecdotal clinical reports and a small number of empirically sound studies, there is an absence of knowledge about the role of the family in the coping process and need for relevant research.

Theories of Family Impact

The richest source of theories about the impact of a family member's illness on the rest of the family has been the field of sociology. One of the best-known theories is that of Talcott Parsons (Parsons & Fox, 1952). A basic assumption of this theory is that the role of the sick person, as it diverges from the normal social role played by that person, has an impact on both the family and on that person. Being ill can have status of sorts, privileges, and (to some extent) obligations, all of which may be different from the conditions that pertain for that particular person when "well." A possible extrapolation is that the assumption by one family member of a role as sick person would, especially when held for a significant period of time, have second-order consequences for the relationships and interactions among other members of the family. For example, when the perceived or real illness of one family member requires special attention, care, or precaution on the part of others at home, this burden may be shouldered readily at first but subsequently become a source of resentment and a very real restriction of freedom. Extrapolations such as these regarding such secondary effects within the family context have not been seriously tested (Crain, Sussman, & Weill, 1966).

The theoretical propositions of family sociologist Reuben Hill (1958) provide another cornerstone of theory regarding mechanisms by which illness has a family-wide impact. One focus of Hill's theory is the initial period following the onset of illness, a period of disequilibrium and crisis during which the family interrelationships may follow a roller-coaster pattern until some new equilibrium is established. Hill does speculate about the characteristics of crises that may influence the adaptation process; of special relevance for the impact of chronic illness is the notion that crises emanating from outside the family itself (e.g., floods, war) are actually more readily accommodated to than are crises from within (e.g., marital infidelity, alcoholism, or the onset of chronic disabling conditions such as the birth of a retarded child or the diagnosis of a chronic disease in one family member). In fact, it has been suggested that exogenous crises may even enhance family integration (Geiger, 1955).

Although theories such as Parsons's or Hill's attempt an explanation of the family as the target of impact from illness, they do little to clarify the role of the family as "impactor" or mediator of the coping processes of the child. The most parsimonious integration of these two concerns may be a systems model. This type of model, best elucidated in relation to illness by Minuchin, Rosman, and Baker (1978), focuses upon the interdependence of parts in a social context. Each part of the family system is seen as organizing and being organized by other parts. The system can be activated at any number of points, and feedback mechanisms operate at many junctions. Behavior is simultaneously caused and causative; beginning and end are defined by arbitrary framing and punctuation. The framework utilized by Minuchin and his colleagues integrates a diversity of factors generally considered the domain of different disciplines, but all related to illness and family functioning. The physiological, endocrine, and biochemical factors contributing to illness are part of a system that includes psychosocial factors stemming from the family, from psychological characteristics of the child that may lead to vulnerability, and from environmental factors ranging from the systems presented by the child to stress-inducing events that impinge upon the family from outside. This model is elucidated in our discussion of the impact of the family on the coping processes of the ill child.

Little else in the way of theory has had direct application to the area of chronic illness within the family context. Perhaps this is just as well; with few exceptions theoretical treatments have been of such a broad and general nature that their relevance for understanding the particularities of the effects of chronic illness on the family—or on the family's role in coping—is rather limited. They do, however, cover some of the major domains of concern that have received the attention of investigators concerned with chronic illness and families. We now turn our attention to the empirical literature that deals with various aspects of this problem.

Impact of Chronic Illness on the Family

Theorists and investigators concerned with chronic illness and families, as noted previously, have focused on family stress as a consequence of illness. In nearly every instance the family has been one with a chronically ill child. Family is almost always construed as a unit with both adults and children, so an adult ill member is also a parent. In short, the literature is clearly child-centered, regardless of who the chronically ill family member happens to be.

FOCI OF CONCERN

The range of chronic illnesses studied includes a wide variety of illnesses that are similar in being chronic and are different in terms of the debilities or regimens of treatment that are entailed. Thus, although the particular illness may influence the role of the family in coping, the stresses on the family, or the way the family might be involved in treatment, the focus of the literature and the focus of this chapter are broader—they are on the commonalities that may be identified across chronic illnesses in the role of the family in coping, as an object of stressors, or as mediators of treatment. Later we consider whether this breadth is reasonable and allows meaningful generalizations. The chronic illnesses that have received attention in the literature include diabetes mellitus, nephrotic (kidney) disorders, cystic fibrosis, arthritis (juvenile and adult), spina bifida, asthma, and malignancies. If common problems such as allergies are considered, a remarkable proportion of families are placed in the position of having one or more chronically ill members. The resolution in the literature has been to focus on those families in which a serious chronic illness is present that causes significant stresses to the family's economic and social well-being and poses problems of treatment that are transferred from external medical sources to the individual or family for self-management.

In addition to concern with the particular family member suffering a chronic illness or the particular chronic disease in question, there has been concern with the various categories of consequences that may (or may not) stem from the occurrence of a chronic illness within the family context. Not surprisingly, one of the concerns that has received a good deal of attention is

the impact of chronic illness on marital discord and likelihood that the family
will be dissolved through divorce.

IMPACT ON PARENTS' MARRIAGE

The impact of a family member's chronic disease on the intactness of the
marriage appears to be quite variable, largely because different chronic
diseases present different stressors. Some investigators have found that the
presence of a chronic illness has little or no impact on divorce rates (Begleiter, Burry, & Harris, 1976; Martin, 1975; Zimmerman, 1980), and others
have found a somewhat reduced incidence of divorce, as though the stress
had a cohesive effect on the solidarity of the marriage (Lansky, Cairns,
Hassanein, Wehr, & Lowman, 1978).

There has been little attempt to systematize findings such as these, although such a synthesis may be possible. The secret seems to be in grouping
chronic illnesses according to aspects–stressors that are similar or are likely
to have the same impact on a particular variable such as divorce. Chronic
diseases in children that require careful and frequent maintenance by a
parent would probably have a greater effect on family functioning than
would a disease whose onset is emotionally stressful (the birth of a handicapped child, the occurrence of an accident that induces a chronic disorder),
but for which there is no lingering imposed family involvement in treatment
(eventual adaptation to limitations imposed by the disorder; maintenance or
remedial treatment assumed by the school system).

A disease with a high probability of genetic recurrence may indirectly
stress a marriage through a rational yet emotionally unacceptable decision to
have no more children. These sorts of stress components associated with
chronic disorders do not seem to increase family disruption rates. Interestingly, however, therapeutic efforts to mitigate these stressful effects
may effectively reduce the rate of disruption in such families to a level below
the norm. Begleiter, Burry, and Harris (1976) reviewed the literature on
families attending genetic counseling clinics and found that the divorce rate
for these families was lower than the overall average for families with children having no genetically transmissible disorders. Begleiter et al. argue
that the genetic recurrence risk of a particular disorder may be a dimension
that mediates its effects on family intactness, with those disorders having a
high-recurrence risk posing more stress on the marital relationship. In their
review of the literature these authors note that the rates of divorce for
couples with children afflicted with low-recurrence risk, such as spina bifida,
or nongenetic disorders, such as leukemia, are lower than the national average; those for parents of children with a high-recurrence risk disorder, such
as cystic fibrosis, are the same as the national average. Although chronic

diseases in children do not automatically increase the likelihood of parental divorce, and under some conditions may actually reduce the likelihood of family disruption, undoubtedly the chronic illness of a family member, particularly a child, imposes stress of some sort on other family members. Joosten (1979) reports, for example, that both parents of families having a child with spina bifida spent more time in child care and were required to depend more on families and neighbors than were parents of a normal child of comparable age. Satterwhite (1978) lists a number of stresses or impositions that are common across many chronic illnesses, including general worry, embarrassment, handling (well-meaning) impositions from relatives, restrictions on parental social life or family travel, and problems relating to siblings such as resentment or parental concerns of sibling neglect.

Cairns and Lansky (1980) were able to discriminate parents of hemophilic children and parents of children with cancer from those of normal children on the basis of their Minnesota Multiphasic Personality Inventory (MMPI) profiles. Waisbren (1980) examined the reactions of parents of developmentally disabled infants (18 months of age or less) in the United States and Denmark. Despite the greater availability of support services in Denmark, the differences between parents from the two cultures were not remarkable. Parents tended to view themselves more negatively after the birth of the child and expressed more negative feelings about the child than did parents of a nonhandicapped infant.

INFLUENCES ON OTHER FAMILY MEMBERS

It is also the case that particular aspects of the disease may exacerbate its impact on family members. For example, Tew and Lawrence (1975) found that mothers of children with spina bifida had higher scores on a malaise inventory (Rutter, Tizard, & Whitmore, 1970) when the child was incontinent, had a severe disability in the area of locomotion, attended a special rather than a normal school, and had an IQ less than 80. Such findings underscore the ways that different chronic illnesses with their varying disabilities and requirements for care from others are likely to vary in their impact on the family, especially on the care givers.

The chronic illness of one family member may affect not only other family members themselves but also their interactions with one another and with the chronically ill individual. For example, Donofrio (1979) found that families with an asthmatic or diabetic child, compared to those with a nondisabled child, showed less ability to reach consensus and less efficient and effective communication, sharing fewer opinions and suggestions and soliciting fewer opinions and suggestions from other family members. On the other hand, Saur (1980) found that families of a young multiply and severely handicapped child were no different from those with a young nonhandicapped child in terms of cohesiveness, expressiveness, conflict, or achievement orientation, nor were there any effects on a social support-network inventory that assessed relationships with friends, co-workers, or professionals. Studying families of children with spina bifida, Nevin and McCubbin (1979) found that families experiencing less stress showed more cohesion and organization and lower conflict than did high-stress families. High-stress families, on the other hand, showed a greater motivation to develop family–community relationships—in short, to enhance social support-system contact. The results of this study suggest that perceived stress may be an important variable in determining the effect of a chronically ill child on other family members, and that the same illness may be more or less stressful for a given family. Overall, however, the evidence is not so clear-cut. Because the various studies in this area have each involved a different chronic illness, there remains the possibility that not all chronic illnesses impose negative effects on family interactions, although some certainly do. It remains for future research to confirm those illnesses that seem to put family interaction patterns "at risk" and to begin to explore what, if any, common characteristics of those illnesses are responsible for the disruptive effects.

As discussed, the first concern of investigators (and probably of professionals also) has been with the parents as the recipients or focus of stress from chronic illness in another family member. There has been less research dealing with the consequences on other children in the family. Lavigne and Ryan (1979) studied the healthy siblings of children with a variety of chronic illnesses including blood disorders, heart problems, and disfigurements, and compared them with healthy children whose siblings were also healthy. Not surprisingly, the siblings of chronically ill children showed greater irritability and social withdrawal, factors that could clearly have an impact on the general adjustment of these children. A study by Burke (1978) reported some interesting findings on the consequences of chronic illness or handicap in one child upon his or her siblings and suggests further that stress may produce multiple and varied (i.e., positive and negative) consequences. Burke proposed that one consequence of stressors is *familial strain*, defined as the propogation of stress throughout the family system. For example, stress on one family member will influence his or her behavior in ways that induce stress on other family members; thus, Burke found that maternal strain was related to both the developmental quotient of the handicapped child and to that of the sibling (Boll & Alpern, 1975), but in different ways. The general presence of a handicapped child was related to reduced developmental levels in siblings. High maternal strain was related to higher developmental quotients in the handicapped child, but to lower ones in the siblings.

Chronic disorders also have an impact on ill individuals themselves. Satterwhite (1978) reports increased instances of maladjustment in chronically ill children, including greater incidence in school of underachievement and referrals to the school psychologist. There are also likely to be different effects on the individual as a function of the specific illness, the debilities or disfigurements it entails, and the particular treatment regimens required. Dorner (1975) reports a study that illustrates the way the characteristics of the individual, such as sex or age, may also influence the impact of the disease. Dorner found that for adolescents afflicted with spina bifida, social isolation and depression were common consequences of impaired mobility associated with the disease; the need for urinary appliances was more stressful for boys than for girls.

SUMMARY

There is little question that the chronic illness of one family member has an impact on other family members and upon the family as a group. There *is* a question, however, about how best to systematize this impact and to understand it. Perceived stress appears to be one dimension of impact that may mediate more specific consequences and therefore merits further attention. Under some conditions, or for some disorders, there is evidence of positive family consequences from a chronic illness; the factors that help determine when an illness or the stress it precipitates will have a positive or negative impact are not known. The questions at hand are theoretical as well as empirical, and concern the development of a more articulated understanding of the processes and factors associated with any chronic disorder that will mediate potential negative and positive impacts.

Role of the Family in the Child's Ability to Cope

We have discussed the role of the family as recipient of stressors attendant to living with a child with a chronic condition. Certainly, however, the family has a reciprocal impact on the child. Although it seems logical that this impact would be highly visible in its influences on the child's ability to cope with his or her condition, there have been few systematic investigations of this topic. The search for nonphysical factors influencing the course of illness originally focused on characteristics of the individual. Initial investigations attempted to identify a personality type—for example, the "diabetic personality" (Bruch, 1948; Menninger, 1935; Meyer, Bollmeier, & Alexander, 1945)—that was associated with the onset and course of the illness. The existence of a specific personality type associated with a particular illness has received little empirical support and the concept can best be relegated to the position of a futile academic exercise.

A second line of investigation of individual characteristics has focused upon the association between health status and psychological adjustment of the ill child. For example, it has been proposed that adequacy of diabetic control may be related to psychological adjustment (e.g., Ack, 1974; Grey, Genel, & Tamborlane, 1980). It is difficult to ignore the family in this context. Once affected primarily by periodic hospitalization, children are now returning with new treatment regimens and increased life expectancies to the community, where the family, not the hospital, is the primary provider. The contextual variable *family* and its role in helping or hindering the child's ability to cope with a chronic condition will therefore be examined here. Three major areas in which it can be hypothesized that family factors would have an impact on the course of the child's illness and on his or her health behaviors are discussed.

PSYCHOLOGICAL AND PHYSICAL HEALTH STATUS

The majority of studies of the psychological and physical health of chronically ill children have investigated the associations between a wide variety of family factors and indices of the emotional and physical status of the child. The most common outcomes of health status utilized are severity of the illness condition, or (as in the case of diabetes) the degree to which the illness was in control and psychological adjustment. An early and classic example of such a line of investigation is the work of Minuchin and his colleagues in Philadelphia (Minuchin *et al.*, 1978). Among their patients was a pool of diabetic children frequently hospitalized for medically unexplained attacks of acidosis. It was noted that these children evidenced difficulties in handling stress, immature coping abilities, and the tendency to internalize anger. Individual therapy instituted to define personality issues and reduce stress factors made no impact. Family therapy, however, led to major changes in roles in the family and amelioration of psychosomatic symptoms that were defined as the emotional exacerbation of already available symptoms. Minuchin noted family functioning factors such as enmeshment, overprotection, rigidity, and lack of conflict resolution—transaction styles that at the extremes are pathological—as key contributors to the adequacy of the child's control of the illness. Family therapy proved impressively successful in ameliorating symptoms immediately and in follow-up.

Minuchin's investigations illustrate the open systems model where child and illness factors and family factors constantly transact to affect the child's ability to cope with the condition. Hospitalizations, a very concrete, definable outcome measure, were greatly reduced. Unfortunately, he provides investigators few criteria for reliably defining or categorizing families as *enmeshed, rigid,* or *overprotective.*

Pless, Roghmann, and Haggerty (1972) placed particular emphasis on the contribution of family life-style as an important variable when assessing the physical and emotional status of chronically ill children. They attempted systematically to study the role of the family in a 1%-probability sample of families with children under 18 years in Monroe County, New York. The authors developed a family functioning index that included components such as marital satisfaction, frequency of disagreements, family happiness, spouse–spouse communications, time spent together, and discussion of problems. At all ages, children who were chronically ill scored lower than nonchronically ill children on self-ratings of self-esteem and parent ratings of behavior symptoms. More importantly, the combination of low family functioning, mild to severe disability, and low self-esteem was the best predictor of deviant behavior.

Most of the literature emphasizes the importance of parental attitudes toward the sick child. Although pre- and post-illness studies have not been conducted, it has been hypothesized that parents change their attitudes toward a child after the child becomes ill (Mattsson, 1977). Some parents become more loving and indulgent; some let up on discipline and rules; others reject, criticize, or neglect the child. Mattsson makes the point that the nature of the specific illness is perhaps less related to the child's ability to cope than are psychosocial factors, of which the parent–child relationship is central. This is of particular import in those illnesses whose control and course are highly influenced by emotional factors (e.g., diabetes and asthma). For example, several investigators have noted how highly emotional factors are related to the control of diabetes and to symptoms such as hypoglycemia and acidosis (e.g., Stein & Charles, 1975; Swift, Seidman, & Stein, 1967). The influence of parental attitudes on the child's ability to cope has been noted in the quality of the parent–child relationship, in families' acceptance of the child with the chronic condition (e.g., Freeman, 1968; Prugh, 1963), and in parents' ability to master their initial reactions of fear and guilt (Green & Solnit, 1964; Mattsson & Gross, 1973; Prugh, 1963; Solnit & Stark, 1961). Children learn and imitate the attitudes and behaviors of their parents. The ways in which they process this information is highly dependent on their immature levels of cognitive ability, and result in unintended behaviors. A child may become passively dependent if he or she senses that the parents' expectations are for vulnerability and probable premature death. Either overprotective or rejecting parental attitudes may result in child rebellion and defiant attitudes that greatly jeopardize his or her condition (Mattsson, 1977).

Unlike many authors who stress only the negative, unproductive parental attitudes conducive to child maladjustment, Mattsson (1977) also delineates some of those parental attitudes and behaviors that help the child to cope with the chronic illness. These include enforcing only necessary and realistic restrictions on the child, encouraging self-care and regular school attendance, promoting reasonable physical activities, using common psychological defenses to cope with the constant strain, remaining calm in crisis situations, maintaining control through cognitive techniques, and lessening their anxiety by becoming more familiar with the child's illness.

Several studies have focused on the ability of the family to maintain its coping ability in order, in turn, to foster coping in the child. Much of this research mentions the family's role in the mediation of stress. For example, Kaplan, Smith, Grobstein, and Fischman (1977) discuss considerations such as what parents, sick children, siblings and extended family members should be told about the course of treatment and the prognosis, who should give the information, what advice should be given to parents about major family changes, what should be done about parents who disagree about handling the illness, and so on. All considerations are aimed at helping adult family members facilitate their own coping processes and those of the sick child. Kupst, Blatterbauer, Westman, Schulman, and Paul (1977) investigated the effects of a variety of intervention techniques on parent understanding of diagnosis, patient satisfaction, and parental anxiety. They recommended a team approach for use in pediatric speciality clinics where time constraints highlighted the need for more personal interaction. It should be noted that, with the exception of the Kupst et al. (1977) study, most research in this area is ancedotal in nature. More carefully designed, controlled studies of parental coping and its influence on the ill child are needed.

ADHERENCE TO TREATMENT REGIMEN

The second major area of concern deals with adherence to a prescribed treatment regimen. Interestingly, despite the importance of this topic, there is a remarkable dearth of concern in the literature regarding the family's role in helping children to cope with their chronic conditions through fostering adherence to treatment regimens. In a recent, comprehensive review of the literature on adherence to health care regimens, Masur (1981) divided coverage of psychosocial variables influencing compliance into "four sections, each of which represents a general category of research variables that have been studied in relation to compliance" (p. 450). These four sections are (a) patient–provider interaction, (b) information–education, (c) behavioral and environmental factors, and (d) the Health Belief Model. In none of these is the role of the family explored.

The investigation of how dimensions of family functioning foster the child's adherence to health regimens and positive health behaviors is an important and potentially exciting future horizon for research in childhood chronic illness. Adequate research paradigms have been established in the child development literature. The next step is to begin to study the relationships of parenting styles, family dimensions, and familial stress to children's adherence to health care regimens.

REHABILITATION

The third area in which it can be hypothesized that the family would play a major role is rehabilitation. At issue are family factors that may promote better adjustment to different and progressive stages of the condition. This is one area of the literature on chronic illness and the family in which the major focus has been on the rehabilitation of adults with chronic conditions, particularly those who have suffered strokes. D'Afflitti and Weitz (1977) reported that 75% of patients look first to their families for support and second to the hospital staff, and that patients appear to be reluctant to engage themselves in a therapy program if they cannot anticipate reentry into a functioning family unit.

The importance of interpersonal relationships in the rehabilitation of chronic disease patients is the dominant theme of the rehabilitation literature (e.g., Litman, 1964). Bruetman and Gordon (1971) discuss rehabilitation in terms of restoring both the physiological and environmental equilibria of the patient and note the great impact of the family on patient expectations and motivations. Robertson and Suinn (1968) report a relationship between stroke patients' rate of progress toward recovery and the degree of empathy between the patient and family members. Greatest improvement was noted when "predictive empathy" was evidenced, that is, when patient and family members could foresee each others' attitudes. D'Afflitti and Weitz (1977) ran family groups for stroke patients, focusing on encouraging patients and family to talk and share feelings and to use appropriate family resources and supports. Although no systematic data are presented, the authors discuss positive outcomes in terms of sharing difficult feelings, recognizing negative feelings, developing realistic expectations, increasing use of community supports, and sharing medical information.

In general, although it is not extensive, the literature on adults with chronic illnesses frequently attends to the role of the family and its beneficial effects on the rehabilitative process. The majority of the literature has focused on stroke, uncommon of course in childhood. It might be, however, that many of the same factors of familial empathy, sharing, openness, and support would operate to enhance childhood rehabilitative processes. This area warrants further investigation.

SUMMARY

The literature suggests that the family plays a significant role in an individual's ability to cope with chronic illness. The positive, or potentially positive, influence of the family on both physical and psychological health of the chronically ill child or adult seems well documented. Evidence regarding the role of the family in fostering adherence to health care regimens and in enhancing the rehabilitative process is less clear; however, logical hypotheses abound and these should be fruitful areas for future research aimed at documenting the role families may play and specifying those factors mediating effective family intervention.

Perhaps more than is preferable, a review of this literature seems to give a sense of promise but not of completion. There are no counterindications to the premise that the family plays an important role in the coping process. However, there is room for further clarification of what this role is or how it may be effectively achieved, primarily with respect to areas of adherence and rehabilitation.

Applications

The integration of current research findings with clinical aspects of comprehensive care is necessary for the development of new programs and progressive policy decisions regarding chronically ill children and their families. In many pediatric, educational, and health care facilities there is an unfortunate trend for comprehensive care programs to develop without thoughtful planning for intervention and attention to research findings (Drotar, Doershuk, Boat, Stern, Matthews, & Boyen, 1981) or research needs.

With respect to the role of families in the treatment of chronic illness, research has been applied in a variety of ways and in many different settings. The development and refinement of clinical techniques such as parent training, genetic counseling, family therapy, and assessment are examples of application that have been informed by available research knowledge and have implications affecting future policy decisions and institutional changes. We now turn to the examination and critical review of some applications of research findings and identify selected gaps in research utilization.

PARENT TRAINING

The range of problems that families of chronically ill children, and parents in particular, must deal with is broad and often behavioral rather than physical in nature. For example, a high incidence of behavior and school problems may develop in both the ill child and healthy siblings. The family may experience difficulties integrating particular medical regimens such as diet and physical therapy into family activities, or may face anxiety around the issue of adherence. Parent training has been utilized as one approach to deal with many of these problems. It generally concentrates on alleviating specific behavior problems by teaching parents child development knowledge and child management skills. While parent training has been shown to be effective in increasing children's compliance to a wide range of school and home behaviors (Cerreto & Miller, 1981; Stevens, 1978), there is as yet no direct evidence of its appropriateness for use with the parents of chronically ill children. However, because many of their problems are similar to those faced by parents of physically healthy children, it is reasonable to assume that parent training structured around specific behaviors would also be successful for parents of chronically ill children (Cerreto, 1980).

It has also been argued that parents of chronically ill children need training in child development (e.g., Slimmer, 1977). Hymovich (1974) pointed out that chronic illness is a crisis superimposed on the normal crisis of development and suggested viewing chronic illness from the perspective of its effects on the accomplishment of common developmental tasks both by the individual family members and the family as a unit. It would be expected that parent–child interactions will improve when parent training also focuses on the child's capabilities and expected conflicts at different stages (Pierre & Cerreto, 1981). Parents' lack of child development knowledge may limit their ability to anticipate and deal with the emotional conflicts arising from such things as the limitations the child experiences from the chronic condition, especially as these change with age. A failure to handle such problems effectively is, in turn, likely to compound parental frustrations and limit parents' ability to participate adequately in the coping process still further. Unfortunately, however, few programs focus on *development* when assisting parents to cope with the child with a chronic illness.

Parent training techniques utilized with handicapping conditions such as emotional disturbance and mental retardation have been slow to enter the domain of chronic illness. There may be several reasons for this. Only recently have new medical advances allowed chronically ill children to return to their homes and communities. Further, the focus in the past has been more on support groups that assist parents to cope with the emotional trauma of possible death than on education that emphasizes control and understanding of the child and the disease. Although it is important to help parents understand and express the pain of having a child with a chronic illness, more attention must be directed toward increasing compliance and positive behavior at home and in the community. Programs have begun to recognize and acknowledge the advances in this area.

GENETIC COUNSELING

Research on parental attitudes toward genetic factors has found that the diagnosis of a genetically transmitted disease can lead to the development of guilt, misconceptions, self-recrimination in the parent who feels responsible for its transmission, or the development of hostile emotions towards the spouse who is held responsible (e.g., McCrae, Cull, Burton, & Dodge, 1973; Pond, 1979; Tarnow & Tomlinson, 1978). Siblings may also develop anxieties about "whether it could happen to me too" or whether their children may be affected. These findings have led professionals who work with chronically ill children and their families to conduct sessions in which the genetic implications of the condition are explained and discussed (Garner & Thompson, 1978).

FAMILY THERAPY

We have discussed the advantages of parent training in the areas of education, child development, and compliance-related behavior problems (e.g., a diabetic child's refusal to take insulin or inappropriate eating). However, the nature of chronic illnesses and their management occasionally produces problems in which systematic psychotherapy is beneficial. Drawing on both the arguments and research dealing with parent training and the family as the treatment context, one might expect family therapy to enhance the family's role and capabilities in coping with chronic illness.

Following a family systems model, Minuchin and colleagues (Baker, Minuchin, Milman, Liebman, & Todd, 1975; Minuchin, 1977; Minuchin et al., 1978) have developed a systems model postulating that family organization is causally related to the development and maintenance of maladaptive emotional and physical responses in diabetic children and that the child's responses in turn play an important role in maintaining the family homeostasis (Minuchin et al., 1978). In support of this model, Minuchin and his colleagues found that in some children with diabetes, stress leads to an increase in arousal and fatty acid production that continues once the interview is terminated (Baker et al., 1975; Minuchin et al., 1978), but that after family therapy these responses decrease (Baker et al., 1975; Minuchin, 1977; Minuchin et al., 1978). Unfortunately methodological problems limit the degree to which this research may be considered conclusive; for example, no appropriate control groups were used. The small number of individual cases also does not clarify what proportion of children with brittle diabetes come from families with the particular characteristics studied (e.g., fatty acid production in response to stress). Issue has also been taken with the causal elements of this model. Johnson (1980), for example, has hypothesized that specific family patterns such as conflict avoidance might develop in response to diabetic children's heightened reactivity, rather than being a cause of it.

Clearly, more extensive evaluation of the use of family therapy to deal with the treatment of chronic illness in children is needed. The benefits, techniques, and outcomes of these therapies require more thorough assessment, as does the applicability of family therapy to a variety of chronic illnesses embodying a range of stressors and management problems. In addition, family therapy acknowledges the family unit, perhaps even more than does parent training. The extent to which it entails more than an elaborated course of parent training that involves the child is not obvious and some attention to the specific elements of effective family therapy is in order.

ASSESSMENT

There is little sense in targeting family factors to enhance coping if we cannot properly assess them first. The refinement of assessment measures also can be highly beneficial to the health provider. In the majority of instances the medical professional may be the sole provider of counseling and supportive services to the family with a chronically ill member. However, time constraints and lack of training often necessitate referrals into the community when treatment problems develop. Health professionals need a comprehensive means of assessing the impact of childhood illness on a family at time of diagnosis and other times of stress (such as adolescence, financial hardships, or marital discord) rather than at a time of crisis or when change in normative family behavior precipitates referral. Future investigators utilizing the knowledge of crises in development need to focus on developing measures predictive of family crisis at different points in time.

Studies of the impact of childhood illness on family functioning and adjustment have only begun to identify and define determinants of family functioning and adjustment and to develop methods of assessment. For example, according to Stein and Riessman (1980), there is no comprehensive measure that can quantify the impact of childhood illness on the family unit and delineate the numerous facets of this complex domain. Several investigators have relied on clinical interviews assessing economic and social resources, change in family life, sibling rivalry, and other areas of concern (Klein, 1974; McAndrew, 1976; Satterwhite, 1976). However, these measures do not have adequate reliability and validity for broad or confident use (Stein & Riessman, 1980).

In order to meet the demand for a comprehensive assessment tool, Stein and Riessman (1980) and Hymovich (1981) have developed scales to measure the impact of childhood chronic disorder on the family. The Stein and Riessman (1980) measure may be used to assess family response at the onset of an illness and over its course. Four dimensions of the measure are salient: (*a*) economic burden, (*b*) social impact: quality and quantity of interaction with those outside the household, (c) familial impact: interaction within the family unit, and (d) subjective distress: the strain experienced by the primary caretaker that is directly related to the demands of the illness. Although this tool is in the stages of preliminary development, it may provide a model for other investigators.

Hymovich's (1981) clinical assessment tool is also in a developmental stage. The conceptual framework on which this tool is based is threefold: (a) developmental tasks of individuals and families; (b) impact variables of perceptions of problems and satisfying situations in the family members' daily lives, resources available to or needed by family members, and coping abilities enabling them to manage stresses imposed by the child's chronic illness; and (c) interventions needed by families of chronically ill children.

HEALTH CARE PRACTICE AND AGENCIES

Medical care, broadly conceived, is almost always in a state of flux. One dimension of the changes relevant to the treatment of chronic illness is a move from the treatment of illness in the individual to the maintenance of health in the family (e.g., Kohut, 1966). Health professionals and agencies are examining the forces that maintain positive health, rather than concentrating on those that lead to illness (Haggerty, 1980). Another dimension of change concerns the focus on treatment or cure rather than on the management of illness. In the past the child with a chronic disorder had a limited life expectancy, and the physician's role was often one of comforting and easing pain rather than treatment. Medical advances have altered this role. With chronically ill children there must now be equal commitments to management and to treatment. This implies an orientation to the whole child in the context of his or her family and its culture (e.g., Harding, Heller, & Kesler, 1979; Hewitt, 1976; Kohut, 1966; Pless & Roghmann, 1971).

For this aspect of the redefinition of health care to be accomplished successfully, the professional and public responsibilities of both the health care facility and the health provider require some reassessment. It has been suggested that exacerbations of the illness that led to hospitalization may be avoided if families receive support prior to hospitalization (Bartmettler & Fields, 1975–1976). Bartmettler and Fields argue that more systematic linkage of the hospital to public health programs, family agencies, schools, and other community caretakers may increase psychosocial adjustment and maintenance and decrease the number of hospitalizations.

POLICY STUDIES

Chronic illness may bring a variety of taxing emotional, financial, and other burdens. While not all stress can be eliminated, public policies and health care facilities can be designed to ameliorate unnecessary stress, enhance the quality of family life, and promote coping in the individual.

Chronically ill children have not received the types of advocacy and types of financial, legislative, educational, and psychological support that children with other handicapping conditions have been given (Hobbs & Perrin, 1980–1982). Except for the provision of medical services to the indigent, families with chronically ill children have been largely neglected (Hobbs & Perrin, 1980–1982). In a presentation to the American Orthopsychiatric Association, L. B. Schorr (1977) clearly stated:

> One of the obstacles to the adoption of [health] policies, which seem so sensible and their need so self-evident, is the lack of understanding—not just among professionals, but in the public at large—that social systems including the health system can be designed to enhance a family's ability to nurture and raise its children. Unless there is a greater recognition of the family context in which children live and through which social programs must operate, these programs will not be effective [p. 6].

Hobbs, McDowell, Cerreto, and Litchfield (1980) explored the public policy implications of stress in families with diabetic children. Preliminary findings indicated that only 33% of the mothers and 9% of the fathers were aware of private and governmental agencies or programs providing services for diabetic children. In general, parents reported needs for better insurance coverage, tax deductions, improved family and public education, and other areas of policy change.

Policy statements are essential to programs affecting familial adjustment to children with chronic conditions; sound empirical investigations are necessary for policy studies to be valid. The conceptual and methodological considerations inherent in conducting such investigations are discussed in the final section of this chapter.

Conceptual and Methodological Concerns

CONCEPTUAL CONCERNS

The further delineation of the role of the family in coping with chronic illness and the use of that knowledge in developing effective treatment interventions are highly dependent on increased attention to conceptual and methodological concerns. These concerns are discussed briefly here; the reader is referred to Watson and Kendall, Chapter 3, for more comprehensive coverage of methodological issues relevant to behavioral medicine in general and chronic illness in particular.

Coping versus Pathology

The use of traditional psychiatric clinical assessment techniques has often contributed to a description of the chronically ill as "pathological" when, in fact, behaviors and attitudes considered abnormal in a "normal" sample are realistic dimensions of daily coping with a chronic condition. For example, consider the use of the MMPI in the evaluation of the chronically ill. The Depression Scale is heavily loaded with statements of somatic concerns that are real components of chronic illnesses. High scores for the chronically ill on the scale thus are probably more a function of the physical concomitants of the illness rather than a reflection of an extreme emotional state or psychodiagnostic category.

Similarly, many of the other assessment tools utilized with the chronically ill have been designed for seriously disturbed psychiatric populations. There has been little establishing of norms for patterns within the chronically ill population, where "normal" and psychologically "healthy" coping may appear pathological when judged by inappropriate standards. Although traditional assessments may have yielded adequate descriptions of subgroups of children who may be at risk for emotional and behavioral problems, they yield little information about individual strengths on which to build intervention programs to enhance coping. Traditional assessment methods have thus contributed to a focus on pathology. The field is ready for its next step, which should be a more concerted effort to look at those attitudinal, emotional, and behavioral factors that can enhance coping.

Commonality of Chronic Illness Conditions across Disease Entities

One of the basic conceptual issues is whether there is some type of commonality across individual chronic illnesses. Life with a child with leukemia is of course different from life with a child with asthma or a child who cannot walk. Differences in the life expectancies, severity, visibility and daily treatment regimens of various illnesses may have very different ramifications on a determination of which factors promote coping. On the other hand, treatment programs such as parent training, family therapy, and so on are themselves nonspecific and can be adapted to individual children, families, and illnesses in specific instances. As long as the differences that do exist across chronic illnesses are not forgotten, there still seems to be merit in aggregating chronic illnesses, at least for such purposes as the derivation of treatment procedures that are appropriate for many types of chronic illness.

A second issue, no less important, is whether there is a single or coherent entity called *stress*. The different demands of individual illness conditions may be balanced by commonalities across all illnesses in how families respond to these demands. Certain patterns of crisis and coping may be similar, regardless of illness condition. For example, are there common familial patterns of reactions such as denial, anger, guilt, or acceptance?

In summary, the investigation of coping with chronic illness is still in the initial stages of development, and the theme of disease-specific versus generic studies will be of prime importance. Currently there appears to be a trend toward the investigation of differences among chronic conditions. However, there are situations and factors which seem common to all or most chronic illnesses—for example, conveying diagnosis to parents, behavioral management of children with chronic conditions, coping with periodic hospitalizations, children's cognitive understanding of health and illness, and parenting styles. Clearly attention to disease-specific issues is appropriate, but the small incidence and prevalence rates of most of the chronic childhood illnesses suggest that the designs of broad intervention programs must to some degree be based on commonalities.

Second-Order Effects

As in the vast literature on the families of mentally retarded and handicapped children (e.g., Gabel, McDowell, & Cerreto, 1983), the term *family* in chronic illness has, for the most part, meant *parents* (mainly mothers) and the *affected child*. Brothers and sisters and extended family members have been sorely neglected. An understanding of the role of the family in coping with chronic illness will not be complete without an examination of how family members, other than parents, affect and are affected by the presence of a chronically ill child.

In some cases this will involve the investigation of direct effects. The few studies of the siblings of chronically ill children (Breslau, Weitzman, & Messenger, 1981; Lavigne & Ryan, 1979) have examined the adjustment of the brothers and sisters themselves. A second line of investigation will be the study of second-order effects, that is, how the sibling or grandparent affects the parent–child dyad and, in turn, the process of coping. Brothers, sisters, and grandparents may very well be untapped resources to enhance the child's capacity to cope with chronic illness.

Developmental Sequences

The small number of children with specific chronic illnesses has resulted in the pooling of age groups for investigation. Because children view their world very differently at different ages and stages of development, coping mechanisms will also vary with time. Additionally, the interaction of the illness with specific developmental tasks of an age group may profoundly affect the methods available to enhance the role of the family. For example, identity, independence, body integrity, privacy, and a desire to be similar to one's peers are all major concerns of adolescence. Each is a factor affected by the daily health regimen of juvenile diabetes. How particular characteristics of the illness interact with particular age-related developmental tasks of childhood is an area warranting further investigation.

It has been proposed that families, too, have a set and series of developmental tasks to accomplish (Duvall, 1977). Different emotional resources are available to families at different stages of the unit's development. The coping techniques necessary when the marriage is new, when children are born, and when children enter school and leave home can be expected to vary and interact with the age-related coping processes of the child. The advantages of this perspective for our understanding of the coping process are being examined.

METHODOLOGICAL CONCERNS

Statements about the role of the family in coping with chronic illness will remain suspect until more faith can be placed in the adequacy of currently utilized research designs and the reliability and validity of measurement techniques. Generalization of findings is limited because of factors such as small subject samples (Begleiter *et al.*, 1976; Hobbs *et al.*, 1980) and lack of representation from all socioeconomic backgrounds (McDowell, 1981; Stein & Charles, 1971, 1975). Many studies rely heavily on clinical observations and anecdotal information (Khurana & White, 1970; Stein & Charles, 1971, 1975) and suffer from lack of adequate control or comparison groups (Litchfield, 1981; Martin, 1975; Hobbs *et al.*, 1980).

Subject Samples

"The choice of subjects in too many studies is determined more by convenience than by the requirements of sound research design [Achenbach, 1978, p. 761]." Although this point is well taken, *convenience* is too pejorative a term. Such convenience becomes a realistic concern when the pool of available subjects is small and the location of sizable samples is confined to large urban areas and medical centers, often the case with children with chronic conditions. Adequate research designs that take into account child variables such as developmental level, intelligence, sex, race, and socioeconomic status and family variables including size, geographic location, formal and informal social networks, and dimensions of interaction are difficult to obtain when the limiting factor is the clinical status of the child. For example, in investigations of the role of siblings in coping with chronic illness, the simultaneous control for variables hypothesized to be of importance—variables such as age, birth order, sex, sibling-affected child–sex match, and number of siblings in the family—is generally impossible. Whether subjects are obtained through the community, university hospitals, clinics, or private practice is also of concern to the generalization of findings.

It is recognized that subject, setting, and sampling variables can seldom be fully controlled; one proposed alternative is the replication of studies across a variety of settings (Achenbach, 1978). Replication permits sounder statements in both the generalization and limitations of specific characteristics of study settings. A complementary alternative is the assembling of a formal, structured network of researchers who ask the same questions in different settings on different samples of families with chronically ill children, utilize the same assessment measures, and share data.

Control and Contrast Groups

Many studies report descriptive findings from a sample of chronically ill children without regard to the consideration of similar variables in samples of healthy children or children with other conditions. The use of adequate controls and contrast groups will help address the issue of whether chronic illness can be treated generically or whether specific conditions must be studied separately.

Measurement

Few assessment techniques have been designed and have had norms established specifically for use with samples of families of chronically ill children. Investigators must choose between using measures that are not entirely appropriate for the goals of the study and devising new measures without adequate attention paid to standardization. Observations of behaviors directly related to the particular illness condition and the use of actuarial prediction techniques have been proposed as alternatives to the use of traditional measures (Bradley, Prokop, & Clayman, 1981).

With specific regard to the measurement of family factors, an abundance of measures have purported to assess similar dimensions such as cohesiveness, adaptibility, or flexibility. However, there are few guidelines available to help determine which measure is appropriate for whom and when. Additionally, there are no data indicating that such dimensions function in similar ways for families of healthy children, families of psychiatrically ill children, and families of chronically ill children. At the very least, future research should attempt to include multiple, convergent measures wherever possible.

Statistical Concerns

Perhaps the most glaring problems and elementary statistical concerns in assessing the role of the family are those inherent in correlational research. Experimental designs are the most powerful means of testing causality but the nature of the important dimensions of chronic illness often make it impossible to control the manipulation of a hypothesized independent variable and assess corresponding changes in the dependent variables. Thus causality is often inappropriately inferred from correlational and parallel findings. Prediction of behavior over time is often confused with the summaries of covariation among variables in multiple regression and discriminant analyses (Achenbach, 1978). The problem is frequently compounded by reference to the independent variables as *predictors*. Again, replication of studies could help to assess cause and effect more accurately.

Additional concerns have been noted by other authors. Among these are regression toward the mean (Achenbach, 1978), proper techniques for measuring changes, and adequate follow-up assessment (Achenbach, 1978; Bradley *et al.*, 1981). It is only when adequate attention is paid to such issues that research findings will contribute to the development of interventions that aid both the child and family to cope with chronic illness.

Conclusion

We have attempted to be critical—reasonably, we hope—in discussing the theory and research dealing with family factors in coping with chronic illness. Our critical stance has been intended to be a thinly disguised exhortation. The first facet of the exhortation is cautionary: methodological limitations and the prevalence of solely clinical observations in this body of literature call for an occasional dose of healthy skepticism and cautious generalization, especially regarding attempts to formulate conclusions or speculations about the roles of *all* families in coping without specifying a given disorder. The second facet deals with the need for continued research, exploring new conceptualizations, using assessment instruments and indices more directly related to the issues at hand and with more rigorously established validity and reliability, and dealing with adults as well as children, and with siblings and extended family members as well as parents and offspring.

If we have been bold in our critical stance, we do not mean to imply that the literature is inconclusive. The family clearly does play a role in the individual child's adjustment to a chronic illness as well as in the course of the disease itself. However, greater specification is needed regarding the processes by which family influence occurs and regarding those factors and interventions that may enhance the ameliorative or therapeutic roles assumed by family members. The best superordinate conceptualization seems to be that of a reciprocal determinism model (Bandura, 1978), broadly conceived (e.g., Minuchin *et al.*, 1978). Illness is a psychological and social phenomenon as well as a physiological one; this observation is perhaps never more true than when the matter in question is a chronic illness viewed from the perspective of the family.

References

Achenbach, T. M. Psychopathology of childhood: Research problems and issues. *Journal of Consulting and Clinical Psychology*, 1978, *46*, 759–776.

Ack, M. Psychological problems in long-standing insulin-dependent diabetic patients. *Kidney International*, 1974, *6*, 141–143.

Baker, L., Minuchin, S., Milman, L., Liebman, R., & Todd, T. Psychosomatic aspects in juvenile diabetes mellitus: A progress report. In Z. Laron (Ed.), *Diabetes in juveniles: Medical and rehabilitation aspects. Modern problems in pediatrics* (Vol. 12). New York: Karger, 1975.

Bandura, A. The self system in reciprocal determinism. *American Psychologist*, 1978, *33*, 344–358.

Bartmettler, D., & Fields, G. L. Using the group method to study and treat parents of asthmatic children. *Social Work in Health Care*, 1975–1976, *1*, 167–176.

Begleiter, M. L., Burry, V. F., & Harris, D. J. Prevalence of divorce among parents of children with cystic fibrosis and other chronic diseases. *Social Biology*, 1976, *23*, 260–264.

Boll, T. J., & Alpern, G. D. The developmental profile: A new instrument to measure child development through interviews. *Journal of Clinical Child Psychology*, 1975, *4*, 25–27.

Bradley, L. A., Prokop, C. K., & Clayman, D. A. Medical psychology and behavioral medicine: Summary and future concerns. In C. K. Prokop & L. A. Bradley (Eds.), *Medical psychology: Contributions to behavioral medicine*. New York: Academic Press, 1981.

Breslau, N., Weitzman, M., & Messenger, K. Psychologic functioning of siblings of disabled children. *Pediatrics*, 1981, *67*, 344–353.

Bruch, H. Physiologic and psychologic interrelationships in diabetes in children. *Psychosomatic Medicine*, 1948, *11*, 200–210.

Bruetman, M. E., & Gordon, E. E. Rehabilitating the stroke patient at general hospitals. *Postgraduate Medicine*, 1971, *49*, 211–215.

Burke, S. O. *Familial strain and development of normal and handicapped children in single and two parent families*. Unpublished doctoral dissertation, University of Toronto, 1978.

Cairns, N. U., & Lansky, S. B. MMPI indicators of stress and marital discord among parents of children with chronic illness. *Death Education*, 1980, *4*, 29–40.

Cerreto, M. C. *Family development program: Impact of service/training model on the families of chronically ill children*. Grant proposal submitted to Department of Health and Human Services, Administration for Children, Youth, and Families, 1980.

Cerreto, M. C., & Miller, N. B. *Siblings of handicapped children: A review of the literature*. Unpublished manuscript, University of Texas Medical Branch, 1981.

Crain, A. J., Sussman, M. B., & Weil, W. B., Jr. Effect of a diabetic child on marital integration and related measures of family functioning. *Journal of Health and Human Behavior*, 1966, 7, 122–127.

D'Afflitti, J. G., & Weitz, G. W. Rehabilitating the stroke patient through patient–family groups. In R. H. Moos (Ed.), *Coping with physical illness*. New York: Plenum, 1977.

Donofrio, J. C. *A comparison of family verbal interaction patterns in families with an asthmatic, diabetic, and non-disabled child*. Unpublished doctoral dissertation, State University of New York at Buffalo, 1979

Dorner, S. The relationship of physical handicap to stress in families with an adolescent with spina bifida. *Developmental Medicine and Child Neurology*, 1975, 17, 765–776.

Drotar, D., Doershuk, C., Boat, T., Stern, R., Matthews, L., & Boyen, W. Psychosocial functioning of children with cystic fibrosis. *Pediatrics*, 1981, 67, 338–343.

Duvall, E. M. *Marriage and family development*. Philadelphia: Lippincott, 1977.

Freeman, R. D. Emotional reactions of handicapped children. In S. Chess & A. Thomas (Eds.), *Annual progress in child psychiatry and child development*. New York: Brunner/Mazel, 1968.

Gabel, H., McDowell, J., & Cerreto, M. C. Family adaptation to the handicapped infant. In *Educating handicapped infants: Issues in development and intervention*. Rockville, Md.: Aspen Systems Corp., 1983.

Garner, A. M., & Thompson, C. W. Juvenile diabetes. In P. Magrab (Ed.), *Psychological management of pediatric problems* (Vol. I). Baltimore: University Park Press, 1978.

Geiger, K. Deprivation and solidarity in the Soviet urban family. *American Sociological Review*. 1955, 20, 57–68.

Green, M., & Solnit, A. J. Reactions to a threatened loss of a child: A vulnerable child syndrome. *Pediatrics*, 1964, 34, 58–66.

Grey, M. J., Genel, M., & Tamborlane, W. V. Psychosocial adjustment of latency-aged diabetics: Determinants and relationships to control. *Pediatrics*, 1980, 65, 69–73.

Haggerty, R. J. Life stress, illness, and social supports. *Developmental Medicine and Child Neurology*, 1980, 22, 391–400.

Harding, R. K., Heller, J. R., & Kesler, R. W. The chronically ill child in the primary care setting. *Primary Care*, 1979, 6, 311–324.

Hewitt, S. Research on families with handicapped children—an aid or an impediment to understanding? *Birth Defects*, 1976, 12, 35–46.

Hill, R. Social stress on the family. *Social Casework*, 1958, 39, 139–150.

Hobbs, N., McDowell, J., Cerreto, M., & Litchfield, P. *Stress in families with diabetic children: Public policy implications*. Annual Report, Vanderbilt University, 1980.

Hobbs, N., & Perrin, J. *Public policies affecting chronically ill children and their families*. Grant funded by Maternal and Child Health and Bureau of Education for the Handicapped, 1980–1982.

Hymovich, D. P. A framework for measuring outcomes of intervention with the chronically ill child and his family. In G. Graves & I. Pless (Eds.), *Chronic childhood illness* (DHEW Publication No. (NIH) 76-877). Washington, D.C.: U.S. Government Printing Office, 1974.

Hymovich, D. P. *Chronic childhood illness: Family impact and parent coping*. Paper presented at the meeting of the Association for the Care of Children's Health, May 1981.

Johnson, S. B. Psychosocial factors in juvenile diabetes: A review. *Journal of Behavioral Medicine*, 1980, 3, 95–116.

Joosten, J. Accounting for changes in family life of families with spina bifida children. *Zeitschrift für Kinderchir Grenzgeb*, 1979, 28, 412–417.

Kaplan, D. M., Smith, A., Grobstein, R., & Fischman, S. Family mediation of stress. In R. H. Moos (Ed.), *Coping with physical illness*. New York: Plenum, 1977.

Kartha, M., & Ertel, I. J. Short-term group therapy for mothers of leukemic children. *Clinical Pediatrics*, 1976, *15*, 803–806.

Khurana, R. C., & White, P. Attitudes of the diabetic child and his parents toward his illness. *Postgraduate Medicine*, 1970, *48*, 72–76.

Klein, S. D. Measuring the outcome of the impact of chronic childhood illness on the family. In G. Graves & I. Pless (Eds.), *Chronic childhood illness* (DHEW Publication No. (NIH) 76-877). Washington, D.C.: U.S. Government Printing Office, 1974.

Kohut, S. A. The abnormal child: His impact on the family. *Physical Therapy*, 1966, *46*, 160–167.

Kupst, M. J., Blatterbauer, M. A., Westman, J., Schulman, M. D., & Paul, M. H. Helping parents cope with the diagnosis of congenital heart defect: An experimental study. *Pediatrics*, 1977, *59*, 266–272.

Lansky, S. B., Cairns, N. U., Hassanein, R., Wehr, J., & Lowman, J. T. Childhood cancer: Parental discord and divorce. *Pediatrics*, 1978, *62*, 184–188.

Lavigne, J. V., & Ryan, M. Psychologic adjustment of siblings of children with chronic illness. *Pediatrics*, 1979, *63*, 616–627.

Litchfield, P. *Social support, patient satisfaction, and the impact of diabetes on the family.* Unpublished doctoral dissertation, George Peabody College for Teachers of Vanderbilt University, 1981.

Litman, T. J. An analysis of the sociologic factors affecting the rehabilitation of physically handicapped patients. *Archives of Physical Medicine and Rehabilitation*, 1964, *45*, 9–16.

Martin, P. Marital breakdown in families of patients with spina bifida cystica. *Developmental Medicine and Child Neurology*, 1975, *17*, 757–764.

Masur, F. T. Adherence to health care regimens. In C. K. Prokop & L. A. Bradley (Eds.), *Medical psychology: Contributions to behavioral medicine*. New York: Academic Press, 1981.

Mattsson, A. Long term physical illness in childhood: A challenge to psychosocial adaptation. In R. H. Moos (Ed.), *Coping with physical illness*. New York: Plenum, 1977.

Mattsson, A., & Gross, S. Social and behavioral studies of handicapped children. *Developmental Medicine and Child Neurology*, 1973, *15*, 524–530.

McAndrew, I. Children with a handicap and their families. *Child Care, Health, and Development*, 1976, *2*, 213–218.

McCrae, W. M., Cull, A. M., Burton, L., & Dodge, J. Cystic fibrosis: Parents' response to the genetic basis of the disease. *Lancet*, 1973, *2*, 141–143.

McDowell, J. *Social support and stress among parents of diabetic children.* Unpublished doctoral dissertation, George Peabody College for Teachers of Vanderbilt University, 1981.

Menninger, W. C. Psychological factors in the etiology of diabetes. *Journal of Nervous and Mental Disease*, 1935, *18*, 1–13.

Meyer, A., Bollmeier, L. N., & Alexander, F. Correlations between emotions and carbohydrate metabolism in two cases of diabetes mellitus. *Psychosomatic Medicine*, 1945, *7*, 335–341.

Minuchin, S. *Psychosomatic diabetic children and their families* (DHEW Publication No. (ADM) 77-477). Washington, D.C.: U.S. Government Printing Office, 1977.

Minuchin, S., Rosman, B. L., & Baker, L. *Psychosomatic families: Anorexia nervosa in context.* Cambridge, Mass.: Harvard University Press, 1978.

Nevin, R. S., & McCubbin, H. Parental coping with physical handicaps: Social policy implications. *Spina Bifida Therapy*, 1979, *2*, 151–164.

Parsons, T., & Fox, R. C. Illness, therapy, and the modern urban America family. *Journal of Social Issues*, 1952, *8*, 31–44.

Pierre, C., & Cerreto, M. C. *The effects of parent training on stress in families of children with juvenile onset diabetes mellitus.* Investigation in progress, 1981.

Pless, I. B., & Roghmann, K. J. Chronic illness and its consequences: Observations based on three epidemiologic surveys. *The Journal of Pediatrics*, 1971, 79, 351–359.

Pless, I. B., Roghmann, K. J., & Haggerty, R. J. Chronic illness, family functioning, and psychological adjustment. *International Journal of Epidemiology*, 1972, 1, 271–277.

Pond, H. Parental attitudes toward children with a chronic medical disorder: Special reference to diabetes mellitus. *Diabetes Care*, 1979, 2, 425–431.

Prugh, D. G. Toward an understanding of psychosomatic concepts in relation to illness in children. In A. J. Solnit & S. A. Provence (Eds.), *Modern perspectives in child development.* New York: International Universities Press, 1963.

Robertson, E. K., & Suinn, R. M. The determination of rate of progress of stroke patients through empathy measures of patient and family. *Journal of Psychosomatic Research*, 1968, 12, 189–191.

Rutter, M., Tizard, J., & Whitmore, K. *Education, health, and behavior.* London: Longmans, 1970.

Satterwhite, B. B. *Impact of chronic illness on child and family: An overview based on five surveys with implication for management.* Paper presented to the annual meeting of the Ambulatory Pediatric Association, St. Louis, April 1976.

Satterwhite, B. B. Impact of chronic illness on child and family: An overview based on five surveys with implications for management. *International Journal of Rehabilitation Research*, 1978, 1, 7–17.

Saur, W. G. *Social networks and family environments of mothers of multiply, severely handicapped children.* Unpublished doctoral dissertation, Florida State University, 1980.

Schorr, L. B. *The family's interface with social institutions.* Paper presented at the meeting of the American Orthopsychiatric Association, April 1977.

Slimmer, L. W. Helping parents cope with their child's seizure disorder. *Journal of Psychiatric Nursing and Mental Health Services*, 1977, 17, 30–33.

Solnit, A. J., & Stark, M. H. Mourning and the birth of a defective child. *Psychoanalytic Study of the Child*, 1961, 16, 523–537.

Stein, S., & Charles, E. A study of early life experiences of adolescent diabetics. *American Journal of Psychiatry*, 1971, 128, 700–709.

Stein, S., & Charles, E. Emotional factors in juvenile diabetes mellitus: A study of early life experiences of eight diabetic children. *Psychosomatic Medicine*, 1975, 37, 237–244.

Stein, R. E., & Riessman, C. K. The development of an impact-on-the-family scale: Preliminary findings. *Medical Care*, 1980, 18, 465–472.

Stevens, J. H. Parent education programs: What determines effectiveness? *Young Children*, 1978, 33, 59–65.

Swift, C. R., Seidman, F. L., & Stein, H. Adjustment problems in juvenile diabetes. *Psychosomatic Medicine*, 1967, 29, 555–571.

Tarnow, J. D., & Tomlinson, N. Juvenile diabetes: Impact on the child and family. *Psychosomatics*, 1978, 19, 487–491.

Tew, B., & Lawrence, K. M. Some sources of stress found in mothers of spina bifida children. *British Journal of Prevention and Social Medicine*, 1975, 29, 27–30.

Waisbren, S. E. Parents' reactions after the birth of a developmentally disabled child. *American Journal of Mental Deficiency*, 1980, 84, 345–351.

Zimmerman, J. L. *The relationship between support systems and stress in families with a handicapped child.* Unpublished doctoral dissertation, University of Virginia, 1980.

15

The Role of the Nurse in Coping with Chronic Disease*

ADA G. ROGERS

Introduction

The nursing profession has undergone dramatic changes during the past few decades, and Florence Nightingale, the founder of modern nursing, would have approved. As a result of these changes, her dream is finally coming true. That is, education and the provision of health care, the two prime interests of her life, are both becoming major activities within nursing. In a paper that was presented in 1893 at the International Congress of Charities, Correction and Philanthropy, Florence Nightingale defined the education of nurses by saying,

> Training is to teach the nurse to help the patient to live. . . . Training is to teach the nurse how God makes health and how He makes disease. Training is to teach a nurse her business—that is, to observe exactly in such stupendous issues as life and death, health and disease. Training has to make her not servile but loyal to medical orders and authorities. True loyalty to orders cannot be without the independent sense or energy of responsibility which alone secures true trustworthiness. Training is to teach the nurse how to handle the agencies within our control which restore health and life in strict intelligent obedience to the physician's or surgeon's power and knowledge; how to keep the health mechanism prescribed to her in gear. Training must show her how the effects on life of nursing may be calculated with nice precision—such care or carelessness; such a sick rate; such a duration of case, such a death rate [Nutting & Dock, 1907, p. 264].

*Supported in part by Grant (DA 01707) from the National Institute on Drug Abuse, Grant (AG 10441) from the National Institute on Aging, and by Core Grant (CA 08748) from the National Cancer Institute.

In essence, Florence Nightingale proposed that nurses should understand and use fundamental health care principles, observe their patients and make appropriate judgments, and show initiative, as well as cooperate with other health professionals. She even suggested that nurses should conduct their own research and use statistical analyses.

This chapter presents the advances that nursing has made in providing its members with education concerning chronic disease and delivering health care to patients with chronic disease. However, in order to understand the advances made by nursing in these areas, it is necessary to examine the history of nursing.

History of Nursing

RELIGION AND SICK CARE

In most primitive and ancient societies, the sick were treated at home, and their care was the responsibility of the women of the household. One exception to the tradition of females providing sick care was practiced by the Greeks, who built temple–hospitals in which care was given primarily by male priests. The early priest–physicians practiced mystic incantations and magic; these practices began to change during the time of Hippocrates, who advocated systematic observation and study of patients, rational experimentation in treatment, and a critical attitude toward traditional theories and methods. He stressed diet, fresh air, exercise, and other hygienic measures for patients. The young male priest apprentices were taught procedures that included giving baths, bedmaking, lifting and handling patients, the use of hot water bags and bran poultices, bandaging, and rubbing. Nevertheless, the Greeks recognized the importance of women in the health and healing arts, although formal education in healing was not available to them.

The concept that women were responsible for tending to the ill prevailed until the formation of the Christian church. In the first and second centuries, the church required that part of the duty of all Christians was to visit the sick and, when necessary, take the poor and the homeless into their own homes. This church mandate eventually weakened, and after the sixth century the monastic orders, which had absolute control over their male and female members, assumed the care of the sick. The great purpose of these orders was the moral and spiritual discipline of its members as well as of those to whom its members ministered. Because of the hard work and distasteful duties associated with nursing, it was considered by the orders to be an effective way to mortify the flesh and develop humility, patience, and other Christian virtues in their members.

Although very little technical or scientific knowledge regarding health care can be attributed to the monastic orders, they did have an influence on modern nursing. For example, the qualifications of a novice entering a woman's order included legitimate age, high social class, honesty, discretion, and moral fitness. Some orders required a knowledge of Latin, literacy in the national language, and the ability to sing. Each novice went through a probationary period under the direction of an older sister who was responsible for her practical training, religious instruction, and deportment. Novices were rotated from one specialized department within the monastic hospital to another, receiving instruction and discipline from those in charge. As the monastic hospitals grew larger, the nursing work became more specialized. Older sisters or brothers were in charge of the wards, a prioress or prior was responsible for housekeeping, laundry, cooking, and other services involving the institution as a whole, and a secular head administered the business of the hospital. These hospitals, then, developed the first nursing specialties and administrative hierarchies.

The Crusades promoted a new type of order that influenced the care of the sick for several hundred years. Beginning with the Christian knights of the first Crusade (1096–1099) who volunteered to help the monks in Jerusalem, several helping orders eventually developed such as the Knights of St. John of Jerusalem, the Teutonic Knights, and the Knights of St. Lazarus. These orders were instrumental in building and maintaining hospitals along the routes traveled by the Crusaders, particularly during the twelfth and thirteenth centuries. The hospitals were so architecturally beautiful and lavishly equipped that they became known as the "palaces of the poor." Female volunteers, who usually were organized under queens or other women of high rank, cared for the female hospital patients as well as the travelers and orphans who were sheltered in the monasteries. Although the helping orders' hospitals declined following the end of the Crusades, the tradition of voluntary service to hospitals has continued, as currently exemplified by the Red Cross and the activities of lay boards of hospitals and other health care institutions (Stewart, 1947, chap. 1).

Between the thirteenth and sixteenth centuries, new religious organizations that were less rigid than the monastic orders provided nursing care to the ill. For example, the Beguines of Flanders lived in small homes rather than monasteries and provided both hospital and visiting nursing to the poor in their communities. Members of the three orders of St. Francis—the Friars, the Poor Clares, and the Tertiaries—not only cared for the sick in their homes but shared their lives (Stewart, 1947, chap. 1).

The years from 1600 to 1850 represent the darkest period in the history of nursing. During the Protestant Reformation many monasteries were closed, and there remained only a few institutions in which religious orders could nurse the sick. The lay hospitals that did exist lowered their standards of care. Nursing, which the religious orders regarded as having special virtues, now was considered by the lay population as similar to domestic work— except that it was more difficult and disageeable. For example, the first U.S. institutions for the care of the sick were a combination of municipal hospital, poorhouse, insane asylum, house of correction, and orphanage. Bellevue Hospital, established in New York City in 1736, was a classic example of this type of institution. The care givers were prostitutes, drunks, and petty criminals (Stewart, 1947, chap. 1).

DEVELOPMENT OF NURSING TRAINING

Because the United States was primarily a Protestant country, the first Catholic hospital was not established in this country until 1828; however, as early as 1751, progressive doctors and some Protestant church groups such as the Quakers did attempt to make some changes in nurses' provision of health care (Yost, 1947). Dr. Valentine Seaman gave the first course of lectures to nurses on this continent in 1798 at the New York Hospital. A Nurse Society, organized in Philadelphia in 1839, received lectures on maternity care from Dr. Joseph Warrington. Further, a number of Lutheran deaconesses who had received some formal scientific and practical nursing training in Kaiserwerth, Germany were brought to Pittsburgh in 1848 by Pastor William A. Passavant to work in a newly opened Lutheran Hospital (Yost, 1947).

The Kaiserwerth training program also produced Florence Nightingale, who in her work with the British and U.S. armies during the Crimean War and the American Civil War became an internationally recognized authority on the care of the ill. Florence Nightingale stressed that sickness could not be treated apart from its causes, which were not only physical but also mental and social in nature. In this regard, she advocated that nurses should be the missionaries of health, teaching the laws of health to both the sick and the well, regardless of their financial resources. She also felt that in order to practice their profession, nurses needed a theoretical background in scientific and medical subjects and practical experience in disease and treatment. In 1860, Florence Nightingale opened her first school of nursing; she incorporated lectures on anatomy, physiology, chemistry, and surgical and medicine topics into the school's curriculum. Practical duties were taught in the hospital setting and arranged in a series of rotating services that offered the students the opportunity to learn about different diseases and their management (Stewart, 1947, chap. 2).

The first nurses' training school to use the Nightingale system was established at Bellevue Hospital in 1873 (Yost, 1947). There were objections to the new type of nursing training, primarily from physicians who suggested that the new nurses would think they knew as much as or more than doctors or would actually try to study medicine (Thompson, 1883). There also were objections to the training being independent of regulation by physicians (Worcester, 1927). Nevertheless, the Nightingale system gained acceptance from the American medical profession and the public by the end of 1892 (Stewart, 1947, chap. 3).

Nurses made a concerted effort to organize and improve their educational standards during the years between 1893 and 1913 (Stewart, 1947, chap. 4). A standard 3-year training program was adopted in 1894 by nursing schools that wished to graduate students with the title of trained nurse.[1] The period between 1893 and 1913 also was characterized by a growing demand among nurses for specialized training in such areas as obstetrics, surgery and operating room work, and public health (Stewart, 1947, chap. 2). However, at least half a century passed before formal education in some of these specialty areas became available and nurses could achieve recognition as clinical specialists. Indeed, it was not until 1954 that Rutgers University prepared the first master's program for clinical specialists in advanced psychiatric nursing (Smoyak, 1976).

In addition to the development of clinical specialist training for nurses, this century has seen the transfer of many duties that were formerly in the exclusive domain of physicians to other health care professionals such as nurses. For example, since 1965 nurse practitioners have assumed the role of primary care providers, in collaboration with physicians, to patients of all age groups and health needs in various delivery settings—such as schools and emergency rooms in rural, suburban, and urban areas. The nurse practitioner provides continuous, comprehensive, and prevention-oriented care to patients that includes attention to the emotional and social aspects of health and illness (Hayden & Rowell, 1982). The nurse practitioner's typical duties include taking medical histories, performing thorough physical examinations, and ordering tests (e.g., complete blood counts, urinalyses, chest X rays, electrocardiograms, and, when indicated, specialized tests such as endocrine studies of patients with weight problems; Kornguth, 1981).

The transfer of duties from physicians to nurses and other health care professionals has been made necessary in part by public demand for new services as well as by physicians' acquisition of new duties as a result of increasing specialization (Smoyak, 1976). For example, penicillin became

---

[1] Similar to the situation that existed in nursing prior to 1894, it is currently possible to attain the title of registered professional nurse by attaining an associate degree (2-year training program), a diploma (3-year program), or a bachelor's degree (a 4–5-year program). Some nursing educators have proposed that by 1985 the title of registered professional nurse should be given only to those with bachelor's degrees; all nurses with education below the bachelor's level would be called technical nurses.

available for civilian use in 1945. At that time, physicians were required to mix and administer penicillin by intramuscular injection, and nurses were prohibited from performing such injections. Physician protest, however, produced a change in nursing policy; nurses were taught to give intramuscular injections and relieved physicians of the responsibility for all injections.[2]

The Role of Nursing in the Management of Chronic Disease

A national survey showed that in 1977 there were 1,401,633 registered nurses; 26,991 of these nurses were male (Moses & Roth, 1979). Employed in nursing were 70% of the female respondents and 77% of the male respondents; 61.4% of those in nursing were working in hospitals. Of the nurses working in hospitals, 63% reported that they held staff level positions and 57% indicated that their duties involved direct patient care. The major activities of the hospital nurses included medication administration, support of persons who are impaired or ill during diagnostic or therapy programs, and instruction of patients in the management of defined illnesses.

These data indicate that hospital nursing duties include several responsibilities that formerly belonged solely in the domain of physicians. Indeed, the provision of patients' basic care is primarily the responsibility of nurses. Until recently, nurses have had to provide care to patients without the benefit of interaction with health professionals other than the attending physicians. However, as medicine and other health-related disciplines have given greater attention to the management of chronic diseases, nurses increasingly have been incorporated as members of multidisciplinary health care teams that may include psychiatrists, psychologists, physical therapists, social service workers, nutritionists, clergy, and pain specialists (Rogers, 1979b, pp. 103–112).

In the team approach to the management of chronic disease, the nurse's role goes beyond the provision of the basic care of patients. The team nurse usually has the most frequent and intensive contact with patients and their families. Because patients with chronic disease are individuals with distinct sets of problems (which may include environmental, family or social, and emotional factors), the nurse may assess and identify the members of the team who can best treat or manage particular problems. In some instances, members of several disciplines may be required to produce a satisfactory

[2]The author was the first student nurse at New Rochelle Hospital to administer the intramuscular injection.

solution to a problem. For example, even the most experienced nurse may find it difficult to implement her or his skills with patients suffering chronic disease who become overdemanding and manipulative. In this situation, the psychologist can aid in the assessment of the behavioral problem and offer pertinent suggestions that may contribute to the nursing management of the patient.

A review of the nursing literature reveals hundreds of articles that indicate the extent of nurses' efforts to help patients and their families to cope better with chronic disease. The diseases that have attracted the greatest attention from nurses are the cardiovascular diseases, cancer, diabetes mellitus, and obesity. Nevertheless, these diseases and their sequelae, such as chronic pain, require greater understanding by nurses. It is encouraging, however, that nurses are investigating methods to help patients and their families cope with their chronic diseases. It is also encouraging that nurses are learning to cope with, understand, and finally gain satisfaction from caring for patients with chronic disease. No longer must nurses feel that their efforts will be wasted on patients who may never get well.

The remainder of the present chapter presents a brief summary of some of the recent literature concerning nurses' efforts to help patients and their families cope with various chronic diseases. It should be noted that there currently exist few controlled studies of chronic disease within the nursing literature. Rather, there are many case studies and reports of pilot studies. This review, then, features primarily the most promising of the recently published pilot and case studies.

CARDIOVASCULAR DISEASE

Coronary Heart Disease

Coronary heart disease (CHD) is responsible for one-third of all deaths in Western societies (Chesney, Eagleston, & Rosenman, 1981). Approximately one-half of all persons with CHD die before they receive any treatment (Herd, 1981). Nonetheless, the rate of death due to CHD has fallen more than 16% since 1970 (National Heart, Lung, and Blood Institute, 1978). One reason for the decline in the death rate has been the formation and increasing sophistication of hospital coronary care units (CCUs) for the treatment of persons suffering acute manifestations of CHD, such as myocardial infarction. The development of the CCU has made it necessary to extend the role of the nurse in coronary care, and, in essence, develop a new nursing specialty. The nurse in a CCU is responsible for the constant surveillance of the patients, using monitoring devices in order to detect early signs of complications, and, if necessary, promptly starting treatment that may prevent death.

Nurses also must be able to assess the needs of the patient to provide physical comfort, safety, and emotional support.

Research concerning the Type A behavior pattern (Friedman & Rosenman, 1959) can be particularly helpful to the CCU nurse. The Type A pattern consists of a complex set of behaviors "primarily characterized by intense ambition, competitive 'drive,' constant preoccupation with occupational 'deadlines,' and a sense of time urgency [Friedman & Rosenman, 1959, p. 1295]." It has been determined that among males the Type A pattern is associated with twice the risk for clinical coronary disease than the Type B (absence of Type A behavior) pattern, independent of the traditional risk factors of age, cholesterol level, systolic blood pressure, and smoking (Rosenman, Brand, Sholtz, & Friedman, 1976). The results of a pilot study (Gibson, 1980) conducted by a CCU nurse suggests that identification of Type A behaviors may help CCU nurses change the behavior of their patients in order to aid prevention of further coronary events. For example, nurses may help patients make realistic estimates of the time span between meals and tests, supply patients with reading materials (particularly those that patients "have not had time to read") to occupy waiting times, discourage multiphasic behavior (e.g., shaving, eating, and talking on the telephone at the same time), and provide rest periods between activities. In order to reduce the risk of recurrent coronary events further, CCU nurses also may teach the families and friends of Type A patients to identify Type A behaviors and to help the patients adopt a less stressful style of behavior.

Hypertension

Hypertension may be considered a "silent" disease, because hypertensive persons cannot use physical cues to monitor changes in blood pressure levels. Thus, the best treatment approach to hypertension may be prevention on a community-wide basis (see Coates, Perry, Killen, & Slinkard, 1981 for a discussion of several prevention programs). Nurses may have a key role in helping physicians and other health professionals design and implement preventive and other treatment programs for hypertension. The recent nursing literature reveals two major models for nurses' participation in the prevention and treatment of hypertension. These are the crisis model and the Neuman model.

The crisis model posits that persons are engaged in a constant process of growth punctuated by developmental hazardous events and situational hazardous events. The developmental hazardous events include the predictable tasks of various stages of life such as school entry during childhood, development of leisure time activities, and the acceptance of (as well as adjustment to) physiological changes during middle age, and the preparation for death during the latter stages of life. The situational hazardous events include unpredictable events such as the death of a loved one, illness, dissolution of relationships, and changes in life style (similar to the stressful life events identified by Holmes & Rahe, 1967).

Thibodeau and Hebert (1981) provided an example of the use of the crisis model in their protocol for the prevention and treatment of hypertension among the patients in a clinic for senior citizens. Hypertension was the most frequently occurring situational hazardous event among the elderly clinic population. The staff used to implement the protocol varied from junior nursing students in a baccalaureate program to doctoral level nurse practitioners and faculty members.

The protocol for hypertension screening included a procedure for the collection of subjective and objective data and a procedure for referrals for positive findings. Each patient proceeded through the entire protocol on the first visit. The subjective data included the general health status (perceived state of wellness) of each patient, developmental hazardous events, situational hazardous events, risk factors (e.g., smoking, stress, diet), history of hypertension, and symptoms (e.g., coordination difficulties, headache). The objective data consisted of the patient's general appearance; blood pressure in both arms; radial pulse rate, rhythm, and quality; and height and weight.

Patients with combined developmental and situational hazardous events were referred for assessment of coping abilities. Patients with risk factors were referred for further data collection and health teaching. Patients with known hypertension were referred for assessment of knowledge and adherence to treatment. All referrals were made to the nurse practitioners, who in turn determined the type or severity of symptoms for further evaluation and the scheduling of visits to the physician.

This protocol standardized data collection, assured a complete data base on all patients, facilitated decision making on referrals, allowed for the evaluation of students' performances, and provided a method of retrieving information concerning the patients. In addition, the protocol generated questions for furture nursing research, including: Is there a relationship between developmental and situational hazardous events and the onset of hypertension? Can nursing care that is directed to helping persons cope effectively with developmental or situational hazardous events reduce the incidence of hypertension or reduce the incidence of morbidity and mortality in elderly patients with hypertension? Although these questions have not yet been answered, the crisis model and protocols similar to those of Thibodeau and Hebert (1981) may assist nurse practitioners in developing prescriptive theory that can guide clinical practice and improve the quality of care.

Unlike the crisis model, the Neuman model (1974) posits three sets of variables that may influence or be affected by stressors and persons' reactions to stress during various developmental stages. These variables may be intrapersonal (events within the individual, e.g., blood pressure levels), interpersonal (events that occur between two or more individuals, e.g., family relationships), or extrapersonal (events that occur outside the individual, e.g., occupational demands) in nature. The Neuman model has been used to develop guidelines for the assessment of and intervention with hypertensive patients at a large medical center (Utz, 1980). Nurses were required to perform their patient assessments using the following guidelines:

1. Intake summary of demographic data, referral source, and related information.
2. Analysis of stressors based on the patient's perceptions.
3. Analysis of stressors based on the nurse's perceptions.
4. Summary of impressions from 2 and 3.
5. Assessment of three major variables: intrapersonal, interpersonal, and extrapersonal.
6. Formulation of the problem: problem list in order of priorities.

Nurses then were required to develop an intervention for the resolution of each problem, goals for each intervention, and a method for evaluating the extent to which the intervention goals were achieved. It should be noted that these guidelines aided the nurses in conceptualizing their goals in terms of primary, secondary, and tertiary prevention. Thus, the nurses were prompted to help their patients make a transition from focusing on the problems associated with illness to coping effectively with those problems and attempting to prevent the development of further difficulties.

DIABETES MELLITUS

Diabetes mellitus is similar to hypertension in that it is a silent disease requiring patients to change their life-styles in order to cope effectively and prevent additional complications (see Turk & Speers, Chapter 8). To maintain health and a symptom-free, active life, patients must regulate their diets and/or medication intake in order to control the disease. The crisis and Neuman models of nursing previously described can be applied to the treatment of diabetic patients. In addition, Gaines (1980) has suggested that nurses may use the SOAP method to aid their treatment planning for patients who suffer complictions (e.g., renal disease) from diabetes. SOAP is an acronym for the four parts of a problem list (Peterson, 1977; Weed, 1964). S stands for subjective data that provide a record of the patient's attitude regarding his or her disease. O stands for objective data including physical findings, laboratory test results and a record of all treatments administered to the patient. A represents assessment of the patient's difficulties (i.e., physical complications as well as behaviors that exacerbate his or her difficulties) based on subjective and objective data. P stands for a treatment plan based on the assessment of the patient's condition. Gaines (1980) described the treatment of a diabetic patient who also suffered from obesity and hypertension. The nurse assigned to the patient hypothesized that the patient had failed to comply with the low-salt, low-calorie diet prescribed for him. The patient's noncompliance was confirmed; in addition, it was discovered that the patient was suffering congestive heart failure. Congestive heart failure is particularly dangerous to a diabetic patient because it can stimulate a stress response that may cause an elevation in blood sugar. With the use of the SOAP method, the nurse was able to evaluate the patient's physical and behavioral responses to treatment. The careful monitoring of the patient's treatments and responses enabled the nurse to establish good rapport with the patient and to use every opportunity to explain to the patient each treatment, what it entailed, and why it was important. After a few days, the patient's condition stablized; however, he could not leave the hospital until he had a teaching session with the nurse who reviewed the medication he would be taking after discharge, the symptoms of high and low potassium, and the need to follow a low-sodium, low-calorie diet strictly. It was anticipated that the reinforcement of what the patient had been taught during hospitalization would improve his compliance with the diet in his home environment.

OBESITY

It has been estimated (Braunstein, 1971) that at least 30% of the adult population in the United States is obese and that the number of obese adults is increasing. However, it is difficult to obtain an accurate estimate of the prevalence of adult obesity, primarily because of the lack of consensus on the criteria for obesity and weight change (Stuart, Mitchell, & Jensen, 1981). For example, insurance companies (American Council of Life Insurance, 1976) generally compare an individual's weight to a standard table of ideal weights stratified by age, sex, height, and frame. It has been suggested (Craft, 1972; Dwyer, Feldman, & Mayer, 1970) that an individual who is at least 20% above optimal weight for age, sex, height, and body frame standards should be considered obese. This criterion, however, does not take into account the ratio between lean body mass and adipose tissue (e.g., Brozek & Kinzey, 1960). In addition to the difficulties associated with the assessment of obesity, there are many problems involved in helping patients who are classified as obese to achieve significant long-term weight losses (see Straw, Chapter 9).

Despite these difficulties, many nurses have become involved in both the assessment and management of obese patients. The assessment of obesity incorporates psychological, physiological, and sociocultural variables. White and Shroeder (1981) have suggested that nurses initially should interview the obese patient in order to determine his or her (a) circumstances at the onset of obesity, (b) usual patterns of weight gain and loss, (c) emotions associated with eating or overeating, (d) desire and ability to change current eating behavior and activity pattern, (e) cognitions concerning behavior change, and (f) eating or activity patterns that may be culturally defined. The information obtained in the initial interview will allow nurses to plan, implement, and evaluate the care of the obese patient. In addition, nurses should perform periodic reassessments that will produce the information necessary for the provision of individualized management plans.

Kornguth (1981) has noted that the role of nurses in the management of obese patients includes (a) education concerning diet; (b) aid in the development of realistic goals for adjustment of caloric intake and weight loss; (c) consultation with or referral to a physical therapist for the development of an exercise program; and (d) psychological support or, if necessary, referral for psychotherapy. Implementation of these duties requires long-term and persistent monitoring of patients. In fact, Kornguth (1981) has suggested that persons involved in the management of obese patients should see each patient at least once every 2 weeks and during follow-up periods should evaluate any chronic health problems that were present at the beginning of treatment. Because nurses tend to have the most frequent and intimate contact with patients in obesity management and other health care programs, they are of paramount importance in promoting weight loss and maintenance of health among obese patients.

CANCER

With the development of new pharmacological and surgical treatments for various forms of cancer during the 1970s and 1980s, the nursing profession has had to recognize cancer nursing as a specialty with unique training requirements (Rogers, 1979b). For example, schools and colleges of nursing have begun to include cancer nursing courses as part of their curricula. Cancer hospitals and cancer units also have had to update information in their in-service education programs to ensure quality in patient care.

The specialized education of cancer nurses is necessary because they must give comprehensive care to patients who have complex physical and emotional needs and who often are in crisis situations (Rogers, 1979a). Cancer nurses also have attempted to meet the needs of their patients better by recognizing that they and the families of their patients may contribute to the patients' difficulties in coping with cancer. Some hospitals, therefore, provide weekly meetings with a psychiatrist or a psychologist to help the cancer nurses air their feelings and frustrations in dealing with a particular patient or patient's family. In turn, the cancer nurses encourage patients and their families to meet with them in order to discuss mutual problems and possible solutions. The nurses also require discharge planning early in a patient's hospitalization. Early discharge planning is necessary to evaluate whether or not family members will be able to cope with the care of the cancer patient, particularly those in the terminal disease stages. Discharge planning also allows cancer nurses to determine the various support systems the family and the patient may require. If home care of the patient seems untenable, hospice care may be necessary. However, as the durations of the patient hospitalizations diminish, nurses eventually may have to provide the bulk of the care to patients who are discharged to their homes.

Future Roles of Nursing in Chronic Disease

It is apparent that the medical profession is characterized not only by specialty areas, such as internal medicine, but also by subspecialty areas such as cardiology, gastroenterology, and hematology. The nursing profession also is developing specialty areas for (a) specific diseases such as cancer; (b) patient classifications such as premature babies, adolescents, and the elderly; and (c) particular services such as those provided by the ostomy nurse and the intravenous (IV) nurse. It is reasonable to assume that nursing specialties will be developed for many of the chronic diseases discussed in this chapter and volume, as has been the case with cancer.

Some of the chronic diseases discussed in the present volume are characterized by chronic pain (e.g., cancer, diabetes, coronary heart disease). A small number of nurses already have relinquished their traditional roles and are devoting their efforts to the management of pain.[3] The need for nurses trained in pain management is particuarly acute because medical specialists who treat diseases associated with chronic pain generally have insufficient knowledge regarding effective management of pain. Hence, clinical nurse specialists and/or nurse practitioners can be—and will become increasingly—valuable in the role of pain managers or pain consultants. The pain manager or consultant may take a complete history of the patient's pain problem, perform a brief physical examination, and evaluate the effectiveness or ineffectiveness of analgesics or other modalities used for the control of the patient's pain. He or she may follow the patient until discharge and recommend whether or not the patient should be seen as an outpatient for

[3]The author knows of one nurse who has obtained a master's degree in chronic pain management from the University of Virginia.

further pain treatment (e.g., in a pain clinic). The pain manager or consultant may also receive telephone calls from the patient after discharge concerning pain or other problems related to the disease and provide appropriate suggestions. The accessibility of the pain manager or consultant to the patient may lessen patient anxiety at discharge and during follow-up as well as free physicians from follow-up care that can be performed equally well by nurses. Finally, the pain manager or consultant may see the patient at follow-up visits before the physician examines the patient. This procedure may give the patient the opportunity to air feelings or complaints to an individual who has been closely involved in the patient's care and thus may best respond to the patient's needs.

The pain manager or consultant may also assist the staff nurses, participate in in-service education programs, and conduct ward conferences. As a member of the treatment team, the pain manager may interact and share knowledge with nurses, medical and surgical house staff, attending medical staff, and other allied health professionals.

In summary, it has been recommended (Bonica, 1974) that all physicians be encouraged to consider chronic pain as a major disease. However, the amount of time and effort required of physicians to provide the proper care of chronic pain patients may be prohibitive. It may be more expedient to increase the number of nurses who are educated in the assessment and treatment of chronic pain and have them function as pain managers or consultants.

Conclusions

Nurses have had great difficulty being accepted—primarily by physicians—as an intrinsic part of the health care delivery system. This has paralleled the struggle of many minority groups in our society. The vision and strength of a few leaders, such as Florence Nightingale, has made it possible for nurses not only to develop new technical skills, but, more importantly, to develop an awareness of their part in human welfare. The advances made in nursing have helped nurses become more involved in helping patients cope with their diseases. Recently, through the use of scientific methods, they have developed new means of approaching problems in chronic diseases. However, it is important for nurses to define clearly their role in health care in order to avoid conflict between nursing and the other health professions and to avoid distorted ideas of nursing among other health professionals.

The future of nurses and nursing depends on the acceptance of nurses' input as health team members. But nurses must also be team players and accept input from others. The ultimate goal is to help the patient understand his or her life processes so that he or she can better control and cope with illness (Carlson, 1972).

Acknowledgments

I wish to thank Elise Frank for her assistance in the literature search and in the preparation of the manuscript.

References

American Council of Life Insurance. *Life insurance fact book.* New York: Author, 1976.

Bonica, J. J. General clinical considerations (including organization and function of a pain clinic). In J. J. Bonica, P. Procacci, & C. A. Pagni (Eds.), *Recent advances on pain: Pathophysiology and clinical aspects.* Springfield, Ill.: Thomas, 1974.

Braunstein, J. J. Management of the obese patient. *Medical Clinics of North America,* 1971, 55, 391–401.

Brozek, J., & Kinzey, W. Age changes in skinfold compressibility. *Journal of Gerontology,* 1960, 15, 45–51.

Carlson, S. A practical approach to nursing practice. *American Journal of Nursing,* 1972, 72, 1589–1591.

Chesney, M. A., Eagleston, J. R., & Rosenman, R. H. Type A behavior: Assessment and intervention. In C. K. Prokop & L. A. Bradley (Eds.), *Medical psychology: Contributions to behavioral medicine.* New York: Academic Press, 1981.

Coates, T. J., Perry, C., Killen, J., & Slinkard, L. A. Primary prevention of cardiovascular disease in children and adolescents. In C. K. Prokop & L. A. Bradley (Eds.), *Medical psychology: Contributions to behavioral medicine.* New York: Academic Press, 1981.

Craft, C. Body image and obesity. *Nursing Clinics of North America,* 1972, 7, 677–685.

Dwyer, J. T., Feldman, J., & Mayer, J. The social psychology of dieting. *Journal of Health and Social Behavior,* 1970, 11, 269–278.

Friedman, M. & Rosenman, R. H. Association of specific overt behavior pattern with blood and cardiovascular findings—blood cholesterol level, blood clotting time, incidence of arcus senilis, and clinical coronary artery disease. *Journal of the American Medical Association,* 1959, 169, 1286–1296.

Gaines, H. P. The multi-problem patient. *The Journal of Practical Nursing,* 1980, 30, 13–16.

Gibson, K. T. The Type A personality: Implications for nursing practice. *Cardiovascular Nursing,* 1980, 16, 25–28.

Hayden, M. L. & Rowell, P. Hospital privileges: Rationale and process. *Nurse Practitioner,* 1982, 7, 42–44.

Herd, J. A. Treatment of cardiovascular disorders. In C. K. Prokop & L. A. Bradley (Eds.), *Medical psychology: Contributions to behavioral medicine.* New York: Academic Press, 1981.

Holmes, T. H. & Rahe, R. H. The social readjustment rating scale. *Journal of Psychosomatic Research,* 1967, 11, 213–218.

Kornguth, M. L. Nursing management. *American Journal of Nursing*, 1981, *81*, 553–554.

Moses, E., & Roth, H. Nursepower. *American Journal of Nursing*, 1979, 79, 1745–1756.

National Heart, Lung, and Blood Institute. *National Heart, Lung, and Blood Institute's fact book for fiscal year 1978* (DHEW Publication No. [NIH]79-1656). Washington, D.C.: National Institutes of Health, 1978.

Neuman, B. Betty Neuman health care systems model: A total person approach to patient problems. In J. Riehl & C. Roy (Eds.), *Conceptual models for nursing practice*. New York: Appleton-Century-Crofts, 1974.

Nutting A., & Dock, L. *History of Nursing* (Vol. 2). New York: Putnam, 1907.

Peterson, G. Problem oriented medical records, Part II. Bringing the SOAP revolution home. *Journal of Practical Nursing*, 1977, *27*, 32–35.

Rogers, A. G. Psychosocial and nursing technique. In J. J. Bonica & V. Ventafridda (Eds.), *Advances in pain research and therapy* (Vol. 2). New York: Raven Press, 1979. (a)

Rogers, A. G. Sociological and nursing aspects of cancer pain. In J. J. Bonica & V. Ventafridda (Eds.), *Advances in pain research and therapy* (Vol. 2). New York: Raven Press, 1979. (b)

Rosenman, R., Brand, R. J., Sholtz, R., & Friedman, M. Multivariate prediction of coronary heart disease during 8.5 year follow-up in the Western Collaborative Group Study. *American Journal of Cardiology*, 1976, *37*, 903–910.

Smoyak, A. Specialization in nursing: From then to now. *Nursing Outlook*, 1976, *24*, 676–681.

Stewart, I. M. *The education of nurses*. New York: Macmillan, 1947.

Stuart, R. B., Mitchell, C., & Jensen, J. A. Therapeutic options in the management of obesity. In C. K. Prokop & L. A. Bradley (Eds.), *Medical psychology: Contributions to behavioral medicine*. New York: Academic Press, 1981.

Thibodeau, A., & Hebert, P. Use of a nursing model to develop a hypertension protocol. *Nurse Practitioner*, 1981, *6*, 21–27.

Thompson, W. G. *Training schools for nurses (Summary of the work of twenty-two schools)*. New York: Putnam, 1883.

Utz, S. W. Applying the Neuman model to nursing practice with hypertensive clients. *Cardiovascular Nursing*, 1980, *16*, 29–34.

Weed, L. L. Medical records, patient care and medical education. *Irish Journal of Medical Science*, 1964, *6*, 271–282.

White, J. H., & Schroeder, M. A. Nursing assessment. *American Journal of Nursing*, 1981, *81*, 550–553.

Worcester, A. *Nurses and nursing*. Cambridge, Mass.: Harvard University Press, 1927.

Yost, E. *American women of nursing*. New York: Lippincott, 1947.

16

The Process of Death and Dying:
Behavioral and Social Factors

SANDRA M. LEVY

Introduction

There is an inherent difficulty in writing a chapter concerned with death and dying. In contrast with a specific disease state such as hypertension that can be managed medically and behaviorally, dying is a process that is physically, psychologically, and philosophically difficult to define.

Although we are accustomed to thinking of development in discrete stages, clearly life is a gradual process of growth and decay. In this sense, death itself is not a single event. Today with the aid of science the gradual process of dying is more evident than ever before—but just *when* the process begins is a matter of social judgment. That is, scientifically we realize that various parts of the body can go on "living" for months after the disintegration of its central organization. On the cellular level, some cell lines can be continued indefinitely. And of course, now the

> constant tinkering of man with his own machinery has made it obvious that death is not really a very easily identifiable event or 'configuration.' . . . death does not come by inevitable appointment, in Samarra or anywhere else. He must sit patiently in the waiting room until summoned by the doctor or nurse [Weir, 1977, p. 60].

To assert that the definition of the dying process is based on social judgment is not to deny that biological changes are marked (e.g., cachexia and wasting in an advanced cancer patient or muscle tissue decay and sloughing in cases of massive myocardial infarction). Nor does this assertion deny the need for symptom control in patients who are dying (e.g., pain or appetite

COPING WITH
CHRONIC DISEASE

management) or deny the need for behavioral intervention for patients and families in order to develop coping strategies. Indeed, such symptom management and coping intervention is the major concern of this chapter. But an understanding at the inception that dying itself is a complex biological–psychological–social process and defining boundaries of concern that are not shared by other topics in this text provide a distinct framework for this chapter.

As the title of this book suggests, the focus of this chapter is on "natural" death, and not on dying by suicide, accident, or natural disaster. As others point out in this volume, the leading causes of natural death in the United States have shifted from acute infection to chronic disease, particularly neoplasia.[1] Even though the percentage of deaths from cancer has drastically increased, cardiovascular disease is still the leading cause of death. This represents a major shift in cause of mortality compared to causes in the death statistics of 1900. At the turn of the century, cerebral vascular accidents and malignant neoplasms together accounted for only 10% of all deaths; influenza, pneumonia, and tuberculosis accounted for 23% of mortality incidence. These same shifts in cause of death can be seen in other industrialized countries (Guberan, 1979).

It is interesting that, despite the rank order of causes of death, most of the literature concerned with death and dying focuses on death from cancer. For example, only approximately 3 out of 40 chapters in a book concerned with dying (Garfield, 1978) dealt with death from causes other than cancer. As Susan Sontag (1979) pointed out, cancer today (in contrast with tuberculosis in the last century) is an inherently mysterious and hence fearful disease. Because it is not readily controllable, it conjures up fantasy, and excessive psychological meaning becomes attached to the disease. Most of the research and writing in the area of death and dying has focused on death from uncontrollable duplication of cells and associated physical wasting. The reader will need to keep in mind this state of affairs as examples from the research literature are discussed.

This chapter is organized into three basic sections. The first section is concerned with the dying patient—both pediatric and adult—and the focus is on symptom control. The second section is concerned with the social structure of dying, including the interpersonal nature of the process as well as forms of social support. The context or place for dying will also be examined. The third section of this chapter considers emerging ethical issues related to dying, including survival by machine and being allowed to die.

---

[1]It should be pointed out, however, that according to age-adjusted figures death from cancer in middle age has remained stable or in fact decreased over the 50 years from the 1930s to 1980s. Cancer is a disease of the elderly, so as more people are living into old age the overall incidence of cancer has gone up. This does not, however, represent a cancer epidemic.

Although this book is primarily concerned with behavioral factors as they contribute to chronic disease processes, because of the complexities already alluded to in the very definition of this present topic, we must return to the conceptual boundaries of dying and consider the complexities again in the light of symptom management and social context.

The Dying Patient: Symptom Control

I am not concerned here with developmental issues related to dying, such as life-span developmental stages (for example, stages in awareness of dying and the concept of death as it develops in childhood and adolescence) or stages of actually dying (for example, Kubler-Ross's [1974] stages of dying, from denial through acceptance). The former will only be touched upon where relevant to symptom management in terminal pediatric patients. The latter stages-of-dying concept has little empirical support and will therefore not be considered further here. Instead, I first explore general issues (for example, truth telling in regard to terminal status), then consider the special issue of pain control, and finally discuss at some length a relatively new approach to symptom management in dying patients—behavioral thanatology (Sobel, 1981).

Very little work has been done with pediatric patients that is specifically directed at managing problems associated with dying. Although considerable attention has been devoted to the general area of stress management in seriously ill children, for the most part this work does not relate directly to problems of dying. Of the work that has been directed toward the dying child, most focuses on the family context Most of the literature has been concerned with the dying adult.

SYMPTOM MANAGEMENT IN THE DYING ADULT

Truth Telling and Psychotherapy

In both an early study (Kelly & Friesen, 1950) with chronically ill patients, half of whom had cancer, and in a more recent study of a random community sample (Kalish & Reynolds, 1976), the data indicated that more people said that they wished to be told if they had cancer or were dying than felt that others like themselves should be told. There were also ethnic differences in response. Specifically, in the Kalish and Reynolds study 60% of the black respondents, 49% of the Japanese–Americans, 37% of the Mexican–Americans, and 71% of the Anglos replied affirmatively that they would tell a friend that the friend was dying. However, more than 70% of each ethnic group except Mexican–Americans responded that they themselves would want to be told. In this study, only 60% of Mexican–Americans reported wanting to know about their own terminal condition.

In a report utilizing the psychological autopsy as a technique for analyzing death awareness and interpersonal response in dying geriatric patients, Kastenbaum (1967) reported that a large proportion of those who were dying were aware of their state, and many spoke openly about their approaching death. In Glaser and Strauss's (1965) qualitative analysis of patients' awareness of dying, their findings suggested that an open awareness (in contrast with mutual pretense or suspicion) was more beneficial for patients and their families. In general, people say they want to know of their disease status and seem to fare better when they do know, although, individual differences exist (Sobel, 1981).

There is still much need for research in this area of truth telling. Although it is very common in the United States to inform patients of their terminal conditions (often within the context of experimental therapeutics and the need for informed consent), the *manner* of communicating, interacting with, for example, ethnic group or cohort differences, needs to be carefully examined.

Traditional Interventions

Before the areas of terminal pain management and behavioral thanatology are addressed, more traditional forms of intervention with dying patients should be mentioned. Shneidman (1978) has written extensively about the nature of psychotherapy with dying patients, and differentiates it from other forms of therapeutic intervention. According to this author, given the "unnegotiable circumstances of the terminal disease [Shneidman, 1978, p. 207]," aspects of psychotherapy with dying patients are unique. For example, in contrast with traditional therapy, the therapist working with a dying patient may deliberately cross personal boundaries and attempt to create a situation of intense emotional involvement. The stark reality is that the patient will die soon, so that ethically speaking, the therapist can afford quickly to become a key, significant figure in the dying person's life [p. 209]."

Findings from the Omega Project (Weisman, Worden, & Sobel, 1980; Worden & Sobel, 1978) suggest that not all dying patients need special therapeutic intervention. These investigators have developed measurements of at-risk status that allow for the identification of patients early in their dying trajectory who are likely to need specialized, professional support. Out of this work at Massachusetts General Hospital has emerged a cognitive–behavioral approach to general symptom management in the dying. We discuss this form of intervention in the section on "Cognitive–Behavioral Thanatology."

Pain Management

Although a great deal of research has been carried out on the management of pain associated with a number of clinical conditions (Melzack, 1973; Melzack & Wall, 1965), little work has been done in the area of pain associated with dying. Questions that need to be addressed include whether the pain associated with terminal illness differs in some way from that associated with a nonterminal condition and if the pain associated with one terminal illness differs from the pain associated with a different terminal illness. For example, phenomenologically and clinically, how does the experience and management of pain associated with terminal cardiovascular disease differ from that associated with multiple myeloma (a painful form of bone cancer where immature white blood cells take over the bone marrow space and burst through the surrounding bone tissue)? Certainly not all dying patients experience pain. But for those who do, more likely than not the experience is characterized by intractability and increasing intensity over time (Oster, Vizel, & Turgeon, 1978).

In a retrospective study of pain intensity in terminal patients, Oster *et al.* (1978) analyzed the nature and dosage of analgesic administration in 90 hospitalized patients in their last week of life. The validity of operationally defining pain by medication dosage might be questioned (obviously, a patient could be in great pain, but too weak or unassertive to report his or her experience and demand help). Nevertheless, using archival data from charts and nursing notes, these researchers found that patients dying with cancer had significantly higher preterminal daily pain ratings and significantly fewer pain-free days than patients dying of cardiac, gastrointestinal, neurological, renal, or pulmonary conditions. However, it should also be noted that approximately 25% of cancer patients apparently die pain-free, at least as evidenced by lack of pain medication administration.

Weakness is the most common symptom in dying patients, but pain, dyspnea, and cough are the symptoms that require immediate management (Twycross, 1978). The use of an opiate with phenothiazine is one of the more effective ways of easing dyspnea and cough and decreasing the associated fear and anxiety that accompany them. Pain itself is typically controlled pharamacologically (e.g., with morphine or dyamorphine), but some types of pain respond better to radiation and nerve blockage than to drugs (Twycross, 1978).

In recent years, Brompton's mixture (Lipman, 1975) has gained attention as a pharamacological method of reducing the experience of intractable pain in the dying. First introduced at St. Christopher's Hospice in England, it has also been used in Canada and on an experimental basis in this country. Melzack, Ofiesh, and Mount (1978) reported an interaction between *place* of care and the use of the Brompton mixture in pain control. They found that patients who received the mixture within the context of a palliative care unit achieved better pain control than patients in a general ward or private care rooms.

Melzack *et al.* interpreted their findings as lending support to the gate-control theory of pain (Melzack & Wall, 1965). Within this theoretical framework, the experience of pain is determined by not only tissue injury, but also by anxiety and expectation. The theory suggests that the amount of input transmitted from peripheral fibers to the brain is determined both by somatic sensory input and by brain activities that exert a descending influence on the gate system. When the amount of input to the brain exceeds a critical level, the resulting pain experience involves the sensory dimension of pain, unpleasant affect, and an evaluative, cognitive dimension (Melzack *et al.*, 1978). Morphine acts at many neural levels (including the brainstem) and both morphine and the phenothiazines decrease anxiety, thus affecting the evaluative component of the pain experience. Again, however, the environmental context was found to contribute to the experience of pain, with a larger proportion of patients within a palliative context achieving pain control (90% versus 75% and 80% for ward and private room patients, respectively). The context itself may have played a role in decreasing negative expectancies and anxiety levels.

Adequate pain control is usually achieved by the use of narcotics, but concern is often expressed about the addictive potential of such drug use (Mount, Ajemian, & Scott, 1978). However, dependence has not been reported as a problem when narcotics are used for the pain of malignant disease (Evans, 1971; Twycross, 1974). In fact, it has been suggested that the excessive concern about the danger of addiction has led to the undertreatment of pain in the hospitalized terminal patient, and that such undertreatment may encourage craving and psychological dependence (Mount *et al.*, 1978).

Some work has been carried out using behavioral means to affect pain experience and expression (Redd, 1982). Based on the early work of Fordyce (1973, 1976), Redd used time out from social stimulation contingent upon crying and other forms of pain expression in a terminal cancer patient. At the same time, he instituted differential social reinforcement for behavior incompatible with pain expression (e.g., talking with family members). Over the 15-day intervention period, crying greatly decreased and was replaced by increased frequency and longer duration of family visits. The frequency of positive statements made by the patient and conversation on his part also increased.

Although Redd discussed the clinical and ethical issues surrounding such an intervention with a dying patient, he failed to consider alternative hypotheses for the shift in behavioral patterns shown by the patient. Rather than the decreased crying and increased socialization being functions merely of social contingencies, other factors could have contributed to the behavioral change. For example, as the patient slipped closer to death (he died shortly after the intervention terminated), he could have experienced an altered sensorium that might have affected his perceptual sensitivity or cognitive interpretation of symptom experience. In addition, the patient could well have had an awareness of impending death, prompting increased communication with family members despite the presence of pain.

Nevertheless, as Kelly (1955) discussed earlier, behavioral change in many cases precedes and alters the construction of events. In addition to the powerful control of terminal pain through the use of narcotics, behavioral and cognitive shaping may also contribute to pain management.

Cognitive–Behavioral Thanatology

In recent years there has been a general rise in the use of cognitive–behavioral techniques not only for the systematic management of clinical conditions ranging from alcoholism to schizophrenia, but also to the management of dying itself (Rebok & Hoyer, 1974; Whitman & Lukes, 1975). For example, Preston (1973) discussed the use of cognitive training to disrupt the disturbing thoughts, feelings, and behaviors of those who are dying, enabling them to concentrate on "images, faces, events, landscapes, or memories with warm, happy, or exciting connotations [p. 65]."

A volume by Sobel (1981) focused entirely on behavior therapy with the terminally ill. In this work, behavioral thanatology is presented as an alternative to traditional approaches to terminal care, including the existential, humanistic, and psychodynamic schools of thought. Paraphrasing the Yale Conference's definition of behavioral medicine (Schwartz & Weiss, 1977), Sobel defines behavioral thanatology as a subfield of behavioral medicine concerned with the development of behavioral science knowledge and techniques relevant to the understanding of terminal illness, life-threatening behavior, and grief. Behavioral thanatology also involves the application of this knowledge and these techniques to the treatment of those who are dying, as well as those who are bereaved, and to the treatment of the patient manifesting life-threatening behavior.

Despite reservations expressed by some professionals that behavioral approaches applied to the terminally ill could be disrespectful or denial-enhancing, Sobel and others present a persuasive case for helping the patient to live realistically and practically with his or her terminal condition:

> The behavioral consultant offers the "death-bored" patient an alternative strategy for living with dying, a strategy that teaches problem-solving in the service of comfort, self-

control, and, to borrow Weisman's (1972) concept, an "appropriate death." An appropriate death does not mean that a patient is maneuvered to die the way we might choose to
die [p. 15].

Sobel adopts a systems perspective (Miller, 1978), and views the patient as
inextricably caught up in a biopsychosocial network. The patient is considered a co-therapist or collaborator (Fischer, 1970) in restoring self-control in
the face of impending death. With emphasis on the role of cognition in self-
control, patients are taught to observe inner and outer events and their
contingencies, to initiate self-administered consequences to specific behaviors, to plan environmental and stimulus modifications, and to maintain,
record, and assess new behaviors or cognitions over time (Beck, 1976; Ellis,
1973).

Although Sobel has provided clinical examples of this form of intervention
with terminal patients, little empirical research has been done utilizing
these techniques for patients who are dying and for their families. As Sobel
pointed out, however, because of the explicit cognitive–behavioral assessment and goal setting that such an approach provides, systematic research
on symptom control in these patients is possible. Certainly, cognitive–behavioral thanatology might prove to be one effective option in the total care
of those who are dying, and might offer a way to restore some dignity in the
form of self-control to those who feel all options being stripped away.

SYMPTOM MANAGEMENT IN THE DYING CHILD

"For every child who dies, many more suffer. Both terminal care and
symptom control in childhood have been neglected areas [Chapman &
Goodall, 1980, p. 753]." In this article, Chapman and Goodall emphasized
the need for adequate symptom control in children who are clearly dying.
They also pointed out that physicians have a difficult time deciding when to
stop intensive medical activity aimed at curing and provide palliation only
for the child. "Science must not blind us to art: What we could do is not
necessarily what we should do [p. 756]." Most of Chapman and Goodall's
focus, in fact, is on pain control in pediatric patients, both with drugs and
also with diversionary tactics of one form or another. Regarding pharmacological control, they pointed out that much more research is needed on
dosages of narcotics for children.

A number of reports (Adams, 1979; Iles, 1979; Peck, 1980) have appeared
on the psychosocial care of the dying child within the family context. Peck
(1980) assumed the position that after repeated relapses have demonstrated
that the disease is incurable, it is important for the parents to make up for
previous neglect of the child's siblings and make the latter aware of the dying

child's state. Peck and others (Garfield, 1978) have counseled the family against being too morbid and instead to try to include the dying child in family life as much as possible. Whether the child dies at home or in the hospital should depend on the parents' wishes and their own assessment of their coping capacities. They may also wish to have a nurse present as death approaches, but Peck advises the parents "to remain alone with the child for awhile after death has occurred [p. 34]."

Awareness of Impending Death

There has been for some years a question of the cognitive awareness of impending death in very young children who are dying (Spinetta, 1974). Chapman and Goodall (1980) provided a case history of a patient who was 9½ years old when first diagnosed as having a sarcoma invading the brachial plexus, and nearly 13 when she died. Toward the end she asked her radiation therapist not to waste time on her because she was going to die.

In a review of the research related to this issue, Spinetta (1974) concluded that there appears to be a genuine awareness in children as young as 6 of the morbidity of their illness. In Bluebond-Langner's (1977) doctoral research on the meaning of personal death to children, she found the child's acquisition of information about his or her terminal condition is a prolonged process involving experiences with the disease and others as well as changes in self-concept. Specifically, she conceptualized five stages of awareness. Stage I is the child's beginning awareness of being seriously ill; Stage II, during remission, is the awareness of being seriously ill with the assumption of getting better. Stage III, after the first relapse, is the child's awareness of always being ill but still with the assumption of getting better. Stage IV, after repeated relapses, is the view of the self as always ill and never getting better. Finally, at Stage V, when learning of the death of a peer, the child realizes that he or she is also, in fact, dying.

An interesting aspect of Bluebond-Langner's (1977) clinical–phenomenological analysis is that the child's awareness is predicated upon his or her ability to integrate and synthesize information that seems to rest on social experience and not merely on cognitive ability or age:

> There are three—and four—year-olds of average intelligence who know more about their prognosis than many intelligent, nine-year-olds. The reason for this is that nine-year-olds may still be in their first remission, have had fewer clinic visits, and hence, less experience. They are only aware of the fact that they have a very serious illness [p. 54]."

Therapeutically, Bluebond-Langner stresses the importance of realizing where the child is in terms of awareness based on his or her own experience. She cautions the clinician to answer only what is asked and to answer in the child's own terms. This researcher also found that children are only selectively open to those around them, and although these dying children seem to want to express their awareness, they do not want to risk being left alone.

Dying Child's Syndrome

The "dying child's syndrome" (i.e., the dying child's sense of isolation and the psychological withdrawal of family members from his or her presence) has been addressed by others (Chapman & Goodall, 1980; Willis, 1974). For example, Spinetta and his colleagues (Spinetta, 1973, 1978; Spinetta, Rigler, & Karon, 1974) have systematically examined the dying child's sense of isolation from family and medical care givers. Utilizing interpersonal distance measures in the form of figurine placements in a three-dimensional space, these researchers found that dying children placed parental and health care figures significantly farther away from the sick child figure than did hospitalized chronically ill controls. A placement of *preferred* distance revealed that fatally ill children not only perceived a growing psychological distance from those around them, but also preferred it that way.

Spinetta and co-workers interpreted their findings within a social learning framework. That is, perceived and preferred interpersonal distance were seen as being a function of the child's prior history of social reinforcement in general, and the reinforcement history associated with the context in which the social distance behavior occurs in particular. That is, the child was more likely to perceive and prefer a greater spatial distance from others as a function of past, as well as current, isolating maneuvers by those around him or her. Although these investigators discussed a number of explanatory possibilities for their findings (including differential medication in the two groups of children), they concluded that there are probably multiple sources of cues eliciting expectancies that combine to shape interpersonal distance behavior. "A differential prior history of nurse, doctor, mother, and father reinforcement for the leukemic children, in the context of the hospital, can explain the increased distance in the placement [of the figures], and can allow for all of the proposed possible explanations, each contributing its own share to the final results (Spinetta *et al.*, 1974, p. 755]."

In addition to social isolation, these investigators also looked at levels of death anxiety by means of projective techniques (Spinetta, 1973). Although Spinetta reported results suggesting greater death anxiety and threat to body function in leukemic children than in controls, he did not describe the control groups sufficiently in this or in the social isolation report. He explained group differences in anxiety as a function of death awareness. However, he did not indicate what specific diseases characterized the control group, or whether group differences were associated with specific treatments rather than diagnosis. For example, differential response—certainly related to anxiety and bodily integrity—could have been a function of more aggressive treatments in the leukemic group rather than a reflection of their death awareness.

Finally, in terms of family communication patterns, Spinetta (1978) reported associations between high levels of openness in communication within the family (as rated by the mother) and the child's satisfaction with self. In addition, in postdeath interviews with the family, Spinetta reported that siblings and parents from homes with a low level of communication expressed regret over lost opportunities to speak with a now-dead child. In this latter study, both the assessment of communication openness and the child's adjustment were rated by the mother, with the opportunity for bias that that method produces.

In summary, there has been little systematic behavioral research related to pediatric thanatology. As our treatments for fatal illness become even more effective, one result will be a lengthening death trajectory with attendant symptom experience—anxiety and distress associated with the disease and its treatment, isolation, boredom, and pain. Certainly research in the area of symptom control and behavioral management strategies should be of high priority.

The Social Structure of Dying

Although my focus so far has been on the individual dying patient, it became apparent in discussing pediatric patients that the dying person exists in a social and environmental context. This context can be viewed at several levels. Most basic is what Berger and Luckmann (1966), as well as others (Gendlin, 1962; Merleau-Ponty, 1967), refer to as the "social construction of reality." That is, our basic perceptions of what is real and the meaning we attach to events are in large part created within a dialectic process arising out of social exchange. According to this view, the significance of dying is created by the participants in the biological event (Glaser & Strauss, 1965).

On a less profound level of examination, the environment for dying can be examined, and places for dying can be compared, in terms of symptom expression in patients and families. Finally, specially formed social support groups for the dying can be considered as a form of potential therapeutic intervention during the process of dying for the patient and afterward for the family. The common theme linking these various analytic levels is that the dying patient is viewed not as an encapsulated entity but as inextricably bound up in an environmental social nexus.

Kastenbaum (1979) and Gorer (1965) have described the cultural milieu within which Americans, in particular, die. Because of our increasing technology and perhaps our decreasing sense of the religious significance of events, until the late 1970s the experience of death itself had become both intolerable and thus hidden away within institutional walls. However, in 1979 Kastenbaum described the sources of a new quest for "healthy dying." That is, as the technology of our death industry has increased, a reaction to this dehumanizing process has set in. An image of a self-actualized death has begun to emerge:

> Increasingly, the person with a life-threatening illness has some kind of positive conception of the death he or she wants to achieve. This is a distinct departure from the interpersonal climate that existed only a few years ago when death was not considered a fit topic of contemplation for either patient or caregiver [p. 192].

I return to this changing expectation in regard to dying in the last section of this chapter in discussing the new death cult. The point stressed here is that there is a shifting social climate—in part a reaction against impersonal technology and a reflection of a growing humanism in medical training. This changing climate is evidenced in new forms of environmental arrangements for dying and new forms of social support systems that have recently proliferated.

PLACES FOR DYING

In projecting population trends, Agate (1973) suggested that there would be increasing numbers of old people—especially women—who would live alone in the community and would most likely end their days in an institution of one form or another:

> It seems almost inevitable that most of these must end their days in geriatric . . . hospitals, or sometimes in residential homes, for lack of sufficient home support. A massive development of social services at home might in theory prevent the admission of lonely old people just to die. . . . In practice this is likely to be but a pious hope [p. 364].

Flynn and Stewart (1979) reviewed 55,288 death certificates in the state of Ohio covering a period of 18 years. They found that for the total period, 65% of the patients died in acute and chronic care hospitals, 15% died in nursing homes, and 20% died at home. Trends over the 18-year period demonstrated a shift from patients dying at home to patients dying in nursing homes.

Sherizon and Lester (1977) studied 22 relatives of six patients who died in an intensive care unit (ICU) of a large midwestern hospital. They found that, for the family, the critical aspect of the patient's situation was not the illness and death per se, but rather the means by which the family was able to become involved with the patient. Highly structured as it was, the ICU became a major constraint on the family's ability to face the death of the patient.

Certainly, in recent years much has been written about the hospice arrangement (Kastenbaum, 1979; Mount et al., 1978; Saunders, 1978; Woodson, 1978). Those involved with the hospice movement claim that the hospice is a system or network of care for the people who have limited life expectancies. Rather than just a "place," a hospice is really a medical and social support system that seeks to maintain continuity of care for the person regardless of his or her location. Most of what has been written has been clinically based rather than founded on empirical data. Dame Cecely Saunders, the founder of St. Christopher's Hospice in England, writes eloquently about the hospice experience and the positive impact of that environment on patients and families alike (Saunders, 1978). The major clinical contribution of the hospice, according to Saunders, is in pain control. She reported data derived from interviews that suggest a significant reduction in the proportion of patients experiencing intractable pain after entering St. Christopher's, in contrast to no reduction in the proportion of patients experiencing pain who eventually died elsewhere.

Saunders (1978) argues for a special place for dying, because staff within acute care facilities are not prepared to manage dying patients. "Often it is not the right place for them nor do their needs match the interest of many of the doctors who look after them. . . . 'satisfactory' patients should get better or at least die without fuss before those treating them have come to the end of their (largely irrelevant) resources [p. 158]."

In contrast, Agate (1973) questions the advisability of establishing numerous "centers for the dying." He suggested that there might be great local opposition to setting up large numbers of such places because they could not all be "centers of excellence"; it would be unlikely that enough skilled people could be found to staff such facilities. In addition, the elderly particularly may have some negative feelings about entering such facilities from which they will most likely never return.

An example of an alternative arrangement—in addition to patients dying at home—is the day-care facility set up specifically to care for patients with preterminal and terminal cancer as well as other chronic diseases. Wilkes, Crowther, and Greaves (1978) reported interview data which suggested that although terminal symptoms were controlled in two-thirds of the patients, the availability of such a facility did not have much of an effect on where those patients died. Of the 190 cancer patients, 83% died within the facility, and only 12% died at home. However, these figures are comparable to those associated with other terminal care arrangements, from nursing homes to acute care facilities.

On the basis of interview data, Hinton (1979) assessed the attitudes and moods in 80 dying patients who were in an acute care hospital ward, in a Foundation Home (a converted Victorian mansion with two attending physicians), or in a hospice with both inpatient and outpatient care. Hinton found few differences in anxiety, depression, or attitude toward the environment between acute hospital and Foundation patients, but the hospice patients were significantly less depressed and anxious. The major distinguishing characteristic between the hospice and the Foundation Home was that the former had an explicit policy of frank, open communication about the dying process. Patients within the hospice openly shared their preference for such communication freedom. Finally, outpatient hospice patients expressed more anxiety than inpatient hospice patients. There were some obvious problems of biased sampling in this study (e.g., patient self-selection into the hospice environment) as well as some not so obvious biasing (e.g., patients were not admitted to the study if they were experiencing physical distress, and the proportion of patients excluded from each facility was not reported). However, the conclusion drawn by Hinton was that although none of the facilities was clearly superior, the open freedom of communication found in the hospice probably contributed to the reports of less distress in these patients.

As Kastenbaum concluded, it does seem fairly clear that symptomatic relief, particularly of pain, is superior in the hospice environment, although even here continued research is needed (Mount *et al.*, 1978; Woodson, 1978). But little is really known of the systematic effects of hospice care on the person's total sense of self—on his or her basic life values. Kastenbaum particularly found lacking any systematic research into the patient's own phenomenological status, or subjective experience, as affected by hospice and nonhospice types of care. In general, we know very little about differential symptom perception and expression, or differential course of dying, as functions of environmental context.

SELF-HELP AND MUTUAL AID GROUPS FOR THE DYING

Levy (1979) reported an analysis of 28 help-giving activities in self-help groups and concluded:

> On the whole, self help groups focus the major portion of their effort on fostering communication between members, providing them with social support, and responding to their needs on both cognitive and emotional levels. Taken as a group, moreover, these activities appear to be non-coercive, non-threatening, and likely to foster group cohesiveness [p. 264].

In recent years, mutual support groups for the seriously ill have proliferated (e.g., Mended Heart Clubs, Ostomy Societies), and at least two groups—

Make Today Count (Kelly, 1978) and the Shanti Project (Garfield & Clark, 1978)—have specifically been organized to improve the quality of life of persons with terminal illness.

As others have discussed (Lieberman & Borman, 1979), there are barriers to carrying out process and outcome research related to self-help or peer-support groups, although Levy (1979) has shown that these barriers are not insurmountable. To the best of this writer's knowledge, however, self-help groups for the dying have not been studied. That is, who they help or do not help, and why, are questions that have yet to be addressed in any systematic fashion.

Some recent work has been reported on the effects of professionally led supportive group therapy with metastatic cancer patients (Spiegel, 1979). Spiegel stressed the importance of direct communication between physicians and dying patients, and reported that within the groups, facing death directly was comforting rather than morbid. Group discussions enabled patients to establish collaborative relationships with their oncologists and to strengthen family support systems. The group sessions also provided opportunities for enhancing the patients' sense of mastery over the final stages of life.

As in Sobel's cognitive–behavioral intervention strategies with individual patients, what seems to be centrally therapeutic in these groups is the enhancement of a sense of control in a life situation where there are few if any options left. However, a more refined understanding of specific techniques affecting differential responsiveness in patient population subgroups has yet to emerge.

Ethics and Dying

I began this chapter by alluding to the complexity of the subject matter— including its very definition. One physician wrote: "It is vital to be absolutely clear about the distinction between prolonging life and prolonging the process of dying, when the latter means simply the temporary postponement of the cessation of heartbeat and respiration by mechanical means after the brain, the essence of the individual, has ceased to function [White, 1977, p. 98]."

As discussed earlier, the perception of dying—of being in a dying state—is in part socially constructed. Because of changes in technology, our perception of dying and of being dead have changed. Earlier, the definition rested on a perceptible heartbeat and respiration. Now, as reflected in White's words, the definition that is coming to be accepted rests on a notion of brain death, or the irreversible loss of human functional quality.

SURVIVAL BY MACHINE AND BEING ALLOWED TO DIE

Morrison (1977) has argued that through the process of reification, the notion of "life" becomes abstracted from signs of living, and making the distinction between life and death becomes a nearly impossible task. In the past, when shortly after cardiac arrest the brain inevitably also ceased to function, determining that a person had died (when "life" was gone) was a relatively easy task. But because in actuality dying (like aging) is a gradual process—and now even more so because of man's tinkering with his own machinery—the distinction between life (being in a living process) and death (the virtual absence of living) may in part rest on more pragmatic grounds. That is, Morrison suggests, because of our growing technological capacity to control graft versus host response and hence our increasing ability to transplant vital organs, the growing need for "parts" has hastened the shift in definition of death from cardiac arrest to brain death.

Kass (1977), on the other hand, has emphasized the need to distinguish between the abstract concept of death (with all its theological, philosophical, and social implications) and the means of measuring the death event. In his response to Morrison's position, Kass suggested that Morrison may have been confusing truth (the state of being alive or dead, operationally defined) with value (i.e., the social value of salvaging viable organs from a now-vegetative existence). It is possible by medical consensus to work toward the establishment of systematic and precise operations that, once executed, provide the objective ground for pronouncing that death has occurred.

In addressing the issue of the social value of body parts, Ramsey (1972) has insisted that declaring death inevitable is not sufficient justification for the premature termination of life:

> To pronounce a condition hopeless is by no means the same as to deduce that a patient has died. For the purpose of organ transplant, or any other purpose, death cannot be reckoned from when it becomes "virtually" certain. This has to be made sun-clear, else the public is justly suspicious that "cannibalizing" organs may be the practice [pp. 68–69].

For Kass (1977), the decision to terminate life-support efforts must be based solely on consideration of the good of the dying person—and not on consideration of those who are waiting. Any other decision base, he argued, points toward murder. He also reminded the reader that this century has already witnessed one such social effort to dispose with useless lives. Kass, like others (Weir, 1977), has fallen back on the Judeo–Christian moral–theological position of not requiring extraordinary means to be followed in the maintenance of a human life (or in the maintenance of living, to avoid reification). However, he stopped short of advocating active euthanasia. Cantor (1977) also took the position that if affirmative medical conduct to end the patient's life is prohibited, the patient must be allowed maximum opportunity to change his or her mind and demand treatment: "The patient declining treatment normally remains alive for a period and thereby retains some opportunity to articulate or demonstrate any change of mind or to eliminate any mistake on the physician's part in comprehending the patient's wishes [p. 268]."

When the patient is not sentient and/or when the patient is suffering excruciating pain, acting in the best interest of the patient becomes more complex. Even the definition of what is an extraordinary life-preserving effort is not so simple a matter to decide. What is extraordinary has never been defined precisely. Although blood transfusions and intravenous feeding are probably generally viewed as ordinary and artificial respirators are not, the total treatment context may alter this distinction. For the patient in an irreversible coma (Ad Hoc Committee of the Harvard Medical School, 1968), the continuation of intravenous feeding may in fact be considered extraordinary.

Paulson's (1973) solution was to suggest that the continuous and active involvement of the family practitioner might be protective of the patient's interest. He argued that legislation is not desirable in the area of medical morals, because legislation cannot solve these (moral) dilemmas: "Even having two physicians decide that a damaged life or the act of dying should be terminated is not necessarily a just solution. Groups rarely act in a more ethical manner than enlightened individuals [p. 136]." In this writing, Paulson developed the notion of a physician–friend. Because it is easier to harm those at a distance than to "destroy a friend," the value of a family friend who is also the attending physician may have some merit. However, emotional investment on the part of both family and professional may preclude other decisions that need to be made on rational grounds. In this area of complex ethics, there may be no perfect solution.

Certainly, there are other issues involved in the question to terminate life than those considered here. One perspective that has not been dealt with is the dying patient's right to refuse further treatment, which rests fundamentally on the concept of informed consent (Ramsey, 1972). Legally, the right to refuse treatment—the right to be "let alone"—has been upheld in the courts, and is based on the principles of self-determination and the right of privacy. Such a right to refuse treatment is not of course absolute, and a state has the right to intervene to protect its interest. For example, if the person refusing treatment has a minor child at home, the courts would have the right to order continuation of treatment in order that the minor child be cared for by the parent as long as possible.

How "informed" is informed consent is a research area relevant to many of the issues that have been addressed here. Based on a model of rational man, the assumption is that a person (or family, if the patient is not competent to decide) is informed of treatment choices, alternatives, and consequences, and then a decision is made on the most reasonable grounds. However, some initial research in this area (Morrow, Gootnick, & Schmale, 1978) has demonstrated that decisions are rarely made so rationally, and patients and families alike base their decisions on affective aspects of the treatment situation, including "trust in their doctors" and "wishing to please." In an early clinically based analysis of decision making in the death process, Miller (1971) analyzed the management of 10 dying patients from the perspective of patient, family, physician, and institutional staff. In only 2 of the 10 cases was there congruency in the decision to suspend or terminate support efforts. (In 7 out of 10 cases the family wished to terminate support, whereas in 9 out of 10 cases the institutional nursing staff wished to continue support services.) This matter of congruency–incongruency in decision making, as well as most of the other topics discussed in this chapter, are increasingly important but as yet underresearched areas.

This discussion of the complex issues surrounding the definition of dying, and the ethical and moral issues involved in terminal care, has only considered in a necessarily superficial manner the issues that are involved. But the reader who is likely to intervene clinically with dying patients and their families—and perhaps with other caregivers as well—should be aware of the relevant major ethical, legal, and social issues.

THE NEW DEATH CULT

Geoffrey Gorer (1965) analyzed what he referred to as the "pornography of death" in our culture. Whereas a generation ago sex was the forbidden topic, now death and dying are not referred to "in front of the children." Yet, like sex, death is an intrinsic aspect of human life, and will be dealt with—if not openly, then surreptitiously. And like pornographic expression of any sort, sensational aspects of the event are exaggerated; death becomes expressed as violence in fiction as well as in life.

But it is not clear that our society relates to death in this manner any longer. Death has come out of the closet, so to speak. As indicated earlier, this has occurred in part because of a backlash against technological control, but this change in attitudes toward death is also a reflection of a larger social movement towards self-actualization rooted in the psychology of Carl Rogers and in European philosophy. In recent years many have embraced the virtues of dying well.

Courses are now given in which people learn to die (Cassell, 1973; Preston, 1973). Associations have sprung up in the United States and in England championing the right to suicide as the ultimate expression of self-actualization and control over one's fate. Guttman (1977), in fact, characterizes this movement as a striving for a sense of personal power and self-esteem that no longer arise in our culture from within or without. Historically, the concept of death has existed metaphorically as sacred power. "Because of the power meanings latent within it, the death experience now grips the contemporary imagination. As part of the hectic search for psychic nutrient, death has been discovered, even eroticized, as the latest power trip [p. 344]."

Whether or not one wants to accept Guttman's thesis, this ascendance of the notion of the death ideal may place a larger expectation on the health care establishment than it can deliver. As Kastenbaum (1979) concluded in his article on healthy dying, it is still an achievement to assist a person to maintain his or her self-integrity and esteem during the terminal phase of illness. A positive quality of life until the end—including the freedom from pain—is a reasonable expectation. But both a demand for a "good death" and the expectation of self-actualization may lead to two unfortunate ends. First, this increasing, socially shared expectancy may place a burden of "correct" death on those who are terminally ill—correct as defined in the care givers' terms. And second, the notion that a self-fulfilling death will compensate for a disappointing life may lead to a neglect of the routine, laborious care of the terminally ill patient and his or her family.

Summary

In considering the "routine and laborious care" of dying patients and their families, I focused on general issues of psychotherapy and truth telling as well as specific issues of pain and self-control through cognitive–behavioral intervention. In discussing the management of the pediatric patient, it was necessary to consider the family structure and the social context of dying. This social and environmental context was the explicit focus in comparing hospice with other places of treatment. And finally, it was necessary to end the chapter as I began it—with a look at ethical issues related to terminal care.

It should be unfortunately apparent to the reader that, as increasingly important as this area of terminal care has become, little systematic research has been carried out on the topics covered here. These issues are becoming even more important as medical technology keeps patients in a dying trajectory for longer periods of time while at the same time treatment options are being decided based on family, patient, and social needs. Among the social issues complicating the decision framework are the need for healthy donor organs and the rising cost of lifesaving efforts.

Behavioral thanatology within a behavioral medicine research framework has much to offer in this complex of treatment issues. Behavioral and social factors contribute across the whole gamut of the disease process, from primary prevention through terminal course. It would seem of the utmost worth to examine, understand, and as much as possible control these contributions in order to alter and improve the quality of dying—however death is ultimately defined.

References

Ad Hoc Committee of the Harvard Medical School. A definition of irreversible coma. *Journal of the American Medical Association*, 1968, *205*, 85–88.

Adams, D. *Childhood malignancy: The psychosocial care of the child and his family*. Springfield, Ill.: Thomas, 1979.

Agate, J. Care of the dying in geriatric departments. *Lancet*, 1973, *1*, 364–366.

Beck, A. *Cognitive therapy and the emotional disorders*. New York: International Universities Press, 1976.

Berger, P., & Luckmann, T. *The social construction of reality*. New York: Doubleday, 1966.

Bluebond-Langner, M. Meanings of death to children. In H. Feifel (Ed.), *New meanings of death*. New York: McGraw-Hill, 1977.

Cantor, N. A patient's decision to decline lifesaving medical treatment. In R. Weir (Ed.), *Ethical issues in death and dying*. New York: Columbia University Press, 1977.

Cassell, E. Learning to die. *Bulletin of the New York Academy of Medicine*, 1973, *49*, 110–118.

Chapman, J., & Goodall, J. Helping a child to live whilst dying. *Lancet*, 1980, *1*, 753–756.

Ellis, A. *Humanistic psychotherapy*. New York: McGraw-Hill, 1973.

Evans, R. Experiences in a pain clinic. *Modern Medicine of Canada*, 1971, *26*, 7.

Fischer, C. The testee as co-evaluator. *Journal of Counseling Psychology*, 1970, *17*, 30–36.

Flynn, A., & Stewart, D. Where do cancer patients die? A review of cancer deaths in Cuyahoga County, Ohio, 1957–1974. *Journal of Community Health*, 1979, *5*, 126–130.

Fordyce, W. An operant conditioning method for managing chronic pain. *Postgraduate Medicine*, 1973, *53*, 123–134.

Fordyce, W. *Behavioral methods for chronic pain in illness*. St. Louis, Mo.: C. V. Mosby, 1976.

Garfield, C. *Psychosocial care of the dying patient*. New York: McGraw-Hill, 1978.

Garfield, C., & Clark, R. The Shanti Project: A community model of psychosocial support for patients and families facing life-threatening illness. In C. Garfield (Ed.), *Psychosocial care of the dying patient*. New York: McGraw-Hill, 1978.

Gendlin, E. *Experiencing and the creation of meaning*. Toronto: Glencoe Press, 1962.

Glaser, B., & Strauss, A. *Awareness of dying*. New York: Academic Press, 1965.

Guberan, E. Surprising decline of cardiovascular mortality in Switzerland: 1951–1976. *Journal of Epidemiology and Community Health*, 1979, *33*, 114–120.

Gorer, G. *Death, grief, and mourning*. London: Cresset Press, 1965.

Guttman, D. Dying to power: Death and the search for self-esteem. In H. Feifel (Ed.), *New meanings of death*. New York: McGraw-Hill, 1977.

Hinton, J. Comparison of places and policies for terminal care. *Lancet*, 1979, *1*, (8106), 29–32.

Iles, J. Children with cancer: Healthy siblings' perceptions during the illness experience. *Cancer Nursing*, 1979, *2*, 371–377.

Kalish, R., & Reynolds, D. *Death and ethnicity: A psychocultural study.* Los Angeles: University of Southern California Press, 1976.

Kass, L. Death as an event: A commentary on Robert Morrison. In R. Wir (Ed.), *Ethical issues in death and dying.* New York: Columbia University Press, 1977.

Kastenbaum, R. The mental life of dying geriatric patients. *Gerontologist,* 1967, *7,* 97–100.

Kastenbaum R. Healthy dying; A paradoxical quest continues. *Journal of Social Issues,* 1979, *35,* 185–206.

Kelly, G. *The psychology of personal constructs* (Vols. I, II). New York: Norton, 1955.

Kelly, O. Living with a life-threatening illness. In C. Garfield (Ed.), *Psychosocial care of the dying patient.* New York: McGraw-Hill, 1978.

Kelly, W., & Friesen, S. Do cancer patients want to be told? *Surgery,* 1950, *27,* 822–826.

Kubler-Ross, E. *Questions and answers on death and dying.* New York: Macmillan, 1974.

Levy, L. Processes and activities in groups. In M. Lieberman & L. Borman (Eds.), *Self-help groups for coping with crisis.* San Francisco: Jossey-Bass, 1979.

Lieberman, M., & Borman, L. (Eds.). *Self-help groups for coping with crisis.* San Francisco: Jossey-Bass, 1979.

Lipman, A. G. Drug therapy in terminally ill patients. *American Journal of Hospital Pharmacy,* 1975, *32,* 270–276.

Melzack, R. *The puzzle of pain.* Harmondsworth, England: Penguin Press, 1973.

Melzack, R., Ofiesh, J., & Mount, B. The Brompton mixture: Effects on pain in cancer patients. In C. Garfield (Ed.), *The psychosocial care of the dying patient.* New York: McGraw-Hill, 1978.

Melzack, R., & Wall, P. Pain mechanisms: A new theory. *Science,* 1965, *150,* 971–979.

Merleau-Ponty, *The phenomenology of perception.* London: Routledge and Kegan Paul, 1967.

Miller, J. *Living systems.* New York: McGraw-Hill, 1978.

Miller, M. Decision-making in the death process of the ill aged. *Geriatrics,* 1971, *26,* 105–116.

Morrison, R. Death: Process or event? In R. Weir (Ed.), *Ethical issues in death and dying.* New York: Columbia University Press, 1977.

Morrow, G., Gootnick, B., & Schmale, A. A simple technique for increasing cancer patients' knowledge of informed consent to treatment. *Cancer,* 1978, *42,* 793–799.

Mount, B., Ajemian, F., & Scott, J. Use of Brompton mixture in treating the chronic pain of malignant disease. In C. Garfield (Ed.), *The Psychosocial care of the dying patient.* New York: McGraw-Hill, 1978.

Oster, M., Vizel, M., & Turgeon, L. Pain of terminal cancer patients. *Archives of Internal Medicine,* 1978, *138,* 1801–1802.

Paulson, G. Who should live? *Geriatrics,* 1973, *28,* 132–136.

Peck, V. Death—the final relief. *Nursing Research,* 1980, *151,* 32–34.

Preston, C. Behavior modification: A therapeutic approach to aging and dying. *Postgraduate Medicine,* 1973, *54,* 67–68.

Ramsey, P. The patient as person. New Haven: Yale University Press, 1972.

Rebok, G., & Hoyer, W. Clients nearing death: Behavioral treatment perspectives. *Omega,* 1974, *10,* 191–201.

Redd, W. Treatment of excessive crying in a terminal cancer patient: A time series analysis. *Journal of Behavioral Medicine,* 1982, *5,* 225–235.

Saunders, C. Terminal care. In C. Garfield (Ed.), *Psychosocial care of the terminally ill.* New York: McGraw-Hill, 1978.

Schwartz, G., & Weiss, S. What is behavioral medicine? *Psychosomatic Medicine,* 1977, *39,* 377–381.

Sherizon, S., & Lester, P. Dying in a hospital intensive care unit: The social significance for the family of the patient. *Omega,* 1977, *8,* 29–40.

Shneidman, E. Some aspects of psychotherapy with dying persons. In C. Garfield (Ed.), *Psychosocial care of the dying patient.* New York: McGraw-Hill, 1978.

Sobel, H. Toward a behavioral thanatology in clinical care. In H. Sobel (Ed.), *Behavioral therapy in terminal care: A humanistic approach.* Cambridge, Mass.: Ballinger, 1981.

Sontag, S. *Illness as metaphor.* New York: Vintage Books, 1979.

Spiegel, D. Psychological support for women with metastatic carcinoma. *Psychosomatics,* 1979, *20,* 780–785.

Spinetta, J. Anxiety in the dying child. *Pediatrics,* 1973, *52,* 841–844.

Spinetta, J. The dying child's awareness of death: A review. *Psychological Bulletin,* 1974, *81,* 256–260.

Spinetta, J. Communication patterns in families dealing with life-threatening illness. In O. J. Sahler (Ed.), *The child and death.* St. Louis, Mo.: C. V. Mosby, 1978.

Spinetta, S., Rigler, D., & Karon, M. Physical space as a measure of a dying child's sense of isolation. *Journal of Consulting and Clinical Psychology,* 1974, *42,* 751–756.

Twycross, R. Clinical experience with diamorphine in advanced malignant diseases. *International Journal of Clinical Pharmacology, Therapy, and Toxicology,* 1974, *9,* 184–198.

Twycross, R. *The management of terminal diseases.* London: Saunders, 1978.

Weir, R. (Ed.). *Ethical issues in death and dying.* New York: Columbia University Press, 1977.

Weisman, A. *On dying and denying.* New York: Behavioral Publications, 1972.

Weisman, A., Worden, J., & Sobel, H. *Psychosocial screening and intervention with cancer patients.* Cambridge, Mass.: A Project Omega–MGH Research Monograph, 1980.

White, L. Death and the physician. In H. Feifel (Ed.), *New meanings of death.* New York: McGraw-Hill, 1977.

Whitman, H., & Lukes, S. Behavior modification for the terminally ill. *American Journal of Nursing,* 1975, *75,* 93–101.

Wilkes, E., Crowther, A., & Greaves, C. A different kind of day hospital for patients with preterminal cancer and chronic disease. *British Medical Journal,* 1978, *2,* 1053–1056.

Willis, D. The families of terminally ill children: Symptomatology and management. *Journal of Clinical Child Psychology,* 1974, *3,* 32–33.

Woodson, R. Hospice care in terminal illness. In C. Garfield (Ed.), *Psychosocial care of the terminally ill.* New York: McGraw-Hill, 1978.

Worden, J., & Sobel, H. Ego strength and psychosocial adaptation to cancer. *Psychosomatic Medicine,* 1978, *40,* 585–592.

17

Prevention, Behavior Change, and Chronic Disease

THOMAS STACHNIK
BERTRAM STOFFELMAYR
RUTH B. HOPPE

Introduction

This chapter is unlike the others in this book because it is not concerned with coping with chronic disease. It instead raises the possibility that the chronic diseases suffered by most people in the United States are preventable and therefore the victims should not have to cope with them. Some might consider this chapter pessimistic, as much of it is an attempt to analyze why more and better preventive efforts relative to the chronic diseases have not been forthcoming. But we contend that substantial pessimism is congruent with the facts: preventive health care services and research in preventive medicine account for less than 5% of all dollars spent for health in the United States (Knowles, 1977). And because that 5% is spread over all diseases, it is apparent how little of our resources are currently addressed to the prevention of chronic diseases per se. It can be argued that the very composition of this book reflects the problem: one chapter on the prevention of chronic diseases and seventeen chapters on how to cope with them.

But the focus of this book on chronic disease is both noteworthy and encouraging in that it recognizes the revolution in the health care requirements of the American people that has occurred in the twentieth century. It is a revolution with which the medical profession itself had just come to grips in the 1970s (Knowles, 1977) and that other Western industrialized societies are also earnestly contemplating (Lalonde, 1975). It is a revolution that will have a profound impact on the training of future physicians, on the role of behavioral scientists in health care delivery, on a host of issues concerning how the resources within our health care system should be distributed, and perhaps most importantly on the priority assigned to the prevention of serious medical problems. This chapter examines all these dimensions of the revolution and concludes with specific suggestions for making chronic disease prevention programs more effective, but first documents the nature of the revolution.

Revolution in Health Care Requirements

At the turn of the twentieth century, the morbidity and mortality rates of Americans were largely related to infectious diseases such as influenza, pneumonia, tuberculosis, gastroenteritis, chronic nephritis, and diphtheria. These are acute illnesses with a fairly abrupt onset and a finite duration—the patient experienced either remission or death within a fairly short period. Today, only influenza and pneumonia from that list (and certain diseases of early infancy) remain as problems of mortality; the remainder have largely been brought under control through improved nutrition and personal hygiene and through the provision of safe water, milk supplies, and sewage disposal. What has replaced them as the major killers are the illnesses almost all of us have come to know through the sickness and/or death of some family friend: heart disease, cerebrovascular disease, respiratory diseases, and cancers of the lung, gastrointestinal tract, breast, uterus, and ovaries. Note that the major health problems now are all chronic illnesses with a gradual onset and an indefinite duration. Patients do not experience remission or immediate death, but rather the illness makes an insidious approach and then lingers a long while, often causing great suffering and financial hardship.

One further distinction between the acute illnesses of the past and the chronic conditions of today is noteworthy: the acute illnesses were largely caused by environmentally imposed risks. When people became ill from influenza or diphtheria it was the result of an inadvertent contact with a virus inflicted on them by a capricious environment, either in isolated instances or as part of an epidemic. They could place the "blame" for the illness on the environment. But with the chronic illnesses that are often the direct result of the life style we live—what and how much we eat and drink, how we exercise, how we deal with daily stresses, how much we smoke, and so on— it is less valid to blame the environment than it was for our forebearers. If blame must be placed, some of it must fall directly on our own instrumental behavior that, over a lifetime, is shaped into an assortment of good and bad habits—mostly the latter, unfortunately for our long-range health prospects. In sum, the most serious medical problems that now plague the majority of Americans are not ultimately medical problems after all, but rather behavior problems, that is, characteristic response patterns that must be altered.

SCOPE OF THE PROBLEM

It may be useful to review briefly a few of the characteristic response patterns that appear most troublesome for Americans and the prevalence of the major chronic diseases to which they are likely related. For example, of the roughly 2 million deaths in the United States in 1969, fully one-half were the result of heart disease (40%) and strokes (10%); 16% were due to various cancers (Knowles, 1977). In addition, the figures for premature death and disability in the same year are perhaps even more appalling: 178,000 people died of heart disease between the ages of 45 and 64, and 1.2 million people in that age group were chronically disabled because of heart disease (Susser, 1975). A decade later the picture had improved somewhat in that deaths from heart disease and stroke had declined in both men and women, but some of those gains were nullified by a concomitant increase in deaths from lung cancer and cirrhosis of the liver (Junge & Hoffmeister, 1981).

Obesity is considered a predisposing condition for degenerative arthritis of the hips, knees, and ankles, as well as for injuries, liver and gall-bladder disease, cancer of the gastrointestinal tract, diabetes, strokes, and heart attacks (Knowles, 1977). Estimates are that 16% of Americans under the age of 30 are obese and about 40% of the total population (80 million people) are 20 or more pounds above their ideal weight. About 30% of all men between 50 and 59 years old are 20% overweight and 60% are at least 10% overweight (Knowles, 1977). A long-term study of cardiovascular disease indicated that each 10% reduction in weight in men aged 35–55 would result in a 20% decrease in coronary disease (Ashley & Kannel, 1974).

High blood pressure is estimated to be a problem for 24 million people in the United States, almost half of whom do not know they have it. Of the remaining 12 million who know about it, only about 4 million are receiving adequate therapy—a dismal situation because high blood pressure is considered the primary cause of 60,000 deaths a year and is a significant causative factor in the more than 1,500,000 heart attacks and strokes suffered annually in the United States (Knowles, 1977). There is also little understanding by the public as to what degree of hypertension warrants treatment. Evidence is now at hand that there is substantial benefit in reducing blood pressure to normal even from the mildly hypertensive range. The incidence of mortality and stroke and the severity of renal failure and congestive heart failure all have been shown to be reduced by adequate antihypertensive therapy. Although the overall situation is discouraging, it should be noted that adults with untreated hypertension declined by 10% from the early 1960s to the early 1970s (U.S. Public Health Service, 1980).

The evidence is compelling that smoking is related to a number of serious health problems. Nevertheless, the consumption of cigarettes in the United States is somewhere around 200 packs annually per person over 18 years of age, reflecting the fact that one-third of all adults still are regular cigarette smokers. One hopeful sign is that the percentage of adult male, adult female, and teenage male smokers declined during the 1970s. A discouraging sign is that the percentage of teenage girl smokers during that period increased by an alarming 51% (U.S. Public Health Service, 1980). What of smoking's relationship to cancer? Based on an assumption that 85% of *lung* cancers are causally related to cigarette smoking, a 20% reduction in deaths from cancer would result if everyone in the United States stopped smoking. Furthermore, although most Americans are aware of the probable relationship between smoking and lung cancer, many do not realize that cigarettes contribute significantly to the incidence of heart disease. Other risk factors being equal, the average smoker is more than twice as likely to have a heart attack as a nonsmoker (Kahn, 1966). Many Americans also do not realize that changing to a cigarette low in tar and nicotine is no solution. Heart disease and strokes appear to be caused by the carbon monoxide and other particles of combustion of cigarette smoke as well as by the nicotine and tar; the safe cigarette is still not here.

If influencing our cigarette smoking seems a formidable task, it will probably prove easy compared to influencing what we eat. Smokers at least have some strong suspicions that they are doing their bodies no service when using cigarettes. Most of us, however, for a variety of reasons, are in no way cognizant that we are slowly, imperceptibly, but surely assaulting our bodies with what we eat in a way that will result in serious, preventable biological problems. In fact, often as a result of misinformation, we even make a special effort to eat certain foods in the belief they are good for us when they very likely are part of the assault. A case in point is the long-standing admonition that a healthy diet includes large amounts of protein from the meat group and the dairy group. Because all foods of animal origin contain cholesterol as part of their cell structure, there is good evidence now that such a diet, which produces high blood levels of cholesterol and saturated fat, hastens the appearance of cardiovascular disease. Studies have also indicated that the effects of such a diet are detectable at an early age. Examination of American soldiers killed in the Korean war revealed that 35% of them had greater than 15% narrowing of their coronary arteries resulting from abnormal collections of cholesterol—and their average age was 22 (Farquhar,

1978a)! Using even younger subjects (5–14 years old), it was shown that children from Wisconsin (home of good and plentiful dairy products) had average blood cholesterol levels almost double those of a group of children of the same age from a rural mountain village in Mexico (Golubjatnikov, Paskey, & Inhorn, 1972). It has even been suggested that the first preventable assault on our arteries begins with the decision to bottle-feed rather than nurse a newborn baby, because cow's milk raises the cholesterol level of an infant higher than does mother's milk.

There are, however, some encouraging trends that should not be overlooked. With respect to nutrition, adult males with high serum cholesterol levels (260 mg/100 ml and over) declined by 12% from the early 1960s to the early 1970s; adult females showed a 22% decline. Furthermore, the percentage of adults who exercised daily increased by 92% during the period 1961–1980. Perhaps most important, when asked if they had "a great deal", "some", "very little", or "hardly any at all" control over their future health, over 50% of those adults surveyed said "a great deal" and over 35% said "some" (U.S. Public Health Service, 1980).

Physical inactivity is another behavioral risk factor often postulated as a contributor to the major chronic diseases. However, it is not discussed here because its independent contribution is unknown, as it usually occurs in combination with the major risk factors. Furthermore, additional discussion of the various risk factors (behaviors) and the extent of their relationship to the chronic diseases is probably unnecessary. Many people are already aware of those relationships and yet continue to behave in ways they know are detrimental to their health. That discrepancy between what people know and how they behave may initially seem an incongruity, but on closer examination is understandable. Research in the behavioral sciences has consistently demonstrated that current behavior is often insensitive to long-range consequences (Honig, 1966). We continue to smoke cigarettes and eat food high in cholesterol and saturated fat because the immediate result of doing so is gratifying. The long-range possibility that it may be "bad for our health" exerts little present control. The ubiquity and power of the gratification principle make it imperative that it be used not only to account for the prevalence of our poor health habits, but that it be incorporated in programs designed to help alter life-styles in more healthful directions. There are of course researchers already engaged in designing and testing such programs, and others are researching basic questions about the relationship between various risk factors (behaviors) and bodily processes. But their relative number is small, it is a fragmented, nonsystematic effort, and there is little evidence that an emphasis on health habit alteration and the attendant research necessary to offer effective programs will arise in the immediate future. What would it take to develop such an emphasis? What stands in the way of mustering a share of our nation's resources commensurate with the magnitude and importance of the problem?

OBSTACLES TO CHANGE

Cultural Forces

There are forces within our health care professions that will resist the emphasis just described and other forces acting on the entire culture that also militate against a changed emphasis. One of those culture-wide forces is an attitude that says, "What's all the fuss about? We all have to die anyway, so it might just as well be of heart disease, stroke, or cancer." What is omitted in that stance, of course, is any reference as to *when* we die or, more importantly, under what circumstances. The changed emphasis called for in this chapter would attempt to make it possible for more Americans to live out their expected life span and to do so in relative good health and spirits. Dropping dead of a heart attack at 48 can be made an unlikely event; it can also be made unlikely that so many people will have to spend the later years of life greatly restricted, perhaps in pain and perhaps incurring enormous medical bills with which the survivors must contend. The argument also ignores the devastated dreams of incapacitated stroke patients who had planned to spend their retirement years traveling, playing with grandchildren, and so on.

A related argument is one that equates health risk factors with the good life. It suggests that life is simply not worth living if a person cannot have pork chops every day, eat unlimited quantities of ice cream, smoke a pack and a half of cigarettes a day, and avoid strenuous physical activity whenever possible. (Asceticism is for constipated cranks who don't know how to live life anyway.) That argument ignores the facts that we have all *learned* to enjoy the life-styles we currently live and that there is no reason we cannot learn to enjoy a more healthful life style just as much (with the attendant rewards later in life). For our children, just in the process of forming life-styles, the argument is particularly specious.

Another culture-wide constraint is a belief by the general public that our salvation from the chronic illnesses rests with our medical technology, a technology that inspires awe in many Americans. Though there have been some spectacular successes with that technology (e.g., organ transplants), they have been achievements that affect a small number of people. Some physicians have contended that the technology is probably overstated and that little change in it has actually occurred:

> Has the effective technology for medical care changed in the past twenty-five years to a degree sufficient to explain the increased cost? Is there in fact a new high technology of

medicine? Despite the widespread public impression that this is the case, there is little evidence for it. The most spectacular technological change has occurred in the management of infectious disease, but its essential features had been solidly established and put to use well before 1950. . . . There have been a few other examples of technology improvement, comparable in decisive effectiveness, since 1950, but the best of these have been for relatively uncommon illnesses. . . . We are left with approximately the same roster of common major diseases which confronted the country in 1950, and, although we have accumulated a formidable body of information about some of them in the intervening time, the accumulation is not yet sufficient to effect either the prevention or the outright cure of any of them [Thomas, 1977, p. 37].

Other physicians have declared categorically that new developments in our medical technology will not upgrade the health of Americans:

Meanwhile, the people have been led to believe that national health insurance, more doctors and greater use of high-cost, hospital-based technologies will improve health. Unfortunately, none of them will. . . . Control of the present major health problems in the United States depends directly on modification of the individual's behavior and habits of living [Knowles, 1977, p. 61].

Although it is gratifying to hear a physician express that point of view, it appears to be a minority view, and thus it would probably be a mistake to assume that medicine will provide the impetus for a different emphasis in health care. In fact, medicine will probably offer some resistance to change—and not necessarily with any malice. It can be reasonably argued that, given the nature of our current health problems, our primary care physicians seldom do what they should be doing. They begin their practice doing what they have been trained to do, and then the contingencies of reinforcement that operate on them make it unlikely that their practice will change significantly. There is a constant supply of money, drama, prestige, and sense of accomplishment (all extremely powerful reinforcers) that all encourage doctors to maintain their current activities without ever addressing the long-range health practices of their patients. It may seem absurd for our medical care apparatus to wait until people are sick, chronically ill, or disabled to be concerned about their health, but it is unrealistic to expect otherwise. Our physicians are products of the same cultural forces that shaped us all; thus, their personal health habits are often no better than those of their patients. Although many physicians have stopped smoking, the care they give to what they eat, the amount they exercise, and their ability to manage stress are all in doubt. Furthermore, there is very little in their medical school training that will encourage them, once in practice, to consider the upstream forces (those that create and maintain ill health) that continuously produce the drowning persons the physician is incredibly busy rescuing downstream. So, if our interest is in finding fault, it must be directed first at some larger social forces that have a vested interest in seeing our current life-styles maintained (e.g., the food, tobacco, alcohol, and advertising industries) and then at our medical school (behavioral sciences) curricula, in which the prevention of serious health problems of our students and their future patients is given short shrift. One public health professional (Blackburn, 1978) sees it this way:

> In the earliest days of preparation for becoming a physician or medical scientist, the student of medicine is imbued with the idea of the Golden Key, the Missing Link, the Magic Bullet, the Serendipitous Breakthrough, and the Holy Grail. Reading from *Microbe Hunters* to *Arrowsmith*, from *The Way of An Investigator* to *The Double Helix*, the student is fascinated with the researcher–master physician model, the cleverness of observation, the elegance of experiment, the doggedness of repetition, the brilliance of deductions, and the glory of the rewards. Medicine has indeed produced great break-throughs by physicians and scientists, eccentric or mad, devoted or humble. They have contributed significantly to mankind's progress in the alleviation of pain and suffering through use of the highest human faculties, plus persistence and more than a little luck. But it appears that with this fervor and this concentration on fundamental mechanisms of disease, a large professional blind spot may have been created to the quite overwhelming role of the environment and culture on individual behavior—behavior which leads in turn to the development of most major disease problems and to the potential for their mass prevention [p. 125].

Forces within the Professions

The culture-wide forces that resist attempts to alter the health habits of Americans are intimidating, but the forces within the health care and behavior change professions precluding a vastly increased effort in that alteration are also very strong. The forces that make it unlikely that physicians will begin attending to the long-range health practices of their patients have already been noted. Unfortunately, the situation regarding the behavior change professions (e.g., psychology) is also far from encouraging. Although the forces acting on those professions are different from those influencing physicians, they exert great control. One such force is scientific conservatism, a stance that has historically served the professions well by slowing the propagation of incomplete or faddist doctrines. In the case at hand, proponents of that conservatism can rightly argue that tight, functional relationships do not exist between the serious, chronic illnesses and the risk factors purported to be causal. They may further point out that some of the most frequently cited evidence concerning those risk factors emanates from cross-cultural research, well known for the interpretative hazards it poses. (The Golubjatnikov *et al.*, 1972 study cited earlier is illustrative. Differences in blood cholesterol levels between Wisconsin children and children from a rural Mexican village were attributed to differences in diet, but it can be cogently argued that those two groups of children differ in many other ways, any one of which might account for the cholesterol discrepancy.) And if in fact there are no valid relationships between the major chronic illnesses and life-style variables, then there is no case to be made for developing the increased emphasis on health habit modification for which this chapter calls.

Nevertheless, it is becoming increasingly difficult to deny the relationship between life-style and the serious chronic illnesses, not so much because of the quality of the present data but because of their compelling quantity. Furthermore, there are limits to the kind of health habit data that can be generated, just as there are limits in other areas of the behavioral sciences (e.g., the effects of punishment on human behavior). Thus the decision about the validity of the life-style–chronic illness relationships may ultimately have to rest on quantity rather than quality. For those who might be persuaded by carefully controlled animal research, some of the data are already in place. One series of studies has shown that the coronary arteries of adult monkeys were narrowed by 60% as a result of being fed diets high in saturated fat and cholesterol over a period of 17 months. The optimistic finding was that two-thirds of the cholesterol deposits melted away in those animals returned to a normal diet for a period of 40 months (Armstrong, Warner, & Connor, 1970). In any event, as decisions are made about whether enough experimental evidence now exists to warrant a commitment to health habit modification, it must be remembered that the decision will perhaps always be an arbitrary one. But this is not an unusual circumstance in the behavioral sciences. Given the nature of the subject matter, professional judgments must often be based on what *probably* constitutes truth.

An additional consideration in the decision-making process should be the importance the American people attach to the issue. In a massive project, Flanagan (1978) interviewed 1000 30-year-olds, 600 50-year-olds, and 600 70-year-olds, asking them to rate the importance in their lives of 15 components drawn from the following categories: physical and material well-being; relations with other people; social, community, and civic activities; personal development and fulfillment; and recreation. Of the 15 components, "health and personal safety—to be physically fit and vigorous, to be free from anxiety and distress, and to avoid bodily harm" was rated more important than any other, easily outstripping such other components as "relationships with your parents, brothers, sisters, and other relatives", and "understanding yourself," areas in which clinicians have traditionally made huge investments of time and skills. Again, the incongruity in that project between what people say they want (good health) and how they behave is striking. But understanding that the absence of immediate, aversive consequences for current high-risk habits augurs poorly for the achievement of long-range health should make that less puzzling.

In 1976, a task force of the American Psychological Association (APA Task Force, 1976) on health research concluded that one of the forces within that discipline most likely to prevent psychologists from becoming involved on a large scale in matters of physical health is the historical prominence of mental health as a focus for applied psychology; that is, their investment in mental health almost completely overshadows other types of health activities. That observation and the importance the task force assigned to the exclusionary effects of that historical prominence seem valid. But portions of the task force report appear constrained by the same exclusive mental health emphasis it says psychology must eschew if other health research is to flower. For example, in discussing the need for increased "psychologic and psychosocial" health-related research, the report largely focuses on earlier descriptive studies of cancer patients and summarizes a number of them, presumably as models for future research. One such study (Blumberg, West, & Ellis, 1956), using data from the Minnesota Multiphasic Personality Inventory and the Rorschach Inkblot Test, found that cancer patients with fast-developing diseases are more defensive and overcontrolled than patients with slow-developing diseases. By combining the results of a number of other studies, the task force (APA Task Force, 1976) was able to state:

> A variety of objective and projective questionnaires and tests were used, and these several different groups arrived independently at a consistent description of the cancer patient as a rigid, authoritarian, inner-directed, and religious person, having ample conflict around sexual and hostile impulses, using excessive repression of affect, and having poor emotional outlets [p. 269].

It must be said, in the strongest possible terms, that more exploration of such typical descriptive mental health variables is not what is needed in the category of health-related psychological and psychosocial research. Additional studies of that kind would have the quality of fiddling while Rome burns. What is required is a massive amount of work directed at modifiable behavior (e.g., smoking as opposed to "rigidity" or "authoritarianism") based on the fundamental question of what can be done to make it less likely that a person will prematurely become a cancer or stroke or heart disease patient. This chapter argues that the answer to that question for behavioral scientists is clear: their expertise must be brought to bear on assisting Americans to alter current habits most likely related to preventable health problems. Again, the emphasis must address those habits that appear most relevant and with which there is a good chance of succeeding (e.g., reducing salt intake to lower blood pressure) rather than attempting to change total behavioral style (e.g., making a person less over-controlled or inner-directed).

A Different Strategy for the Prevention of Chronic Disease

Once it is accepted that the improvement in the health of Americans is synonymous with prevention, there are truisms that must be acknowledged. Risk factors fall broadly into two categories, environmental and behavioral.

The focus of the efforts of clinicians, physicians, and behavioral scientists is the modification of self-imposed risks such as smoking, high-speed driving, lack of exercise, and unbalanced diet, rather than air pollution, water pollution, or hazardous work. Our expertise is of little value when it comes to reducing air pollution or the improvement of occupational safety; in those cases our role is that of the informed citizen willing to participate in the political process. As the improvement of the health of Americans is as dependent on the reduction of environmental hazards as on the alteration of individual behavior, our impact on health will therefore be limited.

Although the ultimate purpose of prevention is the reduction of chronic illness, as clinicians we influence the precursors of chronic illness rather than chronic illness per se. The dependent measure, the index of the success of our work, is smoking rather than cancer or heart disease, or eating rather than obesity. In the choice of behaviors that ought to be modified we rely on the expertise of others, primarily epidemiologists. The list of those behaviors that constitute self-imposed risks, the modification of which has fairly well-established rewards in health, is limited. It always includes smoking, overeating, reckless driving, alcohol abuse, the lack of self-examination for breast cancer, the consultation of medical practitioners for only a limited number of diagnostic procedures (see "The Periodic Health Examination"), inadequate coping with stress, and, at times, inadequate exercise. At this point there are no data suggesting that complete changes in life-style are either possible for most persons or have an effect on health status. For example, there is no evidence whatsoever that a change from a balanced low-fat diet to a vegetarian one, or that the move from a crowded city to the pastoral life of the country, will improve health. If our work is to have any value it must be restricted to the limited set of behaviors that do have established links to health status.

ROLE OF THE BEHAVIORAL SCIENTIST

In the 1970s a multitude of procedures for the modification of health behaviors were developed, researched, and described in the literature. Despite this intense activity, it appears that clinicians have as yet contributed only minimally to the amelioration of the public health problems posed by poor health habits and self-destructive behaviors. For example, according to the National Cancer Institute (1977), only 2% of smokers who have given up the habit have done so with the help of formalized smoking cessation programs; a review of the behavioral treatments of obesity found that these methods, even though they are the most effective ones, are not very powerful in the long run (Foreyt, Goodrick, & Gotto, 1981). However, there is a contradiction: studies evaluating individual programs and techniques found that many of the behavioral treatments do actually help. Smoking cessation programs result in up to 50% abstinence rates (Lichtenstein, 1982), persons who enroll in weight control programs do lose weight (Brownell, 1982), behavioral techniques are helpful in the control of blood pressure (Shapiro & Goldstein, 1982), and so on. We have effective methods but help only a few! The usual response to such a dilemma is to call for more, and of course more sophisticated, research. In the case of health habit modification the call is out for more research on generalization and long-term maintenance. There are, however, alternatives that ought to be considered. It might be that our ineffectiveness does not stem from our inappropriate techniques but from our mode of practice: the problem is our system of service delivery rather than the techniques we employ when working with individuals. If this were true, improvements would not come from further technical sophistication but from changes in our mode of practice.

Most practitioners of a trade or profession assume that their mode of working is a rational response to the problems they set out to deal with. Is that really the case? Might it not be—to take the example of the health professional—that the structure of the service delivery we are part of is responsive to forces only tangentially related to the health problems we set out to cope with? For instance, the decision to hospitalize a patient is not solely dependent on the patient's needs for specialized treatments that can only be given in the hospital, but to a great extent by national policy that determines which treatments are reimbursible. Or, to take an example from behavior therapy, following Wolpe's (1982) development of systematic de-sensitization for the treatment of phobias behavior therapists have for a number of years treated patients exclusively by this method. It entails teaching the patient relaxation techniques and describing to the patient the fear-arousing stimuli. Behavior therapists adhere to this method even though introductory psychology courses have taught everyone the condition under which extinction occurs: unreinforced exposure to the relevant stimuli. Lack of understanding therefore cannot be the explanation for the popularity of office-bound systematic desensitization. But how would it look if highly trained therapists were to go shopping with their patients or were found riding elevators? Only office-based activities are professional work. (By this comment, we in no way want to minimize the importance of systematic desensitization. But there were then and there are now a number of circum-stances where the treatment of choice is *in vivo* exposure to the anxiety-arousing stimuli.)

The framework for the service of most health professionals is private prac-tice and for most of those interested in behavior change that of private practice psychotherapy. Its essence is that the clinician waits in an office to be sought out by persons who have "problems." The clients are responsible for diagnosing themselves as having a problem, finding a therapist, and following the therapist's advice (even the suggestion that a client come for further sessions is "therapist's advice"). Clinicians are responsible for providing treatment to the best of their knowledge and for keeping that knowledge up to date. Whatever the merits of this model for psychotherapy, we propose that it is our professional adherence to it rather than our technical incompetence that has limited our influence on the health habits of Americans. It determines not only where we work—in offices located in professional buildings and medical centers—but also who our clients are (individuals rather than populations at risk found in social systems) and has even influenced our conceptualization of the determinants of the problem behavior and our research and evaluative strategies.

REORIENTATION OF BEHAVIORAL SCIENTISTS

Where Can Prevention Activities Take Place?

Prevention certainly cannot be practiced exclusively in the offices of psychotherapists or behavior therapists, as only a small number of self-diagnosed and referred patients are helped there. Without denying the need for services for self-diagnosed and referred clients, it must be acknowledged that even the most enthusiastic practitioner working with groups of patients will have little impact on the public health problems of smoking, overeating, high-fat diets, high blood pressure, and so on. Poor health habits are widespread and, as we show later, even more of a problem for those who are less likely to contact office-based prevention services. Prevention must occur where large numbers of persons are, or more accurately where large numbers of persons can be reached, because the opportunity exists there for prolonged interaction around health issues. Obvious settings are the office of the primary care physician, the workplace, and such social organizations as churches, clubs, residence halls in colleges, small towns, and neighborhoods in cities. The office of the primary care physician and the workplace offer special advantages. The advantage of the primary care setting is that patients come there for consultation around health concerns. Most of us spend a great deal of time at work and many of our "unhealthy" behaviors are reinforced there and therefore ought to be treated there.

Who Is the Client?

For the office-based practitioner the answer is clear: the individuals who seek him or her out are the clients. This mode of practice would only contribute to prevention (i.e., the amelioration of the public health problems posed by self-destructive behaviors and poor health habits) if it were true that most persons had the choice of leading the healthy life. The fact is, however, that large numbers of Americans have neither the knowledge and the social support to identify the health risks embodied in their own behavior nor the opportunity for change. The chance to self-diagnose smoking, lack of exercise, or high-fat diet as a problem, and the chance to be induced to alter one's health behavior, are all related to level of education, social status, and place of work. In a study of smoking among patients who were admitted to hospital for illnesses unrelated to smoking, it was found that about 50% of manual workers smoked cigarettes, but only 20% of managers and professionals and only 10% of physicians were smokers (Covey & Wynder, 1981). Therefore, to assume that a manual worker and a physician or university professor have equal chances to become nonsmokers is false. The emphasis of our work must therefore shift from the individual to persons at risk. Implied in our discussion up to now is also that we will be effective only if we identify the persons at risk in the context of an established organization.

Roots of the Problem

Most techniques developed for the modification of health behavior focus on individuals. Conditioning and self-control procedures are examples. The individuals have to alter their behaviors because the roots of the problematic behavior are in them. The behaviors to be treated have been learned over the course of a lifetime, and are problematic now only because they have been learned so well. If treatment must occur in an office setting, then this conceptualization of problem behavior is necessary because the alternate explanation—that behavior is maintained by the support it receives from the social environment—would lead the therapist out of the office into the community. However, much that is known about health behavior seems to point to the social environment as its main determinant. The social environment must therefore be mobilized in order to achieve permanent change.

Motivation

Is there a payoff for improving one's health habits? The simple answer ought to be "yes": the payoff is a healthier life. There are, however, a number of problems with this answer. Health behavior is largely determined by the social environment. The social environment provides stimulus control and reinforces many health behaviors directly. We stuff ourselves at our mothers' dinner tables; we smoke with our colleagues during breaks at work; in some work settings we are encouraged to brag about the number of cans of beer we drank over the weekend, and in others about the miles we have run. Not only do the norms of the work place, social class, and neighborhood affect us, but we also smoke, eat, and exercise frequently in the company of colleagues and friends. It follows that improvements in health habits will only come about if the same influences emanating from the social environment that support poor health habits are mobilized for change.

There are two additional points that are important to motivation for change in health behaviors. One is that the effects of changes in life-style are in the distant future, and the other one is that alterations in life-style are exceedingly aversive. The smoker must tolerate withdrawal symptoms, the dieter must forsake his beloved foods, and the sedentary person must leave the comfortable chair. For these reasons changes in health behavior must result in immediate valued feedback, and the incentive value of the reinforcing efforts must be great enough to compete effectively with the pain engendered by change.

Evaluation and Research

Most of the research on health behavior modification has dealt with the development and improvement of specific techniques. The data reported usually come from volunteers, and what we know about a method is that a particular proportion of volunteers succeeded with it. Although such research does allow a comparison of methods, it says nothing about their impact. For example, it might be that a particular smoking cessation program results in an 80% abstinence rate at a 1-year follow-up, but only 5% of all smokers in a given population, for example a factory, are willing to enroll. The goal of prevention is to help as many persons as possible. The appropriate dependent measure is therefore the percentage of all persons at risk who are helped. For example, consider two equal-sized companies with the same number of smokers in each of them, say 100; 80% of all smokers in one company enrolled in a smoking cessation program but only 20% of the smokers in the other enrolled. Even if the second program were 100% successful—all participants were abstinent from cigarettes at a 1-year follow-up—that program would have helped fewer persons than the other one even though it succeeded in helping only 50%. The focus of future research must be on increasing the proportion of persons at risk in a given population who are helped in changing their behavior. Innovations will have to occur not only in program design but also in methods for attracting persons and social organizations to prevention programs.

Our point, then, is that behavior modification and other psychological techniques have, in one sense, as yet not been applied to the problem of prevention. The reason for this is our collective adherence to the private practice model. Our behavior, like that of everyone else, is under reinforcement control; an assured income is always welcome, and following a familiar model reduces anxiety. Ultimately our ineffectiveness in prevention is a political issue. Present-day health policies are such that all rewards come to the office-based, fee-for-service practitioner. (There is no insurance coverage for population-based prevention services.)

Clinicians will only make a contribution to the amelioration of the public health problems presented by self-imposed risk (*a*) if practice and research are moved from the office and lab to the persons at risk; (*b*) if an effort is made to understand problem behaviors in terms of the social context in which they occur (friends, co-workers, and family are the ones who have supported, or at least condoned, the "unhealthy" behavior and it is they who must be induced to encourage the behavior change); (*c*) if the provision of motivation for behavior change becomes part of treatment; (*d*) if persons can make a living by providing effective prevention services; and (*e*) if we use as the dependent measure the percentage of persons at risk who have been helped.

The number of programs that have been designed and evaluated in accordance with these principles is limited. Broad-based heart disease prevention programs and efforts to reduce or prevent smoking in school settings are examples of programs in which the relevant dependent measure has been reported, the programs are brought to the persons at risk, and because the programs are addressed to a community the social system is mobilized for behavior change.

The most interesting and promising school-centered intervention programs are those based on McGuire's (1964) notion of psychological inoculation. Young persons are said to begin smoking in response to social pressure, and the task of prevention programs is therefore to inoculate against those social pressures (Evans, 1976). Results of studies that attempt such inoculations are encouraging. For example, Evans, Rozelle, Mittelmark, Hansen, Bane, and Havis (1978) report that over a period of time 10% of the pupils in an intervention school as opposed to 18% in a control school began to smoke, and McAlister, Perry, and Maccoby (1979) found that after 2 years only 7.1% of pupils in their experimental school, but between 18.8% and 21% in the control school, reported being smokers.

The best-known example of a broad-based intervention program is the Stanford Heart Disease Prevention Program (Farquhar, Maccoby, Wood, Alexander, Breitrose, Brown, Haskell, McAlister, Meyer, Nash, & Stern, 1977; Meyer, Nash, McAlister, Maccoby, & Farquhar, 1980). It was designed to alter, through mass media campaigns and face-to-face contact, behaviors that either contribute to or constitute risk factors for heart disease. Evaluation indicates that it was possible to effect some changes in life-style through mass media campaigns, but even more extensive changes were made through a combination of mass media campaign and face-to-face contact. Other programs that fall into the same category are the Karelia Project in Finland (Puska, Tuomilehto, Salinen, Viirtamo, & Mustaniemi, 1977), and a number of research programs in Europe. The large Multiple Risk Factor Intervention Trial (MRFIT Research Group, 1980) in the United States is often mentioned in the same context as the Stanford Project. The fact is, however, that MRFIT will tell us more about the relationship between changes in health habits and health status than about the planning of prevention programs.

Despite the promising results of the intervention trials, we fear that those endeavors will ultimately be treated as interesting research rather than as models for action. There are neither social structures nor powerful institutions that have prevention as their goal. As long as such institutions are missing, schools will return to the familiar (i.e., traditional health education) and the replications of such programs as the Stanford one will be only pale imitations. For this reason the emphasis of one phase of the Stanford Heart Disease Prevention Program on community structures and community organization is especially important (Farquhar, 1978b).

Any discussion of prevention must include a reference to self-help groups (Caplan & Killilea, 1976). It is possible that their impact outstrips those of all professionals (Stuart & Mitchell, 1978). Such groups have been formed around a variety of tasks ranging all the way from food purchases to the treatment of neurosis. Weight Watchers and Alcoholics Anonymous are two such organizations that concern themselves directly with health behavior. Both of these organizations are standard referral sources for most clinicians, and the influence of Weight Watchers has spread far beyond the Weight Watchers meetings to supermarkets and even the television screen. Weight Watchers and Alocoholics Anonymous, like other self-help movements, gain much of their strength from the group formed for the purpose of treatment. Additionally, participants in self-help groups involve their social environment in the treatment process. Weight Watchers, for example, has made it acceptable for persons to talk about their weight problems, thereby not only eliciting reinforcement for the effort to lose weight but also inducing other members of their circle to appraise their weight and eating habits. Similarly, members of Alcoholics Anonymous will readily tell persons of their alcoholism, which in turn has the effect that their wish not to consume alcohol will be respected. In general it is difficult for professionals to instigate self-help groups, but Weight Watchers is not only supported by professionals, it is also a business venture.

Optimal Settings for Preventive Programs

THE WORK PLACE

Many companies have begun to support prevention programs (Norris, 1981). As yet, however, these efforts at improving health have not been evaluated (Jacobs, 1980). Until now the emphasis has been mostly on fitness (Pyle, 1979), and to a much smaller extent on smoking (Danaher, 1980), hypertension, and obesity. Health clubs and fitness centers have become common although they are provided more often for management than for production workers. The best of those centers are staffed by instructors and provide information on nutrition and stress management. Motivation has rarely received explicit attention, but there are several reports of monetary incentives attached to giving up smoking, and some fitness programs are organized in such a manner as to lend them an air of exclusivity. If this is done, waiting lists for membership develop.

Our own effort in work settings has been to develop programs consistent with the principles outlined earlier. Two pilot studies on smoking cessation programs have been completed (Stachnik & Stoffelmayr, 1981), and an effort to test similar programs for the modification of health behaviors with students living in residence halls is underway. The pilot studies were conducted for two groups of 100 employees of a clerical–technical mix, each group the headquarters staff of a company. The features of the program which we consider to be important follow.

1. Location of program. The programs took place on company premises and meetings were held partially on company time. This reduced the annoyance involved in program attendance and facilitated communication with smokers. The effect was that a large proportion of smokers, about 50% in one program and 70% in the other, took part.

2. Social support. As the programs took place on company premises, co-workers of the smokers became involved also. They provided support and encouragement to the program participants. Although it was possible for participants to stay in touch with each other throughout the day, the following procedures were employed to maximize social support: (a) the program participants were divided into small teams of no fewer than five members whose task was to provide mutual support; (b) contracts with family and friends, in which participants informed between 10 and 20 friends and relatives (excluding other participants in the smoking program) in writing of their intent not to smoke for a given period of time, usually 6 months, resulted not only in the reinforcement of the commitment not to smoke, but also elicited the help and support of those who were contacted; and (c) control procedures. The letter to friends and relatives also indicated the participants' agreement to the following procedure: smoking staff will contact recipients of the letter to inquire about the participants' smoking behavior. On the average, two of the participants' support persons were contacted per week. This procedure not only indicated to the support persons the seriousness of the program, but added to the participants' resolve not to smoke.

3. Monetary incentives. One company put up $50 per participant and the other one $125. Participants themselves contributed $20 and $25. Partici-

pants were required to inform the program staff if they had smoked. If a smoking incident occurred, one-half of the funds in the account of the participant who had smoked was equally divided among the members of teams in which there was no smoking incident. The team with the fewest smoking incidents of course had the largest sum of money in its account at the end of the program. This team also received an additional bonus at that time. These monetary transactions resulted in friendly competition among teams and appeared to enhance group cohesiveness and mutual support.

4. Duration of the program. The two programs each lasted 7 months. One of those months was structured like a usual smoking cessation program, and 6 months were given to the maintenance of abstinence from smoking. A Stop Smoking Day separated the two phases of the program. Regular meetings were held throughout, weekly for the first 3 months and biweekly thereafter. Meeting times were divided into team meetings and time during which all the program participants interacted with each other. Meetings were restricted to 1 hour, and after the stop smoking date included a health education program. This focused not only on smoking, but more broadly on changes in life-style. In one of the programs, attendance at meetings was encouraged by raffling off $50 at each meeting.

5. Evaluation. The data show these programs to be successful in terms of the percentage of population at risk who participated and who were abstinent from cigarettes after 6 months. In one company, 47% of the smokers enrolled in the program and 80% of those who enrolled were abstinent 6 months later; thus the number of smokers in the company was reduced by 37%. In the second company, 70% of the smokers enrolled in the program and 91% of them were abstinent 6 months later; thus the number of smokers in that company was reduced by 65%.

The research questions we face now are: Can this approach be applied to larger social organizations and to behaviors other than smoking? and What will our long-term success rates be? Because participants in our programs are subjected to fairly powerful contingencies, we do not know what the effect of the sudden withdrawal of these contingencies will be.

THE PRIMARY HEALTH CARE OFFICE

Unlike the work place model presented earlier, the primary health care setting attracts individuals who routinely and frequently present themselves for attention to problems related to their health. Because of this large numbers of individuals with adverse health habits enter a system that has potential for helping them, without the patient necessarily having identified the adverse health habit as a problem. As we see, this places an otherwise low success rate of 5–10% in a very different and much more favorable light.

In addition, there is some evidence that an ongoing physician–patient relationship, as well as the perceived stature of the physician, may have a beneficial impact on changing patients' health habits. Smoking clinics that have major medical involvement have been demonstrated in some instances to have higher long-term success rates than those that do not (Delarue, 1973; Kanzler, Jaffe, & Zeiderberg, 1976). Other studies have cited the positive impact of physicians' advice to stop smoking on cessation rates (Burnum, 1974; Porter & McCullough, 1972; Raw, 1976; Russell, Wilson, Taylor, & Baker, 1979). But the fact is that physicians have played only a small role in the prevention of chronic diseases; the reasons for this are not surprising. We have previously indicated that the education and training as well as many contingencies of practice do not facilitate the involvement of primary care physicians in attempts to modify their patients' habits of living. The education of medical students and residents takes place largely in hospital settings where medical activity centers on disease, often in its most severe forms, with little opportunity or reason to focus on potential problems or alteration of risks. Indeed, third-party reimbursement is contingent upon a disease category being identified under which billing may proceed. Smoking or overeating are not classified as diseases.

There are other reasons physicians avoid more direct involvement in preventive health care. For one thing, motivating patients to modify health-risk behaviors is very difficult. Success rates are low and recidivism is high. The rewards, in terms of better patient health, are vague and long-term. Most physicians are oriented, either through disposition or experience, toward more concrete, positive results. Administering an antibiotic to a patient with a urinary tract infection and noting disappearance of bacteria and symptoms is easier and has a higher success rate than altering the eating habits of an obese patient with severe arthritis.

Another impediment is the reimbursement structure of outpatient practice. Third-party groups reimburse physicians for laboratory work, X rays, electrocardiograms, and the performance of minor surgical procedures. The more time-consuming activities of educating and motivating patients are not reimbursed by insurance companies, nor are most patients themselves oriented toward paying the primary care physician, particularly at a level equivalent to reimbursement available for these procedures.

Another factor may be the delivery system itself. Many destructive health habits are established early in life at a time when individuals may be under the care of pediatricians who, by virtue of the age focus of their practice, do not provide care for the chronic diseases that often eventuate. At the other extreme, internists who care for adults disabled by chronic diseases often do not have responsibility for them early in life when the habits begin. To what extent this chronologic division of care hinders physician involvement in preventive practices is not known. Whether family physicians, who have the potential for caring for individuals at both times, can be more effective in modifying health habits remains to be seen.

The Periodic Health Examination

The opportunity for an expanded preventive role for physicians clearly exists. For example, many patients deliberately solicit the primary physician's opinion of their health status by presenting themselves for an annual physical or, using current nomenclature, the periodic health examination. Such visits, after acute upper respiratory illness, constitute the second most frequent reason for consultation with a personal physician in the United States (U.S. National Center for Health Statistics, 1976). In addition, many employers advise or sponsor periodic health examinations for their employees, often in addition to the contributions made to third-party insurance carriers for acute care services. Because of the frequency of such examinations and because of the value placed on them by patients, such visits, if properly focused and conducted, could have a beneficial impact on health habits and reduction of the chronic diseases that these habits precipitate.

Unfortunately, the periodic health examination, as it is currently rendered, may be an example of too little, too late. Indeed, this examination has been criticized, in part because it has a content and frequency that bear little relation to the needs of different age and social groups. There is heavy emphasis in these examinations on *secondary* prevention through screening for occult diseases rather than *primary* prevention through identification of risks that, if modified, can actually prevent development of disease. There is an additional problem of efficacy of screening procedures, many of which have been incorporated into periodic health examinations despite scant evidence that they improve or lengthen life. Indeed, only one published study, that conducted at the Permanente Medical Group in Oakland, suggests a benefit from frequent periodic health examination (Spitzer & Brown, 1975). These investigators found lower mortality and morbidity in a screened as compared to a nonscreened population. A causal role for the screening procedures in explaining their association with lowered morbidity has not been established.

Out of this criticism and re-examination have emerged some new proposals for the periodic health examination. In 1977, Breslow and Somers proposed a lifetime Health-Monitoring Program that advocated incorporation of prevention into day-to-day care and a greater focus on modification of risky health habits, including such nondisease items as car seat-belt usage by adolescents. The Canadian Task Force on the Periodic Health Examination

(Prefontaine and coauthors, 1979) recommended in 1979 that the routine annual checkup be abandoned in favor of a selective approach that considers a person's age, sex, and specific risk status. The American Cancer Society has also modified its recommendations based on new evidence of medical efficacy and cost–benefit analysis (American Cancer Society, 1980). A very small number of adult diseases for which screening is thought to provide some benefit remain: hypertension; breast, cervical, skin, and colorectal cancer; some communicable diseases; glaucoma; and periodontal disease. A number of chronic diseases, among them obstructive lung disease, coronary heart disease, and degenerative arthritis, appear to be most effectively screened by increased attention to the habits that cause them (smoking, high-fat diet, overeating, and, perhaps, insufficient exercise) rather than by application of methods to detect presymptomatic disease (Prefontaine et al., 1979).

Other Possibilities in the Primary Care Setting

There are very few studies that have systematically evaluated the impact, both short- and long-term, of primary physicians on altering the health habits of their patients. There are a few, however, that suggest a positive role for direct physician involvement in changing unhealthy behaviors (Burnum, 1974; Porter & McCullough, 1972; Raw, 1976). One study examined the advice to stop smoking coupled with educational materials and a short period of follow-up visits (Russell et al., 1979). Over 2000 smokers seen in a 4-week period by 28 general practitioners participated in the study. At the end of 1 year the group receiving the advice and support of their physicians had twice as many individuals who quit smoking as the control group. This appeared to be the result of increasing the numbers of people who actually attempted quitting, with a smaller effect on improving the number of relapses during the follow-up period. These data suggest that the physician may be most effective in initiating behavior change in his or her patients, but that perhaps other techniques and/or settings are required to achieve long-term maintenance.

A similar study is underway at Michigan State University to determine the impact of the primary care physician coupled with involvement of the patients' social networks and provision of immediate incentives for changes in health risk behaviors. This study is attempting to determine the relationship between the degree of physician involvement and level of success. It is also comparing the traditional model of affecting such behaviors, referral outside the primary care setting, to a model conducted by the primary physician and his or her staff.

Another model that deserves study is the inclusion within, or closely aligned to, the primary care setting of an individual specifically expert in methods of altering complex human behaviors. Such an individual could be seen as a member of the health care team whose talents in relaxation techniques, cognitive imagery, self-management techniques, contingency management strategies, and group facilitation could aid in achieving better health states. Such a structure would allow treatment packages to be tailored to individual patients and would allow for the combination of several rather than one or two techniques to alter behavior. There is some experimental evidence that such tailoring and combination of methods are associated with higher rates of success (Delahunt & Curran, 1976; Devine & Feenald, 1973).

Health hazard appraisal and health risk assessment are currently being used by many physicians to assess the risk for certain health outcomes in their patients based on computer-weighted scoring schemes (Center for Disease Control, 1980; Goetz, 1980). These techniques relate details of patient history (e.g., family history of coronary disease, hypertension) to epidemiologic data regarding subsequent risk in order to generate a risk score or statement regarding likely attenuation of life expectancy. These tools, although largely unstudied, have the potential for efficiently identifying specific behaviors in need of modification. Unfortunately, this information is often given to patients in written form or supplemented by somewhat casual advice. In order to be effective it most likely needs to be incorporated into a vigorous health habit modification plan, either within the primary care setting or utilizing existing community resources.

In order for the primary care setting to be most effective, physicians ultimately need better information about preventive methods that work. Physicians also need better information regarding resources in their own communities that have been demonstrated to be effective. There needs to be inclusion in traditional medical literature of studies that address techniques of improving health habits. Medical education could also address itself to the possible benefit of providing young clinicians with behavioral skills as specific educational objectives analogous to the successful performance of, for example, sigmoidoscopy.

Such methods, if transportable to varied health settings and if successful in addressing a broad spectrum of adverse health habits, would have the advantage of reaching large numbers of individuals in need of health habit modification. The potential impact of a concerted effort on the part of all primary physicians is much larger than similar methods applied to small, select groups that are frequently self-referred. For example, it has been estimated that if all 2000 or more general practitioners in Great Britain were able to identify smoking as a problem and embark on a program of encouragement and providing information to their patients, even with success rates as low as 4–5% there would be produced more ex-smokers than produced by 10,000 standard smoking clinics each with a success rate of 30% (Russell *et al.*, 1979).

Despite these potential influences by the primary physician, in order to accomplish large-scale change in the health habits of our nation our culture as a whole must also change so as to alter the day-to-day influence of family, peers, and social customs. Even some restriction with respect to the availability of, for example, cigarettes and alcohol may be needed. It is not unreasonable to contemplate the inclusion of incentives, perhaps in the form of reduced insurance premiums, for people who engage in healthful practices. These are complex social changes that will not be easy, in part due to some powerful political obstacles as well as to established habits and customs (Sapolsky, 1980). On the other hand, primary physicians, by virtue of their unique relationship with individuals who consult them regularly regarding other matters relating to health, appear to have both opportunity and potential for making significant contributions to such change.

Summary

An attempt to summarize the present state of affairs relative to the prevention of chronic disease must include the following points:

1. The most serious and prevalent chronic diseases are at least in part related to life-style and thus are ultimately behavior problems rather than medical problems. Acceptance of that proposition has many implications, including greatly changed roles for health professionals and alterations in our health care system.
2. The list of behavioral risk factors that need to be modified in order to reduce significantly the incidence and prevalence of chronic disease is a surprisingly short one. Reductions in just smoking, serum cholesterol levels, and hypertension would have a dramatic impact on the three most common chronic diseases—heart disease, cancer, and stroke.
3. Considered as a whole, people in the United States have scored some notable achievements in chronic disease prevention. And although segments of the population show continued interest in improving their health, it is clear that the benefits of prevention have reached different groups in the population unevenly. Much of the responsibility for the unevenness must fall on untenable assumptions about both people's motivation and opportunity to achieve good health. Prevention programs based on such assumptions will continue to leave large portions of the population unaffected.
4. Chronic disease prevention programs can have far more impact than they have had to date by employing various incentives to increase the number in a target population who are willing to participate, and by abandoning

inappropriate service delivery models in favor of others that capitalize on the use of existing sites and settings for service delivery.

References

American Cancer Society Report on the Cancer-Related Health Checkup. *Ca—A Cancer Journal for Clinicians*, 1980, *30*, 194–240.

APA Task Force on Health Research. Contributions of psychology to health research: Patterns, problems, and potentials. *American Psychologist*, 1976, *31*, 263–274.

Armstrong, M., Warner, E., & Connor, W. Regression of coronary atheromatosis in rhesus monkeys. *Circulation Research*, 1970, *27*, 59–63.

Ashley, F., Jr., & Kannel, W. Relation of weight change to changes in atherogenic traits: The Framingham study. *Journal of Chronic Diseases*, 1974, *27*, 103–114.

Blackburn, H. Prevention of coronary heart disease: The need, potential, strategy, impediments, and implications. In G. Schettler, J. Drews, & H. Greten (Eds.), *Changes in the medical panorama*. Stuttgart: Thieme, 1978.

Blumberg, E. M., West, P. M., & Ellis, F. W. MMPI findings in human cancer. In Welsh, G. S., & Dahlstrom, W. G. (Eds.), *Basic readings on the MMPI in psychology and medicine*. Minneapolis: University of Minnesota Press, 1956.

Breslow, L., & Somers, A. R. The lifetime health-monitoring program. *New England Journal of Medicine*, 1977, *296*, 601–608.

Brownell, K. D. Obesity: Understanding and treating a serious, prevalent, and refractory disorder. *Journal of Consulting and Clinical Psychology*, 1982, *50*, 820–840.

Burnum, J. F. Outlook for treating patients with self-destructive habits. *Annals of Internal Medicine*, 1974, *81*, 387–393.

Caplan, G., & Killilea, M. (Eds.) *Support systems and mutual help*. New York: Grune & Stratton, 1976.

Center for Disease Control. *Risk factor update*. Atlanta, Georgia: U.S. Department of Health and Human Services, 1980.

Covey, L. S., & Wynder, E. L. Smoking habits and occupational status. *Journal of Occupational Medicine*, 1981, *23*, 537–542.

Danaher, B. G. Smoking cessation programs in occupational settings. *Public Health Reports*, 1980, *95*, 149–157.

Delahunt, J., & Curran, J. P. Effectiveness of negative practice and self control techniques in the reduction of smoking behavior. *Journal of Consulting and Clinical Psychology*, 1976, *44*, 1002–1007.

Delarue, N. C. A study in smoking withdrawal. *Canadian Journal of Public Health*, 1973, *64*, 55–79.

Devine, D. A., & Feenald, P. S. Outcome effects of receiving a preferred randomly assigned or non-preferred therapy. *Journal of Consulting and Clinical Psychology*, 1973, *41*, 104–107.

Evans, R. I. Smoking in children: Developing a social psychological strategy of deterrence. *Preventive Medicine*, 1976, *5*, 122–127.

Evans, R. I., Rozelle, R. M., Mittelmark, M. B., Hansen, W. B., Bane, A. L., & Havis, J. Deterring the onset of smoking in children: Knowledge of immediate physiological effects and coping with peer pressure, media pressure and parent modeling. *Journal of Applied Social Psychology*, 1978, *8*, 126–135.

Farquhar, J. W. *The American way of life need not be hazardous to your health*. Stanford, Calif.: Stanford Alumni Association, 1978. (a)

Farquhar, J. W. The community-based model of life style intervention trials. *American Journal of Epidemiology*, 1978, *108*, 103–111. (b)

Farquhar, J. W., Maccoby, N., Wood, P. D., Alexander, J. K., Breitrose, H., Brown, B. W., Haskell, W. L., McAlister, A. L., Meyer, A. J., Nash, J. O., & Stern, M. P. Community education for cardiovascular health. *Lancet*, 1977, *1*, 1192–1195.

Flanagan, J. A research approach to improving our quality of life. *American Psychologist*, 1978, *33*, 138–147.

Foreyt, J. P., Goodrick, G. K. & Gotto, A. M. Limitations of behavioral treatment of obesity: Review and analysis. *Journal of Behavioral Medicine*, 1981, *4*, 159–174.

Goetz, A. A. Health risk appraisal: The estimation of risk. *Public Health Reports*, 1980, *95*, 119–126.

Golubjatnikov, R., Paskey, T., & Inhorn, S. Serum cholesterol levels of Mexican and Wisconsin school children. *American Journal of Epidemiology*, 1972, *96*, 36–39.

Honig, W. K. (Ed.) *Operant behavior: Areas of research and application*. New York: Appleton-Century-Crofts, 1966.

Jacobs, B. Can innovation curb health care costs? *Industry Week*, 1980, *206*, 78–83.

Junge, B., & Hoffmeister, H. Institute for Social Medicine and Epidemiology, Federal Health Office, West Berlin. Personal communication, 1981.

Kahn, H. A. The Dorn study of smoking and mortality among U.S. veterans: Report on 8½ years of observation. In W. Haenszel (Ed.), *Epidemiological approaches to the study of cancer and other chronic diseases* (National Cancer Institute Monograph 19.) Washington, D.C.: U.S. Government Printing Office, 1966.

Kanzler, M., Jaffe, J., & Zeiderberg, P. Long and short term effectiveness of a large-scale proprietary smoking cessation study. *Journal of Clinical Psychology*, 1976, *32*, 661–669.

Knowles, J. The responsibility of the individual. In J. Knowles (Ed.), *Doing better and feeling worse: Health in the United States*. New York: Norton, 1977.

Lalonde, M. *A new perspective on the health of Canadians*. Ottawa: Information Canada, 1975.

Lichtenstein, E. The smoking problem: A behavioral perspective. *Journal of Consulting and Clinical Psychology*, 1982, *50*, 804–819.

McAlister, A. L., Perry, C., & Maccoby, N. Adolescent smoking: Onset and prevention. *Pediatrics*, 1979, *63*, 650–657.

McGuire, W. Inducing resistance to persuasion: Some contemporary approaches. In L. Berkowitz (Ed.), *Advances in experimental social psychology* (Vol. 1). New York: Academic Press, 1964.

Meyer, A. J., Nash, J. D., McAlister, A. L., Maccoby, N., & Farquhar, J. W. Skills training in a cardiovascular health education campaign. *Journal of Consulting and Clinical Psychology*, 1980, *48*, 129–142.

MRFIT Research Group. Primary prevention of heart attacks: the MRFIT. *American Journal of Epidemiology*, 1980, *112*, 185–199.

National Cancer Institute. *The smoking digest. Progress report on a nation kicking the habit*. Bethesda, Md.: Office of Cancer Communications, 1977.

Norris, E. Firms cite victories in battle over rising health care costs. *Business Insurance*, October 5, 1981, pp. 33–35.

Porter, A. M. W., & McCullough, D. M. Counseling against cigarette smoking. *Practitioner*, 1972, *209*, 686–689.

Prefontaine, R., Spitzer, W. O., Bayne, R., Charron, K., Fletcher, S., Frappier-Davignon, L., Goldbloom, R., McWhinney, I., Morrison, B., Offord, D., & Sackett, D. The periodic health examination: Canadian task force on the periodic health examination. *Canadian Medical Association Journal*, 1979, *121*, 1193–1253.

Puska, P., Tuomilehto, J., Salinen, J., Viirtamo, J., & Mustaniemi, H. *Community control of acute myocardial infarction in North Karelia.* Paper presented at the meeting of the International Cardiovascular Congress, Arizona, March 1977.

Pyle, R. L. Corporate fitness programs—how do they shape up? *Personnel,* 1979, *56,* 58–67.

Raw, M. Persuading people to stop smoking. *Behaviour Research and Therapy,* 1976, *14,* 97–101.

Russell, M. A. H., Wilson, C., Taylor, C., & Baker, C. D. Effect of general practitioners' advice against smoking. *British Medical Journal,* 1979, *2,* 231–235.

Sapolsky, H. M. The political obstacles to the control of cigarette smoking in the United States. *Journal of Health Politics, Policy and Law,* 1980, *5,* 277–290.

Shapiro, D., & Goldstein, I. B. Biobehavioral perspectives on hypertension. *Journal of Consulting and Clinical Psychology,* 1982, *50,* 841–858.

Spitzer, W. O., & Brown, B. P. Unanswered questions about the periodic health examination. *Annals of Internal Medicine,* 1975, *83,* 257–263.

Stachnik, T. J., & Stoffelmayr, B. E. Is there a future for smoking cessation programs? *Journal of Community Health,* 1981, *7,* 47–56.

Stuart, R. B., & Mitchell, C. Peer as opposed to professional programming for weight control: Peers hold the edge. *Psychiatric Clinics of North America,* 1978, *1,* 697–712.

Susser, M. Prevention and health maintenance revisited. *Bulletin of the New York Academy of Medicine,* 1975, *51,* 5–8.

Thomas, L. On the science and technology of medicine. In J. Knowles (Ed.), *Doing better and feeling worse: Health in the United States.* New York: Norton, 1977.

U.S. National Center for Health Statistics. *Vital statistics of the United States.* Rockville, Md.: U.S. Government Printing Office, 1976.

U.S. Public Health Service. *Health, United States, 1980* (DHHS Publication No. 81-1232). Washington, D.C.: U.S. Department of Health and Human Services, 1980.

Wolpe, J. *The practice of behavior therapy* (3rd ed.). New York: Pergamon Press, 1982.

18

Coping with Chronic Disease: Current Status and Future Directions

LAURENCE A. BRADLEY
THOMAS G. BURISH

Introduction

The preceding chapters have presented a state-of-the-art summary of the current theoretical and empirical literature regarding patients' efforts to cope with chronic disease. A number of investigators associated with the tradition of psychosomatic medicine (see Adler, Cohen, & Stone, 1979) began to examine the relationship between psychological processes and chronic disease in the 1940s. These investigators, however, were primarily interested in the role of personality factors and life stress in the etiology of chronic disease (Moos, 1979). It has only been since the 1960s that extensive work has been directed toward helping patients to cope better with or to prevent the onset of chronic disease. This chapter summarizes the current status of the literature on coping with chronic disease and discusses on a general level of several promising theoretical, methodological, and conceptual issues that warrant further study.

Theoretical Issues

All of the contributors to this volume have either explicitly or implicitly acknowledged the influence of Richard Lazarus's cognitively oriented model of coping upon their own work (Cohen & Lazarus, 1979; Lazarus & Launier,

1978). Nerenz and Leventhal (Chapter 2), for example, presented a model of patient self-regulation that incorporates patients' cognitive representations of their illnesses, affective responses, and symptomatology. These authors explictly acknowledged Lazarus's work as a major determinant of their own views. The majority of this volume's authors, however, implicitly acknowledged Lazarus's influence by dealing with the issue of how patients' appraisals of their illnesses guide their coping efforts. For example, it was noted that patients often show denial of illness or disability soon after receiving a diagnosis of cancer (Meyerowitz, Heinrich, & Schag, Chapter 6), or suffering a myocardial infarction (MI) (Krantz & Deckel, Chapter 4) or spinal cord injury (Brucker, Chapter 11). It might be hypothesized that patients' use of denial may represent the best means of protecting the self-system from being "engulfed" by the presence of a life-threatening chronic disease during the early stages of the coping process. Denial, therefore, may be adaptive to the degree that it allows patients to process slowly information concerning the nature of their illnesses (e.g., identity, cause, time-line) as well as the potential consequences of their illnesses and associated treatments.

Several theoretical issues were raised by some authors that require further investigation. Two sets of authors (Krantz & Deckel, Chapter 4; Turk & Speers, Chapter 8) noted that it is necessary to determine the specific mechanisms that link psychological processes to the physiological, behavioral, cognitive, and affective aspects of recovery from stroke or MI and of regulation of metabolic activity associated with diabetes. Both sets of contributors provided cognitively oriented models, influenced primarily by Lazarus's work, that may serve as the basis for hypothesis testing and further theoretical refinements.

Another group of authors posed theoretical questions that were more narrowly defined than those already described. Specifically, it was noted that there are several chronic diseases or disorders from which individuals cannot recover, or the symptoms of which cannot be completely controlled. These diseases include epilepsy (Kaplan & Wyler, Chapter 10), pain associated with various chronic diseases (Bradley, Chapter 13), and some spinal cord injuries (Brucker, Chapter 11). There are several behavioral treatment interventions that can be applied to (a) help some persons better control their seizure disorders (electroencephalographic [EEG] biofeedback); (b) reduce the pain associated with spinal cord injury (relaxation training), various forms of arthritis (peripheral skin temperature biofeedback), and phantom limb sensations (electromyographic [EMG] biofeedback and relaxation training); and (c) increase functional outcomes following spinal cord injury (operant and classical conditioning procedures as well as blood pressure biofeedback training). With the exception of the interventions used to increase functional outcomes following spinal cord injury, it is not clear how the majority of the interventions influence patients' physiological functioning and thereby aid patients' coping efforts. For example, it is not known why EEG feedback helps some persons but not others to control their seizure activity, or if skin temperature feedback is effective in reducing arthritic pain because it actually allows rheumatoid arthritics to increase blood flow to affected joints. Further research is necessary to determine the physiological processes that are influenced by the interventions just noted.

Finally, several authors raised theoretical questions regarding the roles of the family and patient support groups in the coping process. Masters, Cerreto, and Mendlowitz (Chapter 14) noted that the majority of work that has been published on family issues consists of poorly controlled investigations of the manner in which nuclear family members are affected by the presence of a chronically ill child or of how the coping of chronically ill children is influenced by various nuclear family members. This literature has not addressed several important issues, such as the benefits of training parents to increase children's compliance with therapeutic regimens and the interaction of various chronic diseases with the specific developmental tasks both of children (e.g., development of autonomy) and of the family (e.g., sending the first child to school). Moreover, the family literature has not carefully examined the potentially beneficial influence of spouses or other family members upon patients' attempts to (a) achieve maximum recovery from MI, stroke, and spinal cord injury; or (b) cope effectively with various cancers, respiratory disorders, diabetes, epilepsy, obesity, and chronic pain. It should be noted that there are several local and national patient support programs designed specifically for patients suffering from cancer, stroke, head injury, obesity, lupus, rheumatoid arthritis, and other chronic disorders. Preliminary evaluations of a small number of these programs are being undertaken. It would be desirable, however, for researchers investigating self-help programs to establish research networks similar to those described by Masters et al. (Chapter 14) so that some uniformity in hypothesis testing and methodological procedures could be achieved. Such uniformity would allow investigators to answer a number of important theoretical and practical questions, including (a) whether patients with various chronic diseases may better perform specific coping tasks as a function of participation in patient support groups, and (b) what specific group factors (e.g., leadership, degree of structure, role of family members) might mediate the observed outcomes.

To summarize, a review of the contributions to the present volume indicates that the literature regarding coping with chronic disease has been greatly influenced by Lazarus's cognitively-oriented model of how people cope with stressful stimuli. In addition, three specific theoretical issues have been addressed by various authors. First, attempts have been made to determine what mechanisms actually link various psychological processes to the physiological, behavioral, cognitive, and affective aspects of recovery from some chronic diseases or attempts to regulate disease activity. The models that have been proposed, however, are preliminary in nature and require a great deal of empirical testing. Second, a small number of investigators have attempted to determine how some behavioral interventions may influence patients' physiological functioning and thus help them to better cope with their illnesses. It has been assumed that several interventions, particularly those involving biofeedback procedures, may have specific effects on the physiological functioning of persons with disorders such as rheumatoid arthritis and epilepsy. However, in many cases these assumptions have not yet received empirical support. Finally, it has been hypothesized that some family characteristics or behaviors may greatly affect patients' reactions to their diseases. It also has been suggested that patient support or self-help groups may positively contribute to patients' coping efforts. Unfortunately, these issues have received only rudimentary investigation.

Methodological Issues

All of the contributors to this volume noted that the coping literature suffers from a paucity of well-controlled investigations. The problems in designing well-controlled outcome studies are often exacerbated by the fact that it is difficult to obtain sufficiently large samples of chronically ill patients to include adequate control groups (see Creer, Chapter 12). It sometimes is possible to recruit sufficiently large subject samples at university medical centers or institutes devoted to the study of certain diseases (e.g., oncology or arthritis research centers); however, the extent to which the results of studies performed with subjects found at these medical centers or institutes may generalize to other patient populations is unknown. For example, Chapman, Sola, and Bonica (1979) demonstrated that there were significant differences between chronic benign pain patients assessed at a university medical center and those examined within private practice settings with regard to self-reports of illness behavior patterns and depression. It would be unwarranted, therefore, to assume that treatment interventions designed on the basis of studies involving patients drawn from university medical centers would necessarily produce optimal results with patients seen in private practice settings (see Kaplan & Wyler, Chapter 10; Masters *et al.*, Chapter 14). The difficulty of conducting well-controlled multigroup studies in chronic disease areas and the need to investigate generalizability from one setting to another suggest the need for greater use of single-subject studies that incorporate adequate placebo control procedures (Kazdin, 1978). The use of single-subject designs among medical center research and private practitioners not only would allow a greater number of investigations to be conducted by researchers and clinicians alike, but also would allow future reviewers to determine the generalizability of various interventions across treatment settings.

Another methodological issue of great importance is the lack of adequate follow-up assessments characteristic of all the research areas discussed in this volume. This lack may be attributed primarily to two factors. First, some chronic diseases are associated with a high rate of mortality or morbidity among subjects (e.g., cancer, cardiovascular disorders), thereby precluding follow-up assessment. In addition, a large proportion of research investigations are performed in university medical centers or specialized institutes that draw people from a large geographic area; it is often difficult to convince patients who live some distance from the institution to return for follow-up assessments. Many investigators, particularly those interested in chronic pain, have resorted to the use of telephone surveys or mailed questionnaires to assess long-term patient functioning. It should be noted, however, that adequate follow-up procedures should include the use of dependent measures that are identical to those employed at the pretreatment and postreatment assessments (Prokop & Bradley, 1981). Thus, in many circumstances telephone surveys or mailed questionnaires are not adequate follow-up procedures.

It is generally recognized that the term *coping* denotes a process that may extend over long periods of time and that is influenced by time-related changes in disease activity. A third methodological issue addressed by several of the contributors, then, is that very few investigators have attempted to assess the efficacy of various coping strategies at different stages of chronic illness (see Meyerowitz *et al.*, Chapter 6; Turk & Speers, Chapter 8; Masters *et al.*, Chapter 14). As several of these authors have suggested, it is necessary to perform situation-specific analyses that identify *at different stages in a particular disease* (a) the adaptive problems experienced by patients, (b) the coping strategies used by or provided to patients, and (c) the relative efficacy of these strategies (see Meyerowitz *et al.*, Chapter 6; Turk & Follick, 1979).

In summary, the major methodological shortcomings in chronic disease research are the lack of well-controlled investigations of treatment outcome, the failure to perform adequate follow-up assessment of patient functioning, and the failure to delineate and assess the efficacy of patients' coping strategies at different disease stages. All of these methodological problems are compounded by the difficulties investigators experience in recruiting sufficiently large subject samples. Unless some alternative methodological procedures are used successfully by some investigators—for example, well-controlled single-subject designs—it is likely that the methodological weaknesses noted will negatively affect the quality of future chronic disease research.

Conceptual Issues

The majority of the investigations described in this volume have focused upon maladaptive patterns of patient coping or the efficacy of interventions designed to improve patient coping. Very little attention has been directed toward the prediction of which persons are likely to cope poorly with various chronic diseases or are most likely to benefit from professional or self-help treatment interventions. Although public and private funding priorities currently favor intervention-outcome studies rather than actuarial or predictive investigations, it is necessary to conduct the types of studies described above in order to understand the coping process more fully and to develop optimal treatment interventions for specific patient groups.

Within the context of intervention studies, nonetheless, several more specific conceptual issues also require attention. First, very little effort has been directed toward the development of cost–benefit ratios associated with various treatment interventions (see Burish & Lyles, Chapter 7; Kaplan & Wyler, Chapter 10). It is suggested that future investigators attempt to determine changes in patients' health care resource utilization on a long-term basis following treatment interventions in order to assess the total benefits of devoting expensive professional staff hours to the provision of those interventions.

Related to the issue of cost and benefits of treatment is the concern with who may best provide interventions to patients with the least expense. Rogers (Chapter 15), for example, noted that nurses have taken on many of the patient care roles that formerly were held by physicians. Similarly, it may be possible to train family members or other chronic disease patients to help some patient groups cope better with their disorders (see Burish & Lyles, Chapter 7; Straw, Chapter 9; Creer, Chapter 12). Thus, it is necessary to compare the cost–benefit ratios associated with treatment provision by various professionals (physicians, psychologists, nurses) and nonprofessionals (family members, patients).

A final conceptual issue that requires attention is the training of health professionals, especially physicians, in the principles of behavioral medicine. Specifically, we advocate the development of programmatic attempts to influence the attitudes and behavior of physicians in training. For example, investigators at Bowman Gray School of Medicine are examining the impact of a 3-year behavioral medicine curriculum on medical students' attitudes regarding the value of behavioral medicine precepts and their application to the treatment of various physical disorders (see Young, Bradley, Hoban, & Pearson, 1983). It is hypothesized that students' attitudes regarding behavioral medicine will become more positive as they progress through their training. If this hypothesis is supported, it will suggest that educating students about behavioral medicine may lead them to show greater willingness than that of current physicians to attend to the behavioral patterns (including health-promotion activities) of patients.

In summary, we have identified two major conceptual issues in chronic disease research. The first issue concerns the need to determine the costs and benefits associated with various treatment interventions and to evaluate whether the cost–benefit ratios of treatments provided by various groups of professional and nonprofessional persons may vary. Second, we have suggested that it would be beneficial to train medically oriented health care professionals in the principles of behavioral medicine. Specifically, we have recommended that medical students be provided with training in health promotion and other aspects of behavioral medicine in order to foster positive attitudes regarding attending to the health-related behaviors of their patients.

Conclusions

The preceding discussion clearly indicates that many theoretical, methodological, and conceptual issues remain unresolved in chronic disease research. The resolution of these issues will be hampered both by practical difficulties (e.g., lack of adequate subject samples) and economic as well as social factors (e.g., scarce research funding, priorities for intervention-oriented rather than predictive research). Nonetheless, we are encouraged by the progress that has been made in helping persons cope with various chronic diseases. The promising results and the suggestions for future research contained in this volume point toward increases both in the quantity and quality of future research on coping with chronic disease. As a result of this research and its clinical implementation, we hope that some day soon there will be fewer patients who will struggle unsuccessfully with the challenge of coping with chronic disease.

References

Adler, N.E., Cohen, F., & Stone, G. C. Themes and professional prospects in health psychology. In G. C. Stone, F. Cohen, & N. E. Adler (Eds.), *Health psychology: A handbook*. San Francisco: Jossey-Bass, 1979.

Chapman, C. R., Sola, A. E., & Bonica, J. J. Illness behavior and depression compared in pain
    center and private practice patients. *Pain*, 1979, *6*, 1–7.
Cohen, F., & Lazarus, R. S. Coping with the stresses of illness. In G. C. Stone, F. Cohen, & N.
    E. Adler (Eds.), *Health psychology: A handbook*. San Francisco: Jossey-Bass, 1979.
Kazdin, A. E. Methodological and interpretative problems of single-case experimental designs.
    Journal of Consulting and Clinical Psychology, 1978, *46*, 629–642.
Lazarus, R. S., & Launier, R. Stress-related transactions between person and environment. In
    L. A. Pervin & M. Lewis (Eds.), *Perspectives in interactional psychology*. New York:
    Plenum Press, 1978.
Moos, R. H. Social-ecological perspectives on health. In G. C. Stone, F. Cohen, & N. E. Adler
    (Eds.), *Health psychology: A handbook*. San Francisco: Jossey-Bass, 1979.
Prokop, C. K., & Bradley, L. A. Methodological issues in medical psychology and behavioral
    medicine research. In C. K. Prokop & L. A. Bradley (Eds.), *Medical psychology: Contri-
    butions to behavioral medicine*. New York: Academic Press, 1981.
Turk, D. C., & Follick, M. J. *Coping with chronic illness: A proposal for a preventative model
    of intervention*. Paper presented at the meeting of the American Psychological Association,
    New York, August 1979.
Young, L. D., Bradley, L. A., Hoban, D., & Pearson, W. S. *Medical students' attitudes toward
    behavioral medicine and psychiatry*. Paper presented at the meeting of the Southeastern
    Psychological Association, Atlanta, March 1983.

Author Index

Numbers in italics refer to the pages on which the complete references are cited.

A

Abeloff, M. D., 145, 152, *156*
Ablin, A. R., 184, *185*
Abitbol, M. M., 165, *185*
Abraham, S., 221, *252*
Abram, S. E., 63, *74*
Abrams, R. D., 139, *158*
Abramson, L. Y., 97, *107*
Achenbach, T. M., 401, 402, 403, *404*
Achterberg, J. 183, *185*, 367, 370, 371, *375*
Ack, M., 389, *404*
Adams, D., 432, *444*
Adams, J., 144, *158*
Adams, J. E., 31, *35*
Adams, K. M., 267, *281*
Adelman, B., 292, *310*
Adler, N. E., 475, *481*
Aelony, Y., 328, *334*
Agate, J., 436, 437, *444*
Agle, D. P., 330, *334*
Agras, W. S., 326, *335*
Ainsworth, K. D., 355, *377*
Ajemian, F., 430, 437, 438, *445*
Akeson, W. H., 46, 52, 53, 61, 71, 72, *80*
Alba, A., 304, *309*, *310*
Alday, E. S., 163, *186*
Alexander, A. B., 50, *74*, 318, *336*
Alexander, F., 388, *406*
Alexander, J. K., 250, *256*, 462, *472*
Allen, G. J., 238, 246, *257*

Allon, N., 225, *252*
Alpern, G. D., 387, *404*
Alperson, B. L., 354, *377*
Alpert, R., 150, *156*
Altmaier, E. M., 173, 174, *188*, *185*
Amir, S., 210, *215*
Amour, J., 198, *213*
Anastasi, A., 60, *74*
Andersen, B. L., 164, 165, 177, *185*
Anderson, B. J., 210, *213*
Anderson, C., 297, *309*
Anderson, E., 89, 90, *108*, 114, *132*
Anderson, J. R., 204, *213*
Anderson, R. A., 63, *74*
Anderson, T. P., 89, 90, *108*, 114, *132*, 344, *375*
Andrasik, F., 48, 50, 51, *74*
Andresen, G. V., 170, 172, *188*
Andrykowski, M. A., 173, *188*
Ang, L., 229, *256*
Aoki, Y., 278, *283*
Arbit, J., 365, 366, *378*
Arky, R. A., 193, *213*
Armellini, F., 223, *253*
Armstrong, M., 455, 456, *471*
Aroskar, M. A., 90, *108*
Arrick, M. C., 52, *80*
Ashby, W. A., 242, *252*
Ashenhurst, E. M., 103, *111*
Ashley, F., Jr., 449, *471*
Atkins, C. J., 332, *334*
Auerbach, S. M., 100, *108*

483

Edwards, D. W., 164, 165, *189*
Efron, B., 50, *76*
Efron, R., 266, *282*
Egbert, L. D., 180, *186*
Ehrlich, G. E., 45, 46, 53, *80*
Eisenberg, H. S., 145, *156*, 162, *186*
Eisenberg, M. G., 296, *309*
Elashoff, J. D., 71, *76*
Eldar, M., 145, *158*
Ellis, A., 432, *444*
Ellis, F. W., 456, *471*
Else, B. A., 57, 63, *76*
Emery, G., 131, *132*
Endress, M. P., 13, *36*
Engel, G. L., 97, *108*
Epstein, L. H., 240, *258*
Epstein, S., 27, *35*
Epting, F. R., 240, 246, *257*
Erikson, M. B. E., 365, *376*
Ertel, I. J., *405*
Esibill, N., 89, *112*
Espmark, S., 86, 89, 104, *109*
Etzwiler, D. D., 196, *214*
Evans, F. M., 196, *214*
Evans, R., 430, *444*
Evans, R. I., 462, *471*
Evans, R. L., 296, *309*
Everhart, D., 13, 17, *36*
Eysenck, H. J., 47, *76*
Eysenck, S. G. B., 47, *76*
Ezrachi, O., 51, 55, 63, 66, 70, 77, 119,
    120, 121, 122, 124, *135*, 146, 155, *156*,
    164, *186*

F

Faglioni, P., 125, 126, *132*, *133*
Falliers, C. J., 317, 320, *334*
Fallstrom, K., 209, *214*
Farquhar, J. W., 250, *256*, 450, 451, 462,
    463, *471*, *472*
Faschingbauer, T. R., 59, *76*
Fedio, P., 275, *281*
Feenald, P. S., 469, *471*
Feibel, J. H., 128, *133*
Feigenson, J. S., 85, *109*, 114, *133*
Feigenson, W., 114, *133*
Feinleib, M., 92, *111*
Feinstein, A. R., 43, 44, 55, *76*
Feldman, J., 419, *423*

Feldman, J. L., 103, 105, *109*
Felig, P., 194, *216*
Ferrans, V. J., 229, *255*
Feuerstein, R. C., 184, *185*
Fields, G. L., 397, *404*
Fikri, E., 230, *254*
Fillenbaum, G. G., 60, *76*
Filskov, S. B., 127, *133*
Finch, C. A., 268, 269, *284*
Fine, P. R., 286, *309*, 364, 365, *378*
Finer, B., 373, *376*
Finesinger, J. E., 139, *158*
Finlay, J., 225, *256*
Finley, W. W., 268, *282*
Fischer, C., 432, *444*
Fischhoff, B., 192, *214*
Fischman, S., 391, *405*
Fisher, E. B., 238, *255*
Fisher, J., 46, *78*
Fisher, S. H., 103, 105, *109*
Fisk, A., 103, 105, *108*
Fitzpatrick, T. E., 128, *133*
Flaherty, L., 365, *379*
Flamm, L., 125, *133*
Flanagan, J., 455, *472*
Fleiss, J., 63, *76*, 139, *156*
Fletcher, S., 468, *472*
Flora, J., 342, *379*
Floreen, A. C., 363, *379*
Flynn, A., 436, *444*
Flynn, W. R., 197, *216*
Foch, T. T., 222, *254*
Folkman, S., 144, *156*
Follick, M. J., 143, 146, 154, *156*, 479, *482*
Folstein, M. F., 104, *109*, 114, *133*
Forbes, G. B., 221, *254*
Fordyce, W. E., 8, *11*, 40, 41, 43, 49, 50,
    51, 53, 55, 57, 61, 62, 63, 64, 65, *76*,
    128, *132*, 287, 299, 300, 301, 302, 303,
    307, *309*, *311*, 340, 341, 345, 353, 362,
    366, 367, *376*, 430, *444*
Forester, B. M., *76*, 139, *156*
Foreyt, J. P., 236, 242, *254*, 457, *472*
Formo, A., 150, *158*
Forster, F. M., 266, *282*
Foster, D., 140, 141, 142, *157*
Foster, S. L., 57, *78*
Fotopoulos, S. S., 373, *376*
Fowler, J. E., 208, 211, *214*
Fowler, R. S., 61, 62, 64, 65, *76*, 300, 301,

Z

Subject Index